Rahul Kumar Sharma
Shailesh Sharma
Ajmer Singh Grewal
Geeta Deswal
Ashwani K. Dhingra
Kumar Guarve
Editors

Natural Solutions for Neurodegenerative Disorders

Exploring Botanical Remedies

nova
Medicine & Health
New York

DOI: https://doi.org/10.52305/DNLX7863

Library of Congress Cataloging-in-Publication Data

ISBN: 979-8-89530-231-6 (Hardcover)
ISBN: 979-8-89530-296-5 (eBook)

Published by Nova Science Publishers, Inc. † New York

Contents

Preface

The book, "Natural Solutions for Neurodegenerative Disorders: Exploring Botanical Remedies," presents an illuminating journey into the world of nature's therapeutic treasures. The growing burden of neurodegenerative disorders demands innovative and effective approaches to prevention and treatment. This book provides a deep dive into the therapeutic potential of plants in combating neurodegenerative disorders, offering a treasure trove of knowledge that promises to transform lives. The aim of this book is to rekindle the appreciation for botanical remedies, showcasing their relevance in modern healthcare, particularly in the prevention and management of neurodegenerative diseases. This book combines ancient wisdom with modern scientific insights, offering a comprehensive exploration of the profound healing potential hidden within plants.

The book opens with a historical perspective on botanical remedies for neurodegenerative disorders, tracing the use of plant-based therapies across various cultures and civilizations. Emerging trends in botanical research for neurodegenerative disorders are then explored, showcasing innovative approaches and the latest advancements reshaping the field. The potential of botanical therapies in managing amyotrophic lateral sclerosis is examined next. The next chapter delves into the latest research on curcumin's role in protecting neurons, reducing inflammation, and mitigating oxidative stress, positioning it as a promising candidate for neurodegenerative disease management. The neuroprotective effects of green tea extracts are discussed, focusing on the bioactive compounds in green tea, such as catechins, and their mechanisms of action in promoting brain health and preventing neurodegeneration. *Bacopa monnieri*, an herb known for its cognitive-enhancing and neuroprotective properties, is thoroughly reviewed. The next chapter provides insights into Ashwagandha's neuroprotective effects, including its ability to reduce oxidative stress and inflammation, which are key factors in neurodegenerative diseases. The potential benefits of ginseng in neurodegenerative disorders are examined. Ginkgo biloba's potential in treating neurodegenerative disorders is discussed, with an emphasis on its antioxidant and anti-inflammatory properties. The chapter on Rhodiola rosea explores its potential in neurodegeneration, highlighting its adaptogenic properties and the scientific evidence supporting its use in enhancing cognitive function and protecting against neuro-degenerative diseases. Catechins, particularly those found in tea, are examined for their neuroprotective properties in the next chapter. Huperzine A, a natural cholinesterase inhibitor, is reviewed for its potential benefits in neurodegenerative disorders such as Alzheimer's disease. Botanical interventions for Parkinson's disease are explored, with a focus on various plants and their bioactive compounds that have shown promise in managing this neurodegenerative condition. The role of botanicals in Alzheimer's disease management is discussed, highlighting various herbs and their neuroprotective effects. This chapter examines the scientific evidence supporting the use of botanical remedies in preventing and managing Alzheimer's disease. The application of nanophytoherbals in Parkinson's therapy is explored, emphasizing the innovative use of nanotechnology to enhance the delivery and efficacy of botanical compounds in treating Parkinson's disease. Adverse effects of botanical interventions are addressed, providing a balanced perspective on the potential risks and safety concerns associated with the use of botanical remedies. Finally, the chapter on phytochemicals and nutraceuticals of *Moringa oleifera* discusses its role in the treatment of neurodegenerative disorders.

This book aims to empower readers with the knowledge needed to harness the healing power of botanicals, fostering collaboration between traditional wisdom and cutting-edge research. By exploring the vast potential of botanical remedies, this book aspires to position these natural solutions at the forefront of brain health and neurodegenerative disease management. We invite healthcare professionals, researchers, and curious minds to join us on this journey of discovery, fostering collaboration between traditional wisdom and cutting-edge research. We hope this book empowers readers with the knowledge needed to tap into nature's potent healing arsenal for the benefit of all.

Rahul Kumar Sharma, PhD
Shailesh Sharma, PhD
Ajmer Singh Grewal, PhD
Geeta Deswal, PhD
Ashwani K. Dhingra, PhD
Kumar Guarve, PhD

Chapter 1

A Historical Perspective on Botanical Remedies for Neurodegenerative Disorders

H. K. Sundeep Kumar[1,*]
Priyadarshini Mishra[1]
Mrityunjay Banerjee[1]
Suman Acharyya[2]
and Bipasha Behera[1]
[1]Institute of Pharmacy and Technology, Salipur, Cuttack, Odisha, India
[2]Netaji Subhas Chandra Bose Institute of Pharmacy, Tatla, Chakdaha, Nadia, West Bengal, India

Abstract

Traditional medical systems like acupuncture, herbal medicine, indigenous traditional medicine, homeopathy, traditional Chinese medicine (TCM), naturopathy, chiropractic, osteopathy, Ayurveda, and Unani medicine represent diverse approaches to health and healing practices worldwide. According to the WHO Global Report on Traditional and Complementary Medicine (2019), these systems reflect millennia of cultural evolution and accumulated knowledge. Herbal medicine, with roots tracing back around 5000 years in Egypt and China, and 2500 years in Greece and Asia, exemplifies this rich history. Traditional Chinese Medicine, a cornerstone of Chinese culture, and Ayurveda, with its extensive practices in India, highlight the depth of these ancient traditions. Kampo medicine, a Japanese system of herbal remedies, has been in use for over 1500 years, demonstrating its

* Corresponding Author's Email: rinkusundeep@gmail.com.

In: Natural Solutions for Neurodegenerative Disorders
Editors: Rahul Kumar Sharma, Shailesh Sharma, Ajmer Singh Grewal et al.
ISBN: 979-8-89530-231-6

longstanding cultural significance. These traditional practices draw on extensive knowledge of medicinal plants and their therapeutic properties, developed over centuries. Despite their historical and cultural value, the rising interest in herbal remedies has brought concerns regarding their safety, legality, and effectiveness. As herbal treatments continue to gain popularity, it is crucial to address these concerns and ensure that the use of such remedies is both safe and effective.

Keywords: traditional medical systems, herbal pharmacopoeias and monographs, herbalism

Abbreviations

AHM	Arab Herbal Medicine
AYM	Ayurvedic Medicine
AYMM	Ayurvedic Materia Medica
CHM	Chinese Herbal Medicine
CMM	Chinese Materia Medica
DSHEA	Dietary Supplement Health and Education Act
HMs	Herbal Materials
HPs	Herbal Preparations
IHM	Indian Herbal Medicine
IM	Indian Medicine
IMM	Indian Materia Medica
TCM	Traditional Chinese Medicine
WHO	World Health Organization

Introduction

Herbal medicine, the oldest form of treatment, has been integral to both developed and developing nations throughout history. Indigenous communities have relied on nature for food, shelter, clothing, and medical care, developing a deep understanding of which plants are beneficial or harmful (Kunle et al., 2012). Literature indicates that over 50,000 plant species possess therapeutic properties. Today, approximately 80% of the global population, particularly in developing countries, relies on herbal medicine as their primary form of treatment (Vujicic and Cohall, 2021). Even in advanced nations like Germany and France, there has been a notable increase in the prescription use of herbs (Wachtel-Galor, 2011; Edzard, 2005). In the United States, the rise in herbal medicine use over the past 20 years can be attributed to dissatisfaction with the cost of prescription drugs and a growing interest in natural or organic alternatives. However, not all herbal remedies are as safe as they might appear (WHO, 2023). In Ethiopia and Uganda, over 80% of the population still relies on medicinal plants, reflecting a long-standing tradition (Asiimwe, 2021; Zemede et al., 2024). The knowledge gained from traditional medicine offers valuable insights into the selection, preparation, and use of herbal treatments. To ensure these remedies are competitive with Western medicine, rigorous clinical and scientific evaluations of their efficacy and safety are essential. Herbal remedies, deeply rooted in both traditional and ethnic practices, remain a valuable resource for medicinal exploration.

Herbal Medicines, Botanical Medicines and Botanical Remedies

Herbal medicine, as defined by the WHO, encompasses the use of herbs, herbal materials (HMs), herbal preparations (HPs), and completed herbal products containing plant parts or combinations of plant materials as active components (WHO, 2023). These herbal products can include components such as leaves, stems, blossoms, roots, and seeds. Active ingredients in herbal medicines consist of plant materials or their processed forms, along with excipients like solvents, preservatives, or dilutions. These active substances, which contribute to the plant's scent, flavor, and color, also serve to protect it from damage and disease. Scientifically, these substances are known as phytochemicals and include various groups such as alkaloids, terpenoids, glycosides, saponins, and flavonoids (Saxena et al., 2013). The efficacy of phytochemicals in improving human health has been established through scientific validation, leading to their commercialization in regions like North America (USA, Mexico, and Canada) (Rojas et al., 2022). For example, aromatic plant species used in remedies may contain essential oils with antibacterial, calming, and anti-spasmodic properties, while high-tannin plant species are employed in treatments for ulcerative colitis and diarrhea due to their antibacterial, astringent, and anti-inflammatory effects (Ndhlala et al., 2011). Table 1 lists the phytochemicals in therapeutic plants that are both biologically active and disease-preventive. Under the U.S. Dietary

Supplement Health and Education Act (DSHEA) of 1994, herbal supplements are classified as dietary supplements and can be marketed without mandatory safety and efficacy testing, although good manufacturing practices must be adhered to during their production.

Table 1. Properties of some major constituents of medicinal plants

Class	Characteristic	Use	Pharmacological activity	Reference
Alkaloids	Organic nitrogenous bases, bitter taste, colorless/yellow, crystalline solids, liquids	Biosynthesis of pharmaceuticals	Anticancer, antimicrobial, amoebicidal, anti-inflammatory	(Kauri and Arora, 2015)
Saponins	Soap-like forming property, bitter taste	Detergent, wetting and emulsifying agent	Antifeedant, antifungal, antiobesity, antioxidant	(Saxena et al., 2013)
Tannins	Water-soluble, leather hides	Used for cationic dyes, production of ink	Antimutagens, anticarcinogens, antimicrobial	(Saxena et al., 2013)
Flavonoids	Free radical scavenger	Prevents microbial infection	Anti-inflammatory, antimicrobial, antibacterial, antioxidant	(Kumar and Pandey, 2013)

Uses and Benefits of Botanical Medicines

Herbal medicines are significant in treating a range of conditions, including infectious diseases, chronic ailments, and various symptoms (Chaughule and Barve, 2024). They are utilized for managing numerous health issues such as premenstrual syndrome, rheumatoid arthritis, fibromyalgia, migraines, menopausal symptoms, chronic fatigue, irritable bowel syndrome, allergies, asthma, eczema, and cancer, as well as for symptomatic relief in conditions like dementia and diabetes (Kumar et al., 2021). Medicinal plants are increasingly recognized as potential sources for new antibacterial drugs, especially in the post-antibiotic era (Abdallah et al., 2023). However, it's crucial to consult with a healthcare professional before starting any herbal remedy, as these treatments can interact with prescription medications and may exacerbate certain medical conditions.

Ginkgo

Ginkgo biloba, known for its active chemicals that enhance circulation and cognitive function, is available in both liquid and solid extracts. Historically, the leaves of the ginkgo plant have been used to treat asthma and cardiovascular conditions, while the seeds have served as an expectorant, antitussive, and anti-asthmatic since 2800 BC. While *G. biloba* is generally considered safe, some common adverse effects include headache, nausea, vomiting, diarrhea, restlessness, cutaneous sensitivity, and dizziness.

Ginseng

Ginseng (*Eleutherococcus senticosus*), the fourth most commonly used Chinese medicinal plant, is widely recognized for its therapeutic benefits. It is used not only to treat diabetes, depression, and hypertension but also as a general tonic to enhance the body's resilience to stress and improve overall energy levels (George, 2011). The whole root of the ginseng plant is utilized in preparations due to its active components, primarily ginsenosides. However, excessive dosages of ginseng can lead to adverse effects such as vaginal bleeding, mastalgia, anxiety, insomnia, and elevated blood pressure (Ekor, 2014; George, 2011).

Kava

Kava (*Piper methysticum*) is renowned for its health benefits, including relief from mental disorders, promotion of relaxation and sleep, weight loss support, and combatting fatigue. It is also used as a stomachic and diuretic and is commonly employed to treat conditions such as gonorrhea, syphilis, rheumatism, fever, headaches, asthma, and urinary infections. However, adverse effects of kava have been reported, including headaches, nausea, dizziness, and localized numbness when taken orally (Ekor, 2014).

St. John's Wort

St. John's Wort (*Hypericum perforatum*) is noted for its calming and astringent properties. Traditionally, it has been used to treat a variety of conditions including sciatica, wounds, depression, anxiety, menopausal neurosis, fibrositis, neuralgia, and excitability. In contemporary medicine, its use as an antidepressant has gained significant attention. Key active ingredients in St. John's Wort include melatonin, hyperforin, and hypericin. Despite its benefits, adverse effects such as weariness, constipation, nausea, vomiting, dry mouth, headaches, dizziness, and photosensitivity have been reported (Ekor, 2014).

Valerian

Valerian (*Valeriana officinalis*) is commonly used as a mild sedative and anxiety reliever. The root of the plant contains various compounds, with valerenic acid (a C15-sesquiterpenoid) and valerena-4,7(11)-diene being particularly noted for their sedative effects (Pyle et al., 2012). Despite its therapeutic benefits, Valerian has been associated with several adverse effects, including ataxia, gastrointestinal issues, headaches, and excitability. Other potential side effects following oral administration include abdominal cramps, fatigue, dizziness, chest tightness, and trembling in the hands and feet.

Ma Huang

Ma-huang (*Ephedra sinica*) is an ancient medicinal herb historically used to treat conditions such as rheumatism, chronic postural hypotension, myasthenia gravis, hay fever, colds, coughs, and enuresis. It contains several alkaloids, including pseudoephedrine and ephedrine, which contribute to its therapeutic effects. However, due to its potential for serious adverse effects, Ma-huang is considered unsafe. Reported negative outcomes include myocardial infarction, premature ventricular contractions, mortality, insomnia, headaches, dizziness, anxiety, stroke, seizures, hypertension, psychosis, and irritability.

A Historical Perspective of Botanical Medicine

Records from ancient Babylonia indicate that the use of plants as medicine dates back 60,000 years. Herbal medicine has been documented for around 5,000 years in Egypt and China, and for 2,500 years in Greece and Asia Minor (Qazi and Molvi, 2016). The methods and ideologies of various herbal therapeutic systems differ based on their regional origins. In China, Traditional Chinese Medicine (TCM) has been practiced since ancient times, with extensive pharmacopoeias and monographs detailing herbal knowledge. Similarly, Ayurveda, developed over 5,000 years ago in India by ancient doctors and saints, includes around 10,000 formulas and 1,500 plants in its Materia Medica. Recognized by the Indian government as a comprehensive healthcare system, Ayurveda contrasts with Western medicine in its holistic approach. Additionally, Kampo, a Japanese herbal remedy developed over 1,500 years ago, features over 148 formulations (Watanabe et al., 2011).

The Utilization of Medicinal Plants in Various Cultures

Traditional Chinese Medicine (TCM)

Traditional Chinese Medicine (TCM) is one of the oldest medical systems, with roots deeply embedded in Chinese culture and history (Patwardhan, 2005). It has evolved independently of external influences, reflecting the rich diversity of China's 56 ethnic groups, each with its own traditional practices, languages, and cultures. The Han people, who pioneered Chinese herbal medicine, primarily utilize plant-based remedies. However, TCM practitioners also incorporate animal parts, insects, minerals, and unrefined synthetic chemicals into their treatments. The term "Chinese herbal medicine" (CHM) encompasses not only the traditional plant-based remedies but also ethnic herbal medicines and folk remedies from various Chinese traditions. Historically, Wang Tao (702–772) contributed significantly to the field with his book Waitai Miyao, which includes around 600 prescriptions based on diagnostic theories involving the tongue's color and condition, reflecting various pathological disorders. Another seminal figure, Li Shizen, authored the comprehensive pharmacopoeia Ben Cao Gang Mu in 1596, which remains a key reference for TCM study and practice. This text, containing 1,894 recommendations, has influenced Chinese medicine and other cultures. It is noteworthy that TCM was traditionally transmitted orally until its formalization into classroom instruction in the 1950s.

Indian Herbal Medicine (IHM)

Traditional health care systems such as Indian medicine (IM), Materia medica (IMM), and herbal medicine (IHM), collectively referred to as Ayurvedic medicine (AYM), are deeply rooted in the philosophy that "everything can be a drug." This approach encompasses a broad spectrum of substances, including plants, herbs, and even animal by-products. Ayurvedic practitioners meticulously document the effects of these substances. Currently, traditional medicine remains the primary healthcare system for about 70% of Indians. The earliest known text in Ayurvedic medicine is the Rasa Vaisesika, authored by Nagarjuna in the fifth century CE. This text, along with the Charaka Samhita, which focuses on therapeutics, forms the foundation of Ayurvedic principles and applications. Notably, around 80% of herbal remedies used in Ayurveda, 46% in Unani medicine, and 33% in allopathic systems are derived from the western Himalayan region. This area is also significant in the British Pharmacopoeia, with 50% of its listed medications connected to local medicinal plants. In India, traditional and folk remedies involve over 25,000 plant-based compositions (Joy et al., 2013). Various traditional systems use different numbers of plant species, including Ayurveda (2,000), Siddha (1,300), Unani (1,000), homeopathic (800), Tibetan (500), contemporary (200), and folk medicine (4,500) (Wakdikar, 2004). Unani medicine, developed by the Islamic physician Avicenna, and Ayurveda both utilize over 7,500 plant species for diverse purposes such as diuretics, expectorants, hepatoprotectants, aphrodisiacs, tonics, antimalarials, and antipyretics (Aggarwal et al., 2011; Kulkarni et al., 2012). These systems also address specific central nervous system disorders and employ specialized herbal concoctions known as Rasayans to promote longevity, delay aging, and rejuvenate the body (Ramakrishnappa, 2013).

Japanese Traditional Medicine (Kampo)

The historical evolution of Japanese traditional medicine reflects its integration and adaptation of Chinese herbal treatments. By the ninth century, Japanese medicine had incorporated natural herbs into its first pharmacopoeia, following the introduction of Kampo from ancient China, either directly or via Korea, along with Buddhism and other cultural elements in the fifth century. The term "Kampo" literally means "method from the Han period" (206 BC to 220 AD), indicating its Chinese origins. During the Edo period, around 1600, Kampo began to develop unique Japanese characteristics. The extensive array of Chinese crude medicines was distilled down to approximately 300 key ingredients, which were then formulated into around 300 prescriptions. Japanese practitioners of Kampo introduced the innovative concept of "abdominal diagnosis," which significantly enhanced diagnostic and therapeutic practices. This approach diverged from the largely theoretical and speculative nature of Chinese medicine, with Japanese medical professionals, such as 18th-century physician Yoshimasu Todo, advocating for a more empirical approach based on direct observation of patients. Todo famously criticized traditional practices by asserting that "in clinical medicine, we should only rely on what we actually have observed by examination of the patient," emphasizing a shift towards practical, evidence-based medicine.

The History of Medicinal Plants in Iran

The ancient medical and pharmaceutical traditions of Iran reflect a rich synthesis of early Mesopotamian practices combined with those of neighboring civilizations such as the Babylonians, Assyrians, and Elamites. Among the revered plants in ancient Iran was Haoma (Ephedra major), which held a sacred status in Zoroastrianism. The Avesta, the holy book of Zoroastrianism, contains significant references to phytotherapy and the medicinal use of plants, notably in one of its sections, the Dorandiyud. Unfortunately, much of Iran's early botanical knowledge was lost due to historical events. The destruction of the Alexandrian library during the Macedonian conquest and the subsequent burning of Ismaili castles and libraries by Hulagu Khan resulted in the loss of many valuable manuscripts and botanical records. In the eighth and ninth centuries, Persian medicine saw remarkable advancements through the work of prominent figures such as Avicenna and Razi. Avicenna's "Canon of Medicine" and Razi's "al-Hawi" are notable contributions to the field. Ibn al-Baitar, another significant figure, compiled a comprehensive treatise in the 13th century detailing the characteristics and uses of approximately 1,400 plants. These works represent crucial contributions to the preservation and development of medicinal knowledge in ancient Iran.

Arabic Herbal Medicine (AHM)

A significant number of plants introduced to pharmacotherapy by Arab scholars have proven to be truly therapeutic and are still featured in global pharmacopoeias today. Many of these plants were imported from India, with which the Arabs had extensive trade connections. Arab physicians were pioneers in integrating dietary management and exercise into medical practice. Notably, Ali Ibn Rabban Al-Tabri (782–855 AD) made substantial contributions; his book Firdous Al Hikmat includes a section dedicated to medicines and poisons, while his Canon, listing over a thousand medications, was highly regarded as a medical textbook in Europe. His other work, Kitab Ash-Shifa, is considered an encyclopedia of scientific knowledge. Additionally, Abu Musa Jabir ben Hayyan authored The Poison and Antidote Book, an extensive treatise on plant toxins and their remedies. The Arabs utilized a variety of plants, such as pepper, cinnamon, rheum, senna, coffee, ginger, strychnos, saffron, and curcuma, and they often substituted potent medications with milder alternatives, like using Sennae folium as a gentle laxative in place of harsher purgatives like Heleborus odorus and Euphorbium.

Other Historical Sources for the Study of Medicinal Plants

Sacred Jewish texts, including the Talmud and the Bible, describe the use of aromatic plants like myrtle and incense in various ceremonial treatments. Hippocrates, the father of Western medicine, listed 300 medicinal plants in his works (459–370 BC), noting their physiological effects: garlic for intestinal parasites; opium, henbane, deadly nightshade, and mandrake as narcotics; fragrant hellebore and haselwort as emetics; sea onion, celery, parsley, asparagus, and garlic as diuretics; and oak and pomegranate as astringents. Theophrastus (371–287 BC), known as the "Father of Botany," laid the foundation for botanical science with his works De Causis Plantarium and De Historia Plantarium. He categorized over 500 medicinal plants and highlighted species such as cinnamon, cardamom, pomegranate, mint, iris rhizome, aromatic hellebore, monkshood, and fake hellebore. Theophrastus also stressed the importance of gradually increasing dosages to acclimate to plant effects. Dioscorides noted the use of chamomile (Matricaria recutita L.), known as chamaemelon, for treating burns, stings, ulcers, and wounds, and its mild carminative action suitable for children. He also described various Mentha species for headaches and stomachaches, oak bark for gynecological issues, white willow for antipyretic effects, and sea onion and parsley bulbs as diuretics. Galen (131–200 AD), the preeminent Roman physician and pharmacist, compiled De succedanus, the first list of interchangeable medications with similar actions, though some of his suggested alternatives are now considered obsolete in modern pharmaceutical practice.

Tapping into Nature and Indigenous Knowledge to Advance Modern Medicine

Combining evolutionary ecology, molecular biology/biochemistry, and ethnopharmacology offers a comprehensive, multidimensional approach to studying medicinal plants, leading to significant scientific insights and improvements in human health and well-being (Davis and Choisy, 2023). Novel drug delivery systems enhance bioavailability and therapeutic efficacy by reducing toxicity and minimizing the need for frequent dosing, thus addressing non-compliance issues (Singh and Gauri, 2023). Recent advances in herbal medicines illustrate these innovations (Roy et al., 2022). For instance, Tu Youyou's team identified artemisinin from sweet wormwood in 1971, a key breakthrough in treating chloroquine-resistant malaria. Similarly, aspirin, derived from willow bark used by the Sumerians and Egyptians over 3,500 years ago, was developed by Bayer chemist Felix Hoffmann in 1897 and continues to benefit millions daily. Shikimic acid, extracted from star anise, is utilized in Tamiflu, an antiviral drug effective against influenza virus types A and B. Additionally, norethindrone, the first active component in contraceptive tablets, is extracted from wild Mexican yam.

Conclusion

Throughout history, the quest for remedies to treat ailments and alleviate discomfort has been a constant pursuit. Many medicinal plants have demonstrated therapeutic properties, which have been recognized and transmitted through generations across different eras and civilizations. As each civilization advanced, it built upon the knowledge of its predecessors, discovering new applications and refining the use of these plants. Today's sophisticated methods of processing and utilizing medicinal herbs are a testament to the enduring and evolving interest in these natural remedies.

References

Abdallah, E. M., Alhatlani, B. Y., de Paula Menezes, R., & Martins, C. H. G. (2023). Back to Nature: Medicinal Plants as Promising Sources for Antibacterial Drugs in the Post-Antibiotic Era. *Plants*, 12(17), 3077.

Aggarwal, B., Prasad, S., Reuter, S., Kannappan, R., Yadev, V., Park, B., Kim, J., Gupta, S., Phromnoi, K., Sundaram, C., Prasad, S., Chaturvedi, M., & Sung, B. (2011). Identification of novel anti-inflammatory agents from Ayurvedic medicine for prevention of chronic diseases: "reverse pharmacology" and "bedside to bench" approach. *Current Drug Targets*, 12(11), 1595–1653.

Asiimwe, S., Namukobe, J., Byamukama, R., & Imalingat, B. (2021). Ethnobotanical survey of medicinal plant species used by communities around Mabira and Mpanga Central Forest Reserves, Uganda. *Tropical medicine and health*, 49(1), 52.

Azaizeh, H., Saad, B., Khalil, K., & Said, O. (2006). The state of the art of traditional arab herbal medicine in the eastern region of the mediterranean: a review. *Evidence-based complementary and alternative medicine*, 3(2), 229–235.

Chaughule, R. S., & Barve, R. S. (2023). Role of herbal medicines in the treatment of infectious diseases. *Vegetos (Bareilly, India)*, 1–11.

Davis, C. C., & Choisy, P. (2024). Medicinal plants meet modern biodiversity science. *Current biology*, 34(4), R158–R173.

Ekor, M. (2014). The growing use of herbal medicines: issues relating to adverse reactions and challenges in monitoring safety. *Frontiers in pharmacology*, 4, 177.

George, P. (2011). Concerns regarding the safety and toxicity of medicinal plants –An overview. *Journal of applied pharmaceutical science*, 1(6), 40-44.

Joy, P. P., Thomas, J., Mathew, S., & Skaria, B. P. (2013). *Medicinal plants.* Aromatic and Medicinal Plants Research Station, Kerala Agricultural University, Odakkali, Asamannoor P. O., Ernakulam District, Kerala, India.

Kauri, R., & Arora, S. (2015). Alkaloids-important therapeutic secondary metabolites of plant origin. *Journal of critical reviews*, 2(3), 1-8.

Kulkarni, R., Girish, K. J., & Kumar, A. (2012). Nootropic herbs (Medhya Rasayana) in Ayurveda: An update. *Pharmacognosy reviews*, 6(12), 147-153.

Kumar, S., & Pandey, A. K. (2013). Chemistry and biological activities of flavonoids: An overview. *The scientific world journal*, 2013, 1-16.

Kumar, S., Mittal, A., Babu, D., & Mittal, A. (2021). Herbal Medicines for Diabetes Management and its Secondary Complications. *Current diabetes reviews*, 17(4), 437–456.

Kunle, O. F., Egharevba, H. O., & Ahmadu, P. O. (2012). Standardization of herbal medicines –A review. *Journal of biodiversity and conservation*, 4(3), 101-112.

Ndhlala, A. R., Stafford, G. I., Finnie, J. F., & Van Staden, J. (2011). Commercial herbal preparations in KwaZulu-Natal, South Africa: The urban face of traditional medicine. *South African Journal of Botany*, 77(4), 830-843.

Pyle, B. W., Tran, H. T., Pickel, B., Haslam, T. M., Gao, Z., MacNevin, G., Vederas, J. C., Kim, S. U., & Ro, D. K. (2012). Enzymatic synthesis of valerena-4,7(11)-diene by a unique sesquiterpene synthase from the valerian plant (Valeriana officinalis). *The FEBS journal*, 279(17), 3136–3146.

Qazi, M. A., & Molvi, K. (2016). Herbal medicine: A comprehensive review. *Journal of Pharmaceutical Research*, 8(2), 1-5

Ramakrishnappa, K. (2013). *Impact of cultivation and gathering of medicinal plants on biodiversity: case studies from India*. FAO. https://www.fao.org/4/y4586e/y4586e09.htm.

Rojas, P., Jung-Cook, H., Ruiz-Sánchez, E., Rojas-Tomé, I. S., Rojas, C., López-Ramírez, A. M., & Reséndiz-Albor, A. A. (2022). Historical Aspects of Herbal Use and Comparison of Current Regulations of Herbal Products between Mexico, Canada and the United States of America. *International journal of environmental research and public health*, 19(23), 15690.

Roy, D., Chakraborty, A., Mukherjee, P., Ghosh B., & Chakraborty, M. (2022). Recent Advances in Herbal Medicines – An Updated Review. *Asian journal of pharmaceutical research and development*, 10(1), 45-48.

Saxena, M., Saxena, J., Nema, R., Singh, D., & Gupta, A. (2013). Phytochemistry of medicinal plants. *Journal of Pharmacognosy and Phytochemistry*, 1(6), 168-182.

Singh, H., & Gauri. (2023). Recent development of novel drug delivery of herbal drugs. *RPS Pharmacy and Pharmacology Reports*, 2, 1-8.

Vujicic, T., & Cohall, D. (2021). Knowledge, Attitudes and Practices on the Use of Botanical Medicines in a Rural Caribbean Territory. *Frontiers in pharmacology*, 12, 713855.

Watanabe, K., Matsuura, K., Gao, P., Hottenbacher, L., Tokunaga, H., Nishimura, K., Imazu, Y., Reissenweber, H., & Witt, C. (2011). Traditional Japanese Kampo Medicine: Clinical Research between Modernity and Traditional Medicine-The State of Research and Methodological Suggestions for the Future. *Evidence-based complementary and alternative medicine*, 2011, 513842.

World Health Organization. (2013). *WHO Traditional Medicine Strategy: 2014–2023*. Available from: https://www.who.int/publications/i/item/9789241506096.

Zemede, J., Mekuria, T., Ochieng, C. O., Onjalalaina, G. E., & Hu, G. W. (2024). Ethnobotanical study of traditional medicinal plants used by the local Gamo people in Boreda Abaya District, Gamo Zone, southern Ethiopia. *Journal of ethnobiology and ethnomedicine*, 20(1), 28.

Chapter 2

Emerging Trends in Botanical Research for Neurogenerative Disorders

Vishnu Mittal[1]
Anjali Sharma[1,*]
and Devkant Sharma[2]
[1]Guru Gobind Singh College of Pharmacy, Yamunanagar, Haryana
[2]Ch. Devi Lal College of Pharmacy, Jagadhri, Yamunanagar, Haryana, India

Abstract

In light of new insights and developments, the field of biology continues to evolve, particularly regarding the study of plant secondary metabolites. These compounds, produced by plants, are not essential for basic life processes but play crucial roles in chemistry, temperature regulation, and health. Ongoing research aims to elucidate how these metabolites function in plant defense systems and to explore their potential for developing novel drugs, functional foods, and agricultural products. Another emerging trend is the integration of contemporary scientific techniques with traditional knowledge. Ethnobotany, which examines the relationship between humans and plants, offers valuable insights into historical plant uses and indigenous knowledge. Collaborating with traditional healers and local communities helps scientists discover new plant species, validate traditional medicinal practices, and investigate sustainable cultivation methods, bridging the gap between traditional wisdom and modern scientific research. This book section highlights the latest advancements in plant science, emphasizing how major themes are significantly influencing the field.

* Corresponding Author's Email: sharma.sharmaa.anjali@gmail.com.

In: Natural Solutions for Neurodegenerative Disorders
Editors: Rahul Kumar Sharma, Shailesh Sharma, Ajmer Singh Grewal et al.
ISBN: 979-8-89530-231-6

Keywords: botanical research, ethnobotany, secondary metabolites, traditional, agricultural products

Abbreviations

ADME	Absorption, Distribution, Metabolism, and Excretion
ALS	Amyotrophic Lateral Sclerosis
AMPA	α-Amino-3-Hydroxy-5-Methyl-4-Isoxazolepropionic Acid
CRISPR	Clustered Regularly Interspaced Short Palindromic Repeats
DNA	Deoxyribonucleic Acid
GABA	Gamma-Aminobutyric Acid
GC	Gas Chromatography
GWAS	Genome-Wide Association Study
HPLC	High-Performance Liquid Chromatography
NMDA	N-Methyl-D-Aspartate
RNA	Ribonucleic Acid
SAR	Structure-Activity Relationship

Introduction

The treatment of brain disorders, a major global health challenge, is significantly advanced by botanical research. The limitations of conventional chemical treatments have prompted a transformation in the study of plant-based therapies. This section explores recent developments in plant research, emphasizing the interplay between information, technology, and scientific advancements (Macro et al., 2021). Data-driven analyses of neurodegenerative diseases reveal economic impacts, therapeutic outcomes, and a growing interest in plant-based medications. The surge in scientific publications and clinical trials concerning natural therapies reflects a shift towards comprehensive, patient-centered approaches. This section underscores the importance of evidence-based plant research, illustrating the progression from financial trends to technical innovations and research developments, which are paving the way for new and effective treatments for neurological disorders (Chen et al., 2023; Wang et al., 2023).

Overview of Neurological Conditions

Neurodegenerative diseases, a rising global health concern, are characterized by a gradual decline in the structure and function of the nervous system. The increasing prevalence of conditions such as Alzheimer's, Parkinson's, Huntington's, and amyotrophic lateral sclerosis (ALS) imposes a growing burden on affected individuals, their families, and healthcare systems. These diseases are influenced by intricate interactions among social, environmental, and genetic factors (Sharma et al., 2023). The economic impact is substantial due to the rising costs of healthcare and the demand for long-term care. Conventional pharmaceutical treatments often manage symptoms but do not address the root causes or halt the progression of these diseases. This limitation has intensified the focus on researching complementary and alternative medicines, including plant-based therapies, to explore potential new approaches for treatment and prevention.

The Significance of Exploring Botanical Solutions

Plant components have unique and potent properties, making the study of botanical treatments within new frameworks essential to botanical research. Valued are the following significant elements:

Synergy and Natural Complexity

For thousands of years, botanicals have produced a diverse range of compounds that have maintained plant health and vitality. Due to their complexity, many bioactive compounds often work together to form a system that may more closely resemble the intricate processes of the human body (Adam et al., 2023).

Diversity of Bioactive Compounds

Terpenoids, flavonoids, polyphenols, and alkaloids are just a few of the many bioactive compounds found in plant species. These compounds exhibit a variety of biological actions, including antioxidant, neuroprotective, and anti-inflammatory effects. Analyzing this diversity reveals numerous potential drugs.

Potential for Disease Modification

Some properties of plant-derived compounds may alter the fundamental mechanisms behind neurological diseases. The potential to modify chronic, degenerative diseases is particularly exciting.

Reduced Side Effects and Safety Profiles

Many plants have safer profiles than newly developed medications, potentially reducing the risk of adverse effects. Traditional use of these plants provides valuable safety information and encourages further research into their therapeutic potential (Angelino et al., 2023).

Sustainable Environmental Practices

The growing attention to botanical medications reflects their increasing global popularity. Pharmacological production has intrinsic benefits when associated with green plant cultivation, aligning with the broader trend towards environmentally and socially conscious healthcare alternatives.

Patient-Centric Approaches

Herbal treatments often appeal to individuals seeking more natural and healthier forms of care. This patient-centric perspective highlights the importance of therapies that support lifestyle choices, as well as overall quality of life and wellness.

Table 1. Some emerging trend in botanical research

Sr. No.	Emerging Trend	Description
1	Genomics and Transcriptomics	Utilizing advanced molecular techniques to study the genomes and transcriptomes of plants, enabling a deeper understanding of their genetic makeup and regulatory processes
2	Metabolomics	Investigating the diverse array of plant metabolites to understand their roles in plant growth, development, and interactions with the environment.
3	Plant-Microbe Interactions	Exploring the complex relationships between plants and microorganisms, including symbiotic and pathogenic interactions, and their impact on plant health.
4	Synthetic Biology	Applying engineering principles to design and construct novel biological systems in plants, potentially leading to the development of enhanced crops.
5	Climate Change Adaptation	Studying how plants respond to climate change, including shifts in growing seasons, temperature, and precipitation, with a focus on developing resilient plant varieties.
6	Phytochemicals and Medicinal Plants	Investigating bioactive compounds in plants for potential therapeutic applications, including the development of new pharmaceuticals.
7	Urban Botany and Green Infrastructure	Examining the role of plants in urban environments, such as green roofs and vertical gardens, for improving air quality, reducing heat islands, and enhancing biodiversity.
8	Plant Phenotyping Technologies	Advancing technologies for high-throughput phenotyping to analyse plant traits, growth patterns, and responses to environmental stimuli on a large scale.
9	Bioinformatics in Plant Biology	Integrating computational tools and techniques to analyse large-scale biological data facilitates the interpretation of complex plant systems.
10	Conservation and Biodiversity	Investigating strategies for the conservation of plant species, including the study of endangered species, seed banking, and habitat preservation
11	Single-Cell Omics	Application of single-cell technologies in studying the genomics, transcriptomics, and metabolomics of individual plant cells, providing insights into cell diversity and responses.
12	CRISPR/Cas-Based Gene Editing	Harnessing CRISPR/Cas technology for precise and targeted genome editing in plants facilitates the development of genetically modified crops with improved traits.
13	Plant-Environment Interactions	Investigating how plants respond to complex environmental factors, including climate change, pollution, and habitat alterations, with a focus on adaptation strategies.
14	Functional Genomics in Non-Model Plants	Extending genomics research to non-model plant species, unravelling the functional genomics of lesser-known plants, and understanding their ecological significance.
15	Plant Synthetic Biology	Engineering plants for specific functions, such as the biosynthesis of pharmaceuticals or biofuels, by designing and constructing synthetic biological circuits within plant systems.

Table 1. (Continued)

16	Data-Driven Plant Breeding	Integration of big data, machine learning, and genomic information to accelerate plant breeding programmes, improving crop yield, quality, and resilience.
17	Mycorrhizal Research	Exploring the role of mycorrhizal fungi in plant nutrition, stress tolerance, and ecosystem functioning, with potential applications in sustainable agriculture.
18	Phenomics and Remote Sensing	Advancing techniques for high-throughput plant phenotyping, incorporating remote sensing technologies to monitor plant health and performance in real-time.
19	Plant Epigenetics and Epitranscriptomics	Investigating the role of epigenetic modifications and RNA modifications in regulating gene expression, development, and stress responses in plants.
20	Circular RNA Research	Exploring the functions and regulatory roles of circular RNAs in plants, shedding light on their involvement in gene expression and response to environmental cues (Bock et al., 2023).

Potential for Personalized Medicine

Customized medication may be feasible due to the wide range of plant compounds available. Personalized therapy approaches could enhance outcomes based on the patient's lifestyle, genetic composition, and specific brain condition (Nikolova, 2022).

Plants offer hope for novel and effective therapies for brain diseases because of their complex biology, potential to modify disease, and patient-centered approaches. Emerging trends in botanical research are shown in Table 1.

Plants in the Context of Emerging Trends

Genomics and Transcriptomics

High-throughput sequencing methods have revolutionized studies in plant genomes and transcriptomics. Researchers are analyzing RNA transcripts and decoding entire plant genomes to gain insights into gene regulation, evolution, and key aspects of plant genomes.

Metabolomics

Metabolomics involves the comprehensive study of plant components. By discovering and measuring a wide range of small molecules in plants, new methodologies illuminate metabolic processes, stress responses, and the production of beneficial substances.

Plant-Microbe Interactions

Exploring the complex interactions between microbes and plants is both valuable and challenging. Understanding how the plant microbiome influences nutrient uptake, stress tolerance, and overall plant health is essential (Abbas et al., 2023).

Synthetic Biology

Synthetic biology applies engineering principles to the creation and modification of new plant traits. This field involves designing artificial biological processes in plants to enhance food production, pest and disease resistance, and nutritional value.

Climate Change Adaptation

Climate change adaptation research focuses on how plants respond to altered environmental conditions caused by climate change. This includes studies on physiological responses, genetic modification, and the development of temperature-sensitive crops.

Phytochemicals and Medicinal Plants

Research in this area centers on the development of new drugs and nutraceuticals, as well as the synthesis and therapeutic applications of phytochemicals.

Urban Botany and Green Infrastructure

This field examines the benefits of green spaces, green roofs, and vertical gardens for improving air quality, reducing urban heat islands, and enhancing wildlife in urban environments (Abdullah et al., 202).

Plant Phenotyping Technologies

Large-scale investigations into plant growth, stress responses, and other physiological aspects are conducted using high-throughput phenotyping, robotics, imaging technologies, and sensor networks.

Conservation and Biodiversity

Research in this area focuses on habitat preservation, biodiversity trends, and the conservation of plant species (Manas et al., 2021).

Genomics and Proteomics in Neuroprotection

Proteomics and genetics breakthroughs have facilitated the identification of complex molecular processes underlying neuroprotection (Yadav et al., 2021). These advancements have yielded new insights into the mechanisms and treatments of brain disorders. Genetic research, particularly through genome-wide association studies (GWAS), has successfully identified genetic variants associated with the risk or protection against brain diseases (Miyoshi et al., 2021). Additionally, pathway analysis methods have revealed interconnected pathways involved in neuroprotection, leading to a systems-level understanding of the biochemical processes at play (Momsen et al., 2022).

Utilizing Omics to Find Botanical Remedies for Neurological Conditions

One novel and versatile approach for identifying plant treatments for brain disorders is the use of omics technology. Omics, which encompasses genetics, transcriptomics, proteomics, metabolomics, and other high-throughput methods, provides a comprehensive understanding of complex biological processes underlying diseases. In the context of plant studies for brain disorders, omics enables the exploration of mechanisms of action, identification of beneficial compounds, and development of novel therapeutic strategies (Joshi et al., 2021). Examples of omics applications include:

Genetics and Genes

- Identification of Susceptibility Genes: Omics-based genetics can identify genetic variants associated with brain diseases. Genome-wide association studies (GWAS) reveal the genetic basis of various conditions by uncovering risk genes.
- Epigenetic Modifications: Epigenomics uses omics methods to reveal modifications that affect gene expression. Identifying epigenetic changes related to brain disorders can enhance understanding of disease origins (Armand et al., 2021).

Transcriptomics: Unravelling Gene Expression Patterns

- Identification of Dysregulated Pathways: Transcriptomics uncovers patterns in gene expression, helping identify genes that are differentially expressed in brain diseases. This understanding of dysregulated pathways provides insight into disease mechanisms.
- Exploring Alternative Splicing: Omics in transcriptomics allows for the examination of alternative splicing events, increasing the understanding of how alternative splicing contributes to brain function (Hasin et al., 2017).

Proteomics: Revealing Protein Profiles

- Identification of Biomarkers of Neurodegeneration: Proteomics focuses on proteins associated with neurodegenerative disorders. Identifying biomarkers aids in diagnosis and provides prognostic information on disease progression.

- Elucidating Protein Networks: Proteomics, combined with genetic information, helps organize protein networks and interactions. Understanding these networks enhances comprehension of disease mechanisms and potential treatments (Collins et al., 2003).

Metabolomics: Profiling Small Molecules

- Profiling Metabolites: Metabolomics profiles molecular patterns related to brain disorders, providing insights into metabolic instability and potential therapeutic targets.
- Screening Botanical Compounds: Metabolomics facilitates the examination of herbal samples for beneficial compounds, helping identify substances with neuroprotective properties (Horner et al., 2010).

Clinical Translation and Therapeutic Development

- Translating Omics Findings to Clinical Applications: Clinical trials validate omics data, integrating these findings into therapeutic development (Ragouussis et al., 2009).

Medicinal Plant Properties with Neuropharmacological Potential

One key aspect of studying the therapeutic properties of plants with neuropharmacological potential is the investigation of natural compounds derived from plants and their effects on the nervous system. This interdisciplinary field integrates concepts from neurology, medicine, and herbal science to identify, understand, and utilize plant-based compounds for addressing mental and brain disorders. Essential components of this research include:

Identification of Bioactive Compounds

- Alkaloids, polyphenols, and terpenes: Beneficial compounds such as alkaloids (e.g., caffeine, nicotine), polyphenols (e.g., vitamins, resveratrol), and terpenes (e.g., essential oils) are found in medicinal plants (Zhao et al., 2022).
- Cannabinoids: Some plants produce cannabinoids that exhibit neuropharmacological effects (Zhao et al., 2022).

Neuroprotective Properties

- Antioxidant effects: Many plant compounds have antioxidant properties that protect neurons from oxidative damage.
- Anti-inflammatory actions: Plant-derived compounds may possess anti-inflammatory properties that reduce neuroinflammation associated with various neurological conditions (Waszkielewicz et al., 2013).

Anti-Anxiety and Anti-Depressant Effects

- GABAergic modulation: Some plants may influence GABAergic circuits, providing calming effects.
- Serotonergic and noradrenergic actions: Plants that modulate serotonin and noradrenaline levels may help alleviate symptoms of depression (Thompson et al., 2008).

Neurotransmitter Receptor Modulation

- NMDA, AMPA, and GABA receptor modulation (neurotransmitter receptors): Interaction with neurotransmitter receptors like GABA, AMPA, and NMDA can affect neurotransmission and brain function.

Anti-Alzheimer's and Anti-Parkinson's Potential

- β-Amyloid and Tau Proteins: Plant-based compounds may inhibit the formation of tau tangles and β-amyloid plaques associated with Alzheimer's disease.
- Dopaminergic Protection: Plant compounds may provide neuroprotection to dopaminergic neurons, potentially altering the course of Parkinson's disease (Lundstrom et al., 2016).

Experimental Models and *In Vitro* Studies

- Cell Cultures: *In vitro* studies enhance understanding of cellular processes and identify potential treatment targets.
- Animal Models: Research using rats and other animals helps assess the safety and *in vivo* effects of plant-based therapies.

Pharmacokinetics and Bioavailability

- Absorption and Metabolism in Pharmacokinetics and Bioavailability: Understanding how plant compounds are absorbed and metabolized influences dosing and effectiveness.
- Blood-Brain Barrier Penetration: The ability of compounds to cross the blood-brain barrier is crucial for their neuropharmacological efficacy (Rao et al., 2023).

Clinical Application and Human Experiments

- Efficacy and security: Translating findings from animal studies to human trials evaluates the effectiveness and safety of plant-based medicines.
- Placebo-controlled trials: Large-scale clinical trials with placebo controls are essential for validating the benefits of neuropharmacological treatments (Dastagir et al., 2023).

Identification and Characterization of Neuroactive Compounds

The process of discovering and characterizing neuroactive compounds involves a complex interplay of various scientific disciplines, including medicine, biology, chemistry, and genetics. Key steps and components in this process include:

- Screening and Identification: Various methods are used to discover new compounds with neuroactive properties. In silico screening employs computational techniques to predict drug neuroactivity based on structure-activity relationships, while high-throughput screening utilizes automated technologies to rapidly test large compound libraries.
- Natural Source Extraction: Compounds can be extracted from natural sources, such as plants with a history of traditional use or marine biodiversity. This approach helps identify molecules with potential neuroactive effects (Hans et al., 2023).
- Chemical Analysis: The identification and quantification of neuroactive chemicals are performed using chromatography techniques, such as gas chromatography (GC) and high-performance liquid chromatography (HPLC), to analyze their chemical properties.
- Functional Testing: Drugs are assessed for their effects on brain activity through functional tests. *In vitro* testing involves growing cells and using electrical measurements to monitor changes in membrane potential or brain activity induced by the compounds.
- Receptor Binding Assays: These tests determine how well drugs interact with specific chemical receptors. Techniques such as radiolabeled ligand binding assays are used to measure the binding affinity of substances to receptors (Alami et al., 2022).
- Behavioral Studies: Animal models are used to evaluate the impact of drugs on memory, mood, and overall function. These studies observe and quantify behavioral responses to neuroactive compounds.
- Structure-Activity Relationship (SAR) Studies: SAR studies explore the relationship between a drug's chemical structure and its neuroactivity. This includes medicinal chemistry optimization to enhance neuroactivity and minimize side effects, as well as cheminformatics, which uses computer-based analysis of chemical data (García-Pérez et al., 2022).

- Pharmacokinetics: The study of pharmacokinetics involves understanding how drugs are absorbed, distributed, metabolized, and excreted in the body, providing insights into their effectiveness and safety (Nenadis et al., 2023).

Implications for Developing Natural Therapies

Precision medicine stands to greatly benefit from targeting neuroactive molecules, as it allows for personalized treatments based on individual genetic profiles. Integrating natural medicines with conventional therapies offers a comprehensive approach that may reduce the side effects associated with commercial drugs. The longevity of natural sources and the inclusion of traditional knowledge into plant studies highlight the importance of socially and culturally sensitive practices (Tupertsev et al., 2023). Community-based methods, along with the accessibility and affordability of natural medicines, present promising opportunities for widespread impact on global health. Continuous research, improvements in preparation methods, and adherence to regulatory standards ensure that plant-based treatments remain of the highest quality and effectiveness. Ultimately, the benefits of studying plants for natural medicine extend beyond symptom relief, offering potential for disease modification, preventive measures, and patient-centered approaches to brain health. The development of natural therapies for neurological disorders is supported by the ongoing advancement in science, technology, and research, fostering the therapeutic potential of neuroactive plant-derived compounds (Macedo et al., 2011).

Challenges and Future Directions

In response to scientific discoveries, social demands, and technological advancements, the field of plant studies remains dynamic and continually evolving. Botanical scientists face both opportunities and challenges due to these changing trends. Key future challenges and goals for plant research include:

Plant Repercussions of Climate Change

Climate change impacts internal processes, regional distribution, and interactions with other species, posing significant threats to plant diversity. Research must focus on identifying resilient species, understanding plant responses to shifting climate conditions, and developing strategies for land conservation and sustainable management.

Plant-Microbe Interactions

Understanding the complex relationships between plants and microbes is crucial for improving nutrient uptake, disease resistance, and overall plant health (Costa et al., 2019). Plant microbiomes play a key role in developing microbial-based solutions for sustainable agriculture and mitigating environmental stress through these interactions.

Functional Ecology and Ecosystem Services

Assessing the contribution of plant species to ecosystem services and identifying their specific roles in various environments can be challenging. Research should prioritize understanding the beneficial functions of plants, including their roles in carbon storage, nitrogen cycling, and environmental stability (Gupta et al., 2017). These studies provide valuable insights for managing and restoring ecosystems.

Medicinal Plants and Phytochemistry

Identifying and characterizing bioactive compounds in plants for medicinal purposes requires detailed chemical analysis and validation. Research should focus on developing sustainable methods for harvesting and utilizing medicinal plants, understanding their chemical contexts, and exploring their potential in pharmaceutical applications.

Conservation and Restoration Ecology

Balancing land use with the need to protect endangered plant species is a major challenge. Effective conservation strategies, biodiversity restoration, and the integration of innovative conservation techniques with traditional biological knowledge are essential for preserving plant diversity (Prasansuklab et al., 2013).

Conclusion

In conclusion, the study of emerging trends in plant research, particularly in the context of brain diseases, reflects a dynamic field characterized by significant advancements in scientific methodologies. The shift toward natural medicine, especially for neurological conditions, highlights the potential of plant-based treatments to address diseases and promote longevity. Advances in technologies such as genomics and omics, combined with enhanced collaboration among researchers, have deepened our understanding of therapeutic processes. Data-driven approaches are paving the way for innovative and sustainable healthcare solutions, including dynamic models of plant interactions and the identification of biomarkers. The integration of cutting-edge technology with traditional plant knowledge holds the promise of transforming the treatment of brain diseases, offering novel and effective therapeutic options. Ongoing use of omics technology is steering research towards clinical applications, increasing the potential for discovering new and impactful drugs in the future.

References

Abbas, M. T., Batool, Z., Ahmad, C. A., Khan, H. A. A., & Akhter, A. (2023). Application of modern biotechnology and bioinformatics approaches in agricultural sciences: A systematic review. *World Journal of Biology & Biotechnology*, 8(2), 13-17.

Abdullah, Z., Muhammad, R., Govender, N., Harun, S., Azlan, N., Muhammad, N., Zainal, Z. Z., & Mohamed-Hussein, Z. (2022). Multi-omics approaches and resources for systems-level gene function prediction in the plant kingdom. *Plants*, 11(19), 2614.

Adam, H., Gopinath, S. C. B., Arshad, M. K. M., Adam, T., Subramaniam, S., & Hashim, U. (2024). An Update on Parkinson's Disease and its Neurodegenerative Counterparts. *Current Medicinal Chemistry*, 31(19), 2770-2787.

Alami, M. M., Ouyang, Z., Zhang, Y., Shu, S., Yang, G., Mei, Z., & Wang, X. (2022). The Current Developments in Medicinal Plant Genomics Enabled the Diversification of Secondary Metabolites' Biosynthesis. *International Journal of Molecular Sciences*, 23(24), 15932.

Carta, A., Astuti, G., Franzoni, J., Giacò, A., Tiburtini, M., Pinzani, L., Peruzzi, L., & D'Antraccoli, M. (2023). A comprehensive approach to improving endemic plant species research, conservation, and popularization. *Journal of Zoological and Botanical Gardens*, 4(2), 490-506.

Armand, E. J., Li, J., Xie, F., Luo, C., & Mukamel, E. A. (2021). Single-cell sequencing of brain cell transcriptomes and epigenomes. *Neuron*, 109(1), 11-26.

Bock, D. G., Cai, Z., Elphinstone, C., González-Segovia, E., Hirabayashi, K., Huang, K., Keais, G. L., Kim, A., Owens, G. L., & Rieseberg, L. H. (2023). Genomics of plant speciation. *Plant Communications*, 4(5), 100599.

Bockaert, J., & Pin, J. P. (1999). Molecular tinkering of G protein-coupled receptors: An evolutionary success. *EMBO Journal*, 18(7), 1723-1729.

Collins, F. S., Morgan, M., & Patrinos, A. (2003). The human genome project: Lessons from large-scale biology. *Science*, 300(5617), 286-290.

Costa, I. M., Lima, F. O. V., Fernandes, L. C. B., Norrara, B., Neta, F. I., Alves, R. D., Cavalcanti, J. R. L. P., Lucena, E. E. S., Cavalcante, J. S., Rego, A. C. M., Filho, I. A., Queiroz, D. B., Freire, M. A. M., & Guzen, F. P. (2019). Astragaloside IV supplementation promotes a neuroprotective effect in experimental models of neurological disorders: A systematic review. *Current Neuropharmacology*, 17(7), 648–665.

Dastagir, G., Hussain, F., & Ul Uza, N. (2023). Anatomical and histochemical characterization of some highly medicinal plants as a tool for quality control. *Microscopy Research & Technique*, 86(8), 966–990.

Gupta, V., & Sharma, B. (2017). Forensic applications of Indian traditional toxic plants and their constituents. *Forensic Research & Criminology International Journal*, 4, 00101.

Maia, M. A., Maia, M. A., & Sousa, E. (2019). BACE-1 and γ-secretase as therapeutic targets for Alzheimer's disease. *Pharmaceuticals*, 12, 41.

Hasin, Y., Seldin, M., & Lusis, A. (2017). Multi-omics approaches to disease. *Genome Biology*, 18(1), 83.

Horner, D. S., Pavesi, G., Castrignanò, T., De Meo, P. D. O., Liuni, S., Sammeth, M., Picardi, E., & Pesole, G. (2010). Bioinformatics approaches for genomics and post-genomics applications of next-generation sequencing. *Briefings in Bioinformatics*, 11(2), 181–197.

Nikolova, I. (2022). Botanical products in Acyrthosiphon pisum (Harris) management in Pisum sativum L. *Journal of Environmental Science & Health – Part B: Pesticides, Food Contaminants, & Agricultural Wastes*, 57(11), 905-915.

Joshi, A., Rienks, M., Theofilatos, K., & Mayr, M. (2021). Systems biology in cardiovascular disease: A multiomics approach. *Nature Reviews Cardiology*, 18(5), 313–330.

Lundstrom, K. (2016). Unlocking the therapeutic potential of plant extracts. *Future Medicinal Chemistry*, 8(3), 245–248.

Macêdo, Y., Filho, A. R. G., & Gil, E. S. (2021). Drug identification by electroanalysis with multiple classification approaches. *Chinese Journal of Analytical Chemistry*, 49(11), 47-53.

Manas, R., Mathur, R., Kumar, T. P., Upadhyay, D., Lal, N., Khatik, D., & Sharma. (2021). Advances in genomics and proteomics in agriculture. In *Crop improvement* (1st ed., pp. 1–13). CRC Press.

D'Antraccoli, M., Carta, A., Astuti, G., Franzoni, J., Giacò, A., Tiburtini, M., Pinzani, L., & Peruzzi, L. (2023). A comprehensive approach to improving endemic plant species research, conservation, and popularization. *Journal of Zoological and Botanical Gardens*, 4(2), 490–506.

Momsen, J., Bray Speth, E., Wyse, S., & Long, T. (2022). Using systems and systems thinking to unify biology education. *CBE Life Sciences Education*, 21(2), es3.

Miyoshi, E., Morabito, S., & Swarup, V. (2021). Systems biology approaches to unravel the molecular and genetic architecture of Alzheimer's disease and related tauopathies. *Neurobiology of Disease*, 160, 105530.

Nenadis, N., Pyrka, I., & Tsimidou, M. Z. (2023). The Contribution of Theoretical Prediction Studies to the Antioxidant Activity Assessment of the Bioactive Secoiridoids Encountered in Olive Tree Products and By-Products. *Molecules*, 28(5), 2267.

García-Pérez, P., Lozano-Milo, E., Zhang, L., Miras-Moreno, B., Landin, M., Lucini, L., & Gallego, P. P. (2022). Neurofuzzy logic predicts a fine-tuning metabolic reprogramming on elicited Bryophyllum PCSCs guided by salicylic acid. *Frontiers in Plant Science*, 13, 991557.

Chen See, P., & Baum, N. (2023). Use of botanicals in modern healthcare. *Healthcare Administration Leadership & Management Journal*, 1(1), 27-30.

Prasansuklab, A., & Tencomnao, T. (2013). Amyloidosis in Alzheimer's Disease: The Toxicity of Amyloid Beta (A β), Mechanisms of Its Accumulation and Implications of Medicinal Plants for Therapy. *Evidence-Based Complementary & Alternative Medicine*, 2013, 413808.

Ragoussis, J. (2009). Genotyping Technologies for Genetic Research. *Annual Review of Genomics & Human Genetics*, 10, 117-133.

Rao, A., Kumari, S., Laura, J. S., & Dhania, G. (2023). Qualitative phytochemical screening of medicinal plants using different solvent extracts. *Oriental Journal of Chemistry*, 39(3), 621–626.

Sharma, S., Priya, T., Goel, N., Kashyap, D., & Garg, V. K. (2023). Overview of neurodegenerative disorders. In *Cognitive technologies* (pp. 3–12).

Thompson, M. D., Percy, M. E., McIntyre, B. W., & Cole, D. E. C. (2008). G protein-coupled receptors disrupted in human genetic disease. *Methods in Molecular Biology*, 448, 109–137.

Tupertsev, B., Osipenko, S., Kireev, A., Nikolaev, E., & Kostyukevich, Y. (2023). Simple *In Vitro* 18O Labeling for Improved Mass Spectrometry-Based Drug Metabolites Identification: Deep Drug Metabolism Study. International Journal of Molecular Sciences, 24(5), 4569.

Waszkielewicz, A. M., Gunia, A., Szkaradek, N., Słoczyńska, K., Krupińska, S., & Marona, H. (2013). Ion channels as drug targets in central nervous system disorders. *Current Medicinal Chemistry*, 20(10), 1241–1285.

Wang, X., Chan, Y. S., Wong, K., Yoshitake, R., Sadava, D., Synold, T. W., Frankel, P., Twardowski, P. W., Lau, C., & Chen, S. (2023). Mechanism-Driven and Clinically Focused Development of Botanical Foods as Multitarget Anticancer Medicine: Collective Perspectives and Insights from Preclinical Studies, IND Applications and Early-Phase Clinical Trials. *Cancers*, 15(3), 701.

Yadav, A. K., Banerjee, S. K., Das, B., & Chaudhary, K. (2022). Editorial: Systems biology and omics approaches for understanding complex disease biology. *Frontiers in Genetics*, 13, 896818.

Zhao, L., Shi, Y., Lau, H. C.-H., Liu, W., Luo, G., Wang, G., Liu, C., Pan, Y., Zhou, Q., Ding, Y., Sung, J. J.-Y., & Yu, J. (2022). Uncovering 1058 novel human enteric DNA viruses through deep long-read third-generation sequencing and their clinical impact. *Gastroenterology*, 163(3), 699-711.

Chapter 3

Amyotrophic Lateral Sclerosis (ALS) and Botanical Therapies

Arushi[1]
Kavita Munjal[2,*]
Hitesh Chopra[3]
Vinod Kumar Gauttam[1]
Chetan Vashist[4]
Pratinav Pandey[2]
and Mayank Goyal[5]

[1]Shiva Institute of Pharmacy, Bilaspur, Himachal Pradesh, India
[2]Amity Institute of Pharmacy, Amity University, Noida, Uttar Pradesh, India
[3]Department of Biosciences, Saveetha School of Engineering,
Saveetha Institute of Medical and Technical Sciences, Chennai, Tamil Nadu, India
[4]IITM College of Pharmacy, IITM Group of Institutions, Sonipat, Haryana, India
5IES Institute of Pharmacy, IES University, Bhopal, Madhya Pradesh, India

Abstract

Amyotrophic lateral sclerosis (ALS) currently has limited treatment options and no known cure, prompting both patients and researchers to explore complementary and alternative therapies, including ethnobotanical remedies. Botanical therapies, which encompass phytochemicals, plant-derived compounds, and various herbal extracts, have gained attention due to their neuroprotective and anti-inflammatory properties. Compounds such as resveratrol, curcumin, and cannabinoids

* Corresponding Author's Email: kavitamunjal915@gmail.com.

In: Natural Solutions for Neurodegenerative Disorders
Editors: Rahul Kumar Sharma, Shailesh Sharma, Ajmer Singh Grewal et al.
ISBN: 979-8-89530-231-6

have shown promise in preclinical studies, indicating they may help alleviate symptoms and slow disease progression in ALS. However, comprehensive clinical trials are essential to confirm the efficacy and safety of these botanical treatments for ALS. Issues related to dosing, regulation, and potential drug-herb interactions must be carefully addressed. Caution is necessary when using these therapies, and consultations with medical professionals are crucial, as they may not offer a cure or significant benefits and could potentially cause side effects or interact with other medications. Botanical remedies present a promising avenue for ALS research and treatment, reflecting the potential of plant-based substances in mitigating ALS pathogenesis. Further research and well-designed clinical studies are recommended to explore these options thoroughly, as they may offer hope for those seeking alternative treatments for this debilitating condition.

Keywords: amyotrophic lateral sclerosis, ALS, neurodegenerative, neuroprotective, herbals, botanicals, therapies

Abbreviations

ACTs	artemisinin-based mixture treatment
ASO's	Antisense oligonucleotides
ALS	Amyotrophic lateral sclerosis
AST-IV	Astragaloside IV
DPPH	2,2-Diphenyl-picrylhydrazyl
EGCG	Epigallocatechin gallate
LDH	Lactate Dehydrogenase
LMNs	Lower motor neurons
MLDs	Motor neuron diseases
NfL	Neurofilament light chain

Introduction

Charcot disease, also known as ALS, is a severe neuromuscular disorder that impacts motor neurons. There are two primary forms of the disease, with the most common type (90-95%) being sporadic and lacking a clear genetic inheritance (Oskarsson et al., 2018). Individuals with Charcot disease experience a progressive loss of their ability to walk, breathe, and eat. This debilitating adult-onset neurodegenerative condition results in the loss of UMNs and LMNs that control muscles in the spinal cord and brain. These motor neurons are essential for transmitting critical mobility-related signals from the brain to the muscles. When these nerve cells are damaged or fail to function properly, the brain loses its ability to initiate and control voluntary movements such as walking, chewing, and speaking. Consequently, voluntary skeletal muscles throughout the body progressively weaken and twitch. In the advanced stages of the disease, this can lead to severe paralysis and respiratory failure, ultimately resulting in death (Salzinger et al., 2024).

Plant-Derived Natural Compounds for Amyotrophic Lateral Sclerosis Treatment

Synthetic chemistry is heavily utilised in medication design and discovery, but natural products still have a significant impact. There are 252 essential medications on the WHO list, and 11% of them are plant-based (Oskarsson et al., 2015) (Figure 1).

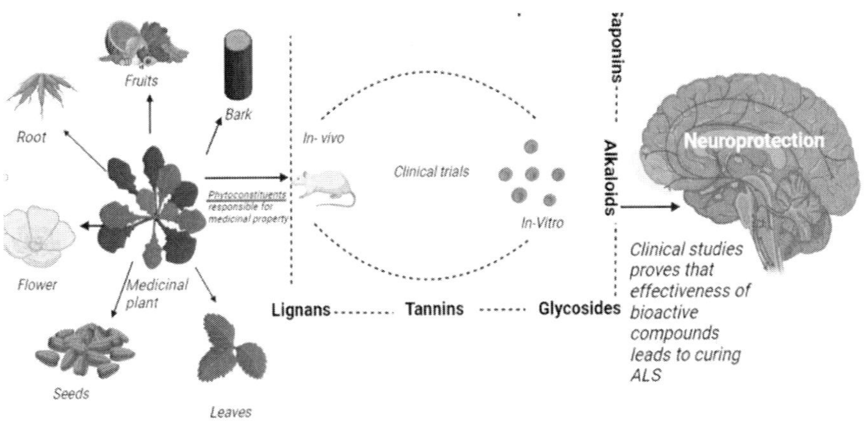

Figure 1. Phytoconstituents role in ALS treatment.

Alkaloids

Alkaloids are secondary metabolites found in plants (Munjal et al., 2023). Annotinine, a lycopodium alkaloid isolated from the Lycopodium annotinum plant of the Lycopodiaceae family, exhibits antioxidant activity by scavenging free radicals through DPPH and inhibiting dityrosine synthesis (Cucovici et al., 2021). It is also beneficial for treating ALS by reducing oxidative stress and maintaining its levels in patients (Brown et al., 2017). Montanine, an isoquinoline alkaloid extracted from Hippeastrum vittatum of the Amaryllidaceae family, possesses anti-convulsant properties. Extracts from Rhodolirium speciosum and Rhodophiala pratensis have shown efficacy in inhibiting acetylcholinesterase (Sena et al., 2024). Piperine, found in long pepper (Piper longum) and black pepper (Piper nigrum) within the Piperaceae family, is known for its pungent nature and has neuroprotective, anti-inflammatory, antifungal, antioxidant, and antidepressant effects (Benjaminsen et al., 2018). Its derivative, 'HJ105,' has demonstrated anti-inflammatory properties, reducing inflammation, apoptosis, and oxidative stress by inhibiting the formation of the Keap1-Nrf2 complex, thereby offering neuroprotective effects in SH-SY5Y cells stimulated by Aβ1-42 (Alhudaithi et al., 2024; Gauttam et al., 2022). Nantenine, an aporphine alkaloid derived from the Nandina domestica fruit of the Berberidaceae family, exhibits sedative and anticonvulsant properties. It modulates neuronal activity by addressing hyper-excitability due to calcium influx caused by calcium signaling (Antona et al., 2021). Nantenine is beneficial in ALS treatment as it reduces calcium influx into cells, mitigating neuronal hyperexcitability. The Table 1 below summarizes various plant-derived alkaloids, their sources, study types, and mechanisms by which they offer protection to ALS patients.

Table 1. Mechanism of different Alkaloids used for ALS treatment

Alkaloids	Source	Study type	Mechanism	Reference
Annotinine	*Lycopodium amotinum*	*In- vitro* PC 12 cells	By reducing iron ascorbate induced damage	(Vuong, 2008)
Montanine	*Hippeastrum Vittatum*	*In- vitro* SH- SY5Y cells	Raises the cellular GSH level and reduce the levels of LDH	(Uher et al., 2022)
Piperine	*Piper nigrum* and *Piper longum*	In cell line	Suppress the formation of Keap1- Nrf2 complex.	(Gjorgieva et al., 2023)
Nantenine	*Nandina domestica*	*In- vitro* PC 12 cells	Reduce the calcium influx into cells.	(Riberio et al., 2003)

Flavonoids

Phenolic compounds, which occur naturally in various vegetables, fruits, and plants, include a diverse group of flavonoids known for their health benefits (Hasnat et al., 2024). Ampelopsin, also called dihydromyricetin, is a flavanonol-type flavonoid isolated from Ampelopsis grossedentata of the Vitaceae family. Research has demonstrated its neuroprotective effects against H_2O_2-induced apoptosis in PC12 cells (Brown et al., 2021). Ampelopsin has been shown to inhibit the p38 signaling pathway activated by H_2O_2 (Chen et al., 2022). Additionally, ampelopsin activates the ERK and Akt signaling pathways, leading to the expression of heme oxygenase-1, which can be nearly completely blocked by inhibitors of these pathways (Carrera et al., 2020). Anthocyanins, a group of water-soluble flavonoids found in red, blue, and purple fruits and vegetables, are noted for their antioxidant properties and potential health benefits (Amico et al., 2021). They help reduce spinal cord astrogliosis and maintain neuromuscular junction integrity and muscle activation. Epigallocatechin gallate (EGCG) is another flavonoid used in ALS treatment (Park et al., 2015). Table 2 summarizes various flavonoids, including their sources, study types, and mechanisms by which they offer protection to ALS patients.

Table 2. Phytoconstituents used in ALS treatment

Flavonoids	Source	Study type	Mechanism	Reference
Ampleopsin	*Ampelopsis grossedentata*	*In- vitro* PC 12 cells	Suppress ROS production and upregulating the expression of HO-1	(Christensen, 2018)
Anthocyanins	Purple, blue and red vegetables and fruits	hSOD1 G93A Transgenic mouse model of ALS	Reduce spinal cord astrogliosis	(Winter et al., 2018).
EGCG	Green tea	*In-vivo* Transgenic mice SOD1-G93A	Upregulation of Bcl-2 gene	(Goncalves et al., 2021)

Saponins

Saponins are nonvolatile, surface-active compounds known for their detergent, hemolytic, and neuroprotective properties (Yu et al., 2014). They are utilized in the treatment of ALS due to these beneficial effects.

Madecassoside, a triterpenoid saponin found in Centella asiatica, exhibits anti-inflammatory, antioxidant, and neuroprotective properties. It enhances antioxidant activity, protecting neurons from damage caused by free radicals. Additionally, madecassoside reduces neurotoxicity induced by lipopolysaccharide in rats by stimulating the Nrf2-HO pathway (Arthur et al., 2016; Wolf et al., 2014).

Astragaloside IV (AST-IV), a pentacyclic triterpenoid saponin derived from Astragalus membranaceus, offers neuroprotective, antiviral, immunomodulatory, and anti-inflammatory effects (Logroscino et al., 2019; Godos et al., 2020). Ginsenosides, steroid-like saponins extracted from Panax ginseng of the Araliaceae family, are known for their neuroprotective properties. They act by reducing the production of TNF-α and CD14 in the TLR4 signaling pathway. Ginsenoside Re, in particular, has been shown to decrease motor neuron loss, reduce Iba-1 expression, and lower levels of phospho-p38 protein and antioxidant HO1, which contribute to its antioxidative effects (Kellogg et al., 2018).

Tannins

Tannins are polyphenolic compounds found in the leaves, roots, and fruits of various plants, known for their antioxidant and astringent properties. Epicatechin, a type of flavanol within the broader tannin family, is particularly abundant in cocoa beans. It is celebrated for its strong antioxidant qualities, which aid in neutralizing harmful free radicals in the body (Hayashi et al., 2016). The cardiovascular benefits often associated with chocolate may, in part, be due to its high epicatechin content. Gallotannins, another form of tannins, are found in the bark of numerous plants, including oak trees. These tannins are utilized in leather tanning due to their astringent properties. In traditional medicine, oak bark has been recognized for its potential anti-inflammatory and antibacterial effects.

Terpenoids

Terpenoids are a diverse group of molecules with various biological functions. Menthol, derived from peppermint and spearmint (Mentha spicata), interacts with cold-sensitive receptors in the skin to produce a cooling sensation. It is commonly used in products such as cough drops and topical pain relievers

(Wang et al., 2024). Limonene, a terpenoid with a fruity and citrus aroma, is typically found in the peels of citrus fruits like oranges, lemons, and limes. It has anticancer, antioxidant, and anti-inflammatory properties and is often used as a flavoring agent and in cologne stabilizers (Wang et al., 2024). Artemisinin, extracted from the Artemisia annua plant, is a key component of artemisinin-based combination therapies (ACTs) used to treat malaria and has potential applications in cancer.

Lignans

Phenolic compounds are formed through the oxidative dimerization of two phenylpropanoid units and are used in the treatment of neurological diseases, particularly via the peroxidation dismutase-SOD1 pathway (Mueed et al., 2024). Notable examples include:

- Pinoresinol, sesamine, and secoisolariciresinol.
- Sesamine, derived from *Zanthoxylum fagara* and *Sesamum indicum*, exhibits neuroprotective, anti-inflammatory, antioxidant, and anti-diabetic properties in neuronal cells such as PC12.
- Secoisolariciresinol, found in flaxseed and converted into enterolignans, shows antioxidant properties and may offer additional health benefits such as hormone balancing and support for menopause and hormone-related conditions (Singh et al., 2024).

The Role of Botanical Therapies

Herbal remedies, which include phytoconstituents such as flavonoids, glycosides, polyphenols, terpenoids, and alkaloids, play a significant role in the potential treatment of ALS by mitigating oxidative stress and reducing free radical generation in neurons. These phytoconstituents help slow disease progression and prevent motor neuron degradation, acting as neuroprotective agents in ALS management (Esterhuizen et al., 2019). In addition to their neuroprotective effects, some phytoconstituents possess anti-inflammatory properties, which are crucial for ALS treatment. Chronic inflammation is a key factor in ALS progression, and compounds like curcumin and resveratrol have been studied for their ability to modulate inflammatory responses in the central nervous system, potentially alleviating the inflammation associated with the disease (Satyavert et al., 2021). Phytoconstituents may also impact mitochondrial function. For example, creatine has been explored for its role in supporting mitochondrial health and energy production, which could positively affect motor neuron survival in ALS patients. Although research into phytoconstituents for ALS is ongoing, their natural origins and relatively low toxicity profiles make them promising candidates for complementary or adjunctive therapies alongside conventional treatments (Martin et al., 2021). It is important to note that ALS is a complex and poorly understood condition. The full benefits and mechanisms of phytoconstituents in managing ALS require further investigation through clinical trials and rigorous scientific studies. Patients considering the use of phytoconstituents should consult with healthcare professionals to ensure safe and informed decisions (Scott et al., 2017).

Dietary Supplements for ALS

Dietary supplements have garnered interest as potential adjunctive therapies for managing ALS. These supplements include a diverse range of vitamins, minerals, amino acids, and other compounds that are often available over the counter. Although they are not considered primary treatments for ALS, they may offer supportive benefits for the health and well-being of individuals living with the disease (Marchi and Tondo, 2024):

Nutritional Support

ALS can cause difficulty with swallowing and impaired nutrient absorption, potentially leading to malnutrition. Dietary supplements can help bridge this gap by providing essential vitamins and minerals that patients might struggle to get from their regular diets. This includes B-complex vitamins, vitamin D, as well as minerals like calcium and magnesium.

Weight Maintenance

For ALS patients, maintaining a healthy body weight is crucial to support their energy levels and overall well-being (Ahmad et al., 2016). Protein supplements and high-calorie shakes can assist individuals in maintaining or gaining weight.

Muscle Function

Creatine, a widely used dietary supplement, has been investigated for its potential to improve muscle function and provide energy to muscles affected by ALS. Although results have been mixed, some individuals with ALS may find benefits from creatine supplementation (Huisman et al., 2015).

Antioxidant Protection

Antioxidant supplements, such as vitamin E, may help mitigate oxidative stress associated with ALS. By targeting and reducing the damage caused by free radicals, these supplements aim to support overall cellular health.

Pain and Symptom Management

Certain dietary supplements, such as fish oil and omega-3 fatty acids, may offer anti-inflammatory benefits that could help alleviate ALS symptoms, such as muscle pain and stiffness (Ahmed et al., 2016). However, ALS remains a complex and rapidly progressing condition with no known cure (Scott et al., 2017). While these supplements might provide some benefits, they should not replace standard medical treatments and therapies prescribed by healthcare professionals. It is crucial for individuals with ALS to consult with their healthcare team before adding dietary supplements to their treatment regimen. Ongoing research is necessary to fully understand the potential advantages and risks of these supplements in managing ALS.

Clinical Studies and Evidence

Clinical studies and evidence-based research are crucial in ALS research and care (Huisman et al., 2015). They offer valuable insights into the underlying causes of the disease, explore potential treatment options, and help improve the quality of life for individuals with ALS.

Understanding ALS: Pathophysiology and Genetics

To effectively address ALS, it is essential to understand its pathophysiology and genetic basis (Goutman et al., 2022). While most cases of ALS are sporadic (SALS) and do not have a family history, approximately 5–10% of cases are familial (FALS) and are linked to specific genetic mutations.

C9orf72 Hexanucleotide Repeat Expansion

The hexanucleotide repeat expansion in the C9orf72 gene is the most common genetic cause of frontotemporal dementia (FTD) and ALS. Research aims to uncover the mechanisms through which this repeat expansion leads to neurodegeneration (Babic et al., 2019). Recent studies have investigated potential therapeutic strategies to target this genetic mutation, including the use of antisense oligonucleotides (ASOs) and small molecules.

Sporadic ALS and Genetic Susceptibility

Although a specific genetic cause for sporadic ALS (SALS) has not been identified, genome-wide association studies (GWAS) have identified genetic variations associated with an increased risk of developing the disease. These genetic risk factors offer valuable insights into potential disease mechanisms and pathways (Ajroud et al., 2015).

Biomarkers and Diagnostic Advances

Accurate and early diagnosis of ALS is essential for effective patient care and participation in clinical trials. Research into biomarkers and diagnostic tools has been extensive, aiming to improve the precision of ALS diagnosis (Benatar et al., 2016).

Neurofilament Light Chain (NfL) as a Biomarker

NfL, a protein released into cerebrospinal fluid and blood during neuronal damage, has emerged as a promising biomarker for ALS (Benatar et al., 2016). Elevated NfL levels are associated with disease progression and can assist in both diagnosis and monitoring of disease progression.

Advanced Imaging Techniques

Advanced neuroimaging techniques such as DTI and fMRI offer valuable insights into ALS-related changes in brain structure and connectivity. These imaging biomarkers are essential for understanding disease mechanisms and assessing the effects of treatments (Ghaderi et al., 2023).

Disease Progression and Clinical Trials

Clinical trials represent a critical avenue for evaluating potential treatments and interventions for ALS (Kiernan et al., 2021). Understanding disease progression is vital for designing effective trials.

Clinical Trial Design

Recent advancements in trial design, such as adaptive trial methodologies and the development of more sensitive outcome measures, have enhanced the efficiency and precision of clinical trials for ALS (Fournier, 2022).

Assistive Devices and Technology

The integration of robotic assistance and eye-tracking communication technologies has greatly improved the quality of life for ALS patients, allowing them to maintain independence and enhance their ability to communicate (Memon, 2024).

End-of-Life Support and Palliative Care

To address the psychological and emotional needs of ALS patients and their families, palliative care plays a crucial role (Ziegler et al., 2018). This includes end-of-life planning and discussions about ventilatory support and advance directives.

Conclusion

In conclusion, the study of ALS involves a complex interplay of scientific research, clinical exploration, and compassionate care. This relentless neurodegenerative disorder continues to challenge researchers and healthcare providers alike. However, the combined efforts of the scientific community have shed light on various aspects of this enigmatic disease. These discoveries have not only deepened our understanding of ALS but have also led to the development of targeted therapies, such as antisense oligonucleotide treatments, offering new hope for patients. The search for biomarkers and diagnostic tools has produced promising candidates like neurofilament light chain (NfL), which enable earlier diagnosis and more accurate monitoring of disease progression. Advanced imaging techniques and electrophysiological assessments have further refined our grasp of ALS pathophysiology. Clinical trials have evolved with innovative designs and more sensitive outcome measures, paving the way for emerging treatments, including ASOs, gene therapies, and stem cell-based approaches, which hold the promise of significant breakthroughs in disease modification. The approach to ALS care has also become more comprehensive, incorporating not only medicinal therapies but also multidisciplinary clinics, assistive technologies, and palliative care to enhance the quality of life for individuals with ALS, allowing them to maintain independence and dignity. Patient-centered research, driven by collaboration between patients, advocates, and scientists, continues to accelerate progress. While ALS remains a challenging and devastating disease, the synergy of research, clinical care, and patient advocacy offers a hopeful path toward better understanding, treatment, and ultimately, overcoming ALS.

References

Ahmed, R. M., Caga, J., Devenney, E., Hsieh, S., Bartley, L., Highton-Williamson, E., E., Ramsey, E., Zoing, M., Halliday & Kiernan, M. C. (2016). Cognition and eating behavior in amyotrophic lateral sclerosis: effect on survival. *Journal of neurology*, *263*(8), 1593-1603.

Ajroud-Driss, S., & Siddique, T. (2015). Sporadic and hereditary amyotrophic lateral sclerosis (ALS). *Biochimica et Biophysica Acta (BBA)-Molecular Basis of Disease*, *1852*(4), 679-684.

Alhudaithi, S. S., Kalam, M. A., Binobaid, L., Ali, R., Almutairi, M. M., Qamar, W., Hithlayn, H. B., Almutairi A. & Alshememry, A. K. (2024). Sorafenib and Piperine co-loaded PLGA nanoparticles: Development, characterization, and anti-cancer activity against hepatocellular carcinoma cell line. *Saudi Pharmaceutical Journal*, *32*(5), 102064.

Arthur, K. C., Calvo, A., Price, T. R., Geiger, J. T., Chio, A., & Traynor, B. J. (2016). Projected increase in amyotrophic lateral sclerosis from 2015 to 2040. *Nature communications*, *7*(1), 12408.

Aye, M., Jarrahpour, A., Haghighijoo, Z., Heiran, R., Pournejati, R., Karbalaei-Heidari, H. R., Sinou, V., Brunel, J. M., Akkurt, M., Ozdemir N. & Turos, E. (2024). Novel Benzotriazole-β-lactam Derivatives as Antimalarial Agents: Design, Synthesis, Biological Evaluation and Molecular Docking Studies. *Chemistry & Biodiversity*, *21*(2), e202301745.

Babić Leko, M., Župunski, V., Kirincich, J., Smilović, D., Hortobágyi, T., Hof, P. R., & Šimić, G. (2019). Molecular mechanisms of neurodegeneration related to C9orf72 hexanucleotide repeat expansion. *Behavioural neurology*, *2019*(1), 2909168.

Benatar, M., Boylan, K., Jeromin, A., Rutkove, S. B., Berry, J., Atassi, N., & Bruijn, L. (2016). ALS biomarkers for therapy development: state of the field and future directions. *Muscle & nerve*, *53*(2), 169-182.

Benjaminsen, E., Alstadhaug, K. B., Gulsvik, M., Baloch, F. K., & Odeh, F. (2018). Amyotrophic lateral sclerosis in Nordland County, Norway, 2000–2015: prevalence, incidence, and clinical features. *Amyotrophic Lateral Sclerosis and Frontotemporal Degeneration*, *19*(7-8), 522-527.

Brown, C. A., Lally, C., Kupelian, V., & Flanders, W. D. (2021). Estimated prevalence and incidence of amyotrophic lateral sclerosis and SOD1 and C9orf72 genetic variants. *Neuroepidemiology*, *55*(5), 342-353.

Brown, R. H., & Al-Chalabi, A. (2017). Amyotrophic lateral sclerosis. *New England Journal of Medicine*, *377*(2), 162-172.

Carrera-Juliá, S., Moreno, M. L., Barrios, C., de la Rubia Ortí, J. E., & Drehmer, E. (2020). Antioxidant alternatives in the treatment of amyotrophic lateral sclerosis: a comprehensive review. *Frontiers in physiology*, *11*, 63.

Chen, B., Zhao, J., Zhang, R., Zhang, L., Zhang, Q., Yang, H., & An, J. (2022). Neuroprotective effects of natural compounds on neurotoxin-induced oxidative stress and cell apoptosis. *Nutritional neuroscience*, *25*(5), 1078-1099.

Christensen, L. P. (2018). The role of direct and indirect polyphenolic antioxidants in protection against oxidative stress. In *Polyphenols: Mechanisms of action in human health and disease* (pp. 147-179), Academic Press.

Cucovici, A., Fontana, A., Ivashynka, A., Russo, S., Renna, V., Mazzini, L., Gagliardi I., J., Martinelli, I., Lisnic, V. & Leone, M. A. (2021). The impact of lifetime alcohol and cigarette smoking loads on amyotrophic lateral sclerosis progression: a cross-sectional study. *Life*, *11*(4), 352.

D'Antona, S., Bertoli, G., Castiglioni, I., & Cava, C. (2021). Minor Allele Frequencies and Molecular Pathways Differences for SNPs Associated with Amyotrophic Lateral Sclerosis in Subjects Participating in the UKBB and 1000 Genomes Project. *Journal of Clinical Medicine*, *10*(15), 3394.

D'Amico, E., Grosso, G., Nieves, J. W., Zanghì, A., Factor-Litvak, P., & Mitsumoto, H. (2021). Metabolic Abnormalities, Dietary Risk Factors and Nutritional Management in Amyotrophic Lateral Sclerosis. *Nutrients*, *13*(7), 2273.

De A Ribeiro, R., do Carmo, L. G., Vladimirova, I., Jurkiewicz, N. H., & Jurkiewicz, A. (2003). Nantenine blocks muscle contraction and Ca2+ transient induced by noradrenaline and K+ in rat vas deferens. *European journal of pharmacology*, *470*(1-2), 37-43.

De Marchi, F., & Tondo, G. (2024). Food, Dietary Supplements and Nutraceuticals in Aging and Neurodegenerative Diseases. *CNS & Neurological Disorders-Drug Targets*, *23*(5), 543-544.

Esterhuizen-Londt, M., & Pflugmacher, S. (2019). Vegetables cultivated with exposure to pure and naturally occurring β-N-methylamino-L-alanine (BMAA) via irrigation. *Environmental research*, *169*, 357-361.

Fournier, C. N. (2022). Considerations for amyotrophic lateral sclerosis (ALS) clinical trial design. *Neurotherapeutics*, *19*(4), 1180-1192.

Gauttam, V. K., Munjal, K., Singh, V., Sharma, I., & Sahpuriya, P. (2022). Phytochemicals for metabolic syndrome. In *Natural Products for Treatment of Metabolic Syndrome* (pp. 235-245). Springer.

Ghaderi, S., Fatehi, F., Kalra, S., & Batouli, S. A. H. (2023). MRI biomarkers for memory-related impairment in amyotrophic lateral sclerosis: a systematic review. *Amyotrophic Lateral Sclerosis and Frontotemporal Degeneration*, *24*(7-8), 572-588.

Gjorgieva Ackova, D., Maksimova, V., Smilkov, K., Buttari, B., Arese, M., & Saso, L. (2023). Alkaloids as natural NRF2 inhibitors: Chemoprevention and cytotoxic action in Cancer. *Pharmaceuticals*, *16*(6), 850.

Godos, J., Currenti, W., Angelino, D., Mena, P., Castellano, S., Caraci, F., Galvano, F., Del Rio, D., Ferri, R., & Grosso, G. (2020). Diet and mental health: Review of the recent updates on molecular mechanisms. *Antioxidants*, 9(4), 346.

Gonçalves, P. B., Sodero, A. C. R., & Cordeiro, Y. (2021). Green tea epigallocatechin-3-gallate (EGCG) targeting protein misfolding in drug discovery for neurodegenerative diseases. *Biomolecules*, *11*(5), 767.

Goutman, S. A., Hardiman, O., Al-Chalabi, A., Chió, A., Savelieff, M. G., Kiernan, M. C., & Feldman, E. L. (2022). Emerging insights into the complex genetics and pathophysiology of amyotrophic lateral sclerosis. *The Lancet Neurology*, *21*(5), 465-479.

Hasnat, H., Shompa, S. A., Islam, M. M., Alam, S., Richi, F. T., Emon, N. U., Ashrafi, S., Ahmed, N. U., & Ahmed, F. (2024). Flavonoids: A treasure house of prospective pharmacological potentials. *Heliyon*.

Hayashi, Y., Homma, K., & Ichijo, H. (2016). SOD1 in neurotoxicity and its controversial roles in SOD1 mutation-negative ALS. *Advances in biological regulation*, *60*, 95-104.

Huisman, M. H., Seelen, M., van Doormaal, P. T., de Jong, S. W., de Vries, J. H., van der Kooi, A. J., de Visser, M., Schelhaas, H. J., van den Berg, L. H., & Veldink, J. H. (2015). Effect of Presymptomatic Body Mass Index and Consumption of Fat and Alcohol on Amyotrophic Lateral Sclerosis. *JAMA neurology*, *72*(10), 1155–1162.

Kciuk, M., Mujwar, S., Rani, I., Munjal, K., Gielecińska, A., Kontek, R., & Shah, K. (2022). Computational bioprospecting guggulsterone against ADP ribose phosphatase of SARS-CoV-2. *Molecules*, *27*(23), 8287.

Kellogg, J., Bottman, L., Arra, E. J., Selkirk, S. M., & Kozlowski, F. (2018). Nutrition management methods effective in increasing weight, survival time and functional status in ALS patients: a systematic review. *Amyotrophic Lateral Sclerosis and Frontotemporal Degeneration*, *19*(1-2), 7-11.

Kiernan, M. C., Vucic, S., Talbot, K., McDermott, C. J., Hardiman, O., Shefner, J. M., Al-Chalabi, A., Huynh, W., Cudkowicz M., & Turner, M. R. (2021). Improving clinical trial outcomes in amyotrophic lateral sclerosis. *Nature Reviews Neurology*, *17*(2), 104-118.

Logroscino, G., & Piccininni, M. (2019). Amyotrophic lateral sclerosis descriptive epidemiology: The origin of geographic difference. *Neuroepidemiology*, 52(1-2), 93-103.

Martin, R. M., Bereman, M. S., & Marsden, K. C. (2021). BMAA and MCLR interact to modulate behavior and exacerbate molecular changes related to neurodegeneration in larval zebrafish. *Toxicological Sciences*, *179*(2), 251-261.

Memon, Q. A. (2024). A Comprehensive Review of Current Assistive Technology Research for Paralyzed People. *Current and Future Trends on Intelligent Technology Adoption: Volume 2*, 287-305.

Mueed, A., Ibrahim, M., Shibli, S., Madjirebaye, P., Deng, Z., & Jahangir, M. (2024). The fate of flaxseed-lignans after oral administration: A comprehensive review on its bioavailability, pharmacokinetics, and food design strategies for optimal application. *Critical Reviews in Food Science and Nutrition*, *64*(13), 4312-4330.

Munjal, K., Ahmad, S., Gupta, A., Haye, A., Amin, S., & Mir, S. R. (2020). Polyphenol-enriched fraction and the compounds isolated from Garcinia indica fruits ameliorate obesity through suppression of digestive enzymes and oxidative stress. *Pharmacognosy Magazine*, *16*(70).

Munjal, K., Gautam, V. K., Goel, Y., Ahamad, J., and Mir, S. R. 2023. Qualitative Diagnostic Features of Alkaloidal Spices. In *Analysis of Food Spices* (pp. 135-150): CRC Press.

Nieves, J. W., Gennings, C., Factor-Litvak, P., Hupf, J., Singleton, J., Sharf, V., Oskarsson, B., Fernandes Filho, J. A. M., & Mitsumoto, H. (2016). Association between dietary intake and function in amyotrophic lateral sclerosis. *JAMA neurology*, *73*(12), 1425-1432.

Oskarsson, B., Gendron, T. F., & Staff, N. P. (2018, November). Amyotrophic lateral sclerosis: an update for 2018. In *Mayo clinic proceedings* (Vol. 93, No. 11, pp. 1617-1628). Elsevier.

Oskarsson, B., Horton, D. K., & Mitsumoto, H. (2015). Potential environmental factors in amyotrophic lateral sclerosis. *Neurologic clinics*, *33*(4), 877-888.

Park, Y., Park, J., Kim, Y., Baek, H., & Kim, S. H. (2015). Association between nutritional status and disease severity using the amyotrophic lateral sclerosis (ALS) functional rating scale in ALS patients. *Nutrition*, *31*(11-12), 1362-1367.

Salzinger, A., Ramesh, V., Das Sharma, S., Chandran, S., & Thangaraj Selvaraj, B. (2024). Neuronal Circuit Dysfunction in Amyotrophic Lateral Sclerosis. *Cells*, *13*(10), 792.

Satyavert, Gupta, S., Choudhury, H., Jacob, S., Nair, A. B., Dhanawat, M., & Munjal, K. (2021). Pharmacokinetics and tissue distribution of hydrazinocurcumin in rats. *Pharmacological Reports*, *73*, 1734-1743.

Scott, L. L., & Downing, T. G. (2017). A single neonatal exposure to BMAA in a rat model produces neuropathology consistent with neurodegenerative diseases. *Toxins*, *10*(1), 22.

Sena, S., Kaur, H., & Kumar, V. (2024). Lycorine as a lead molecule in the treatment of cancer and strategies for its biosynthesis using the *in vitro* culture technique. *Phytochemistry Reviews*, 1-28.

Singh, R., Saffeullah, P., Ahmad, S., & Umar, S. (2024). Linseed (Linum usitatissimum L.) accessions depict genetic variations in growth and yield characteristics, biochemical parameters, antioxidant potential, and secoisolariciresinol diglucoside content. *Genetic Resources and Crop Evolution*, 1-24.

Uher, M., Hroch, M., Peřinová, R., Havelek, R., Křoustková, J., Řezáčová, M., Muthna, D., Koutova D, Kunes, J. & Cahlikova, L. (2022). Semisynthetic derivatives of haemanthamine and their *in vitro* antiproliferative activity evaluation against a panel of human cell lines. *Arabian Journal of Chemistry*, *15*(5), 103746.

Vuong, Q. V. (2008). Utilisation of bioactive compounds from agricultural and food waste. *Clin. Cancer Res.*, *11*, 4627-4633.

Wang, X., Xin, J., Sun, L., Sun, Y., Xu, Y., Zhao, F., Niu, C., & Liu, S. (2024). Exploring the Biomedical Potential of Terpenoid Alkaloids: Sources, Structures, and Activities. *Molecules*, *29*(9), 1968.

Winter, A. N., Ross, E. K., Wilkins, H. M., Stankiewicz, T. R., Wallace, T., Miller, K., & Linseman, D. A. (2018). An anthocyanin-enriched extract from strawberries delays disease onset and extends survival in the hSOD1G93A mouse model of amyotrophic lateral sclerosis. *Nutritional Neuroscience*, *21*(6), 414-426.

Wolf, J., Wöhrle, J. C., Palm, F., Nix, W. A., Maschke, M., Safer, A., Becher, H., & Grau, A. J. (2014). Incidence of amyotrophic lateral sclerosis in Rhineland-Palatinate, Germany. *Amyotrophic Lateral Sclerosis and Frontotemporal Degeneration*, *15*(3-4), 269-274.

Yu, Y., Su, F. C., Callaghan, B. C., Goutman, S. A., Batterman, S. A., & Feldman, E. L. (2014). Environmental risk factors and amyotrophic lateral sclerosis (ALS): a case-control study of ALS in Michigan. *PloS one*, *9*(6), e101186.

Ziegler, L. E., Craigs, C. L., West, R. M., Carder, P., Hurlow, A., Millares-Martin, P., Hall, G. & Bennett, M. I. (2018). Is palliative care support associated with better quality end-of-life care indicators for patients with advanced cancer? A retrospective cohort study. *BMJ open*, *8*(1), e018284.

Chapter 4

Curcumin for Neuroprotection: An Update

Ashna Gupta
Priyanka Kriplani*
and Bhawna Chopra
Guru Gobind Singh College of Pharmacy, Yamunanagar, Haryana, India

Abstract

Curcumin, the active compound in turmeric, has garnered substantial interest for its potential neuroprotective properties. Neuroprotection, which involves maintaining and enhancing neuronal structure and function, is crucial in combating various neurodegenerative disorders such as Alzheimer's disease, stroke, and Parkinson's disease. Derived from the rhizome of turmeric (Curcuma longa), curcumin exhibits a range of mechanisms that contribute to its neuroprotective effects, including antioxidant, anti-inflammatory, and anti-amyloid properties. It modulates key signaling pathways like NF-κB and PI3K/Akt to combat neuronal damage and improve synaptic plasticity. Additionally, curcumin promotes autophagy and inhibits apoptosis, supporting neuronal survival. The compound's impact on neuroinflammation and oxidative stress further enhances its neuroprotective capacity. Both preclinical and clinical studies have shown promising results, demonstrating curcumin's efficacy in improving cognitive function, memory retention, and motor skills in various experimental models and human subjects. Curcumin's ability to neutralize free radicals and reduce inflammation underscores its potential in mitigating neuronal damage.

* Corresponding Author's Email: priyanka15n@gmail.com.

In: Natural Solutions for Neurodegenerative Disorders
Editors: Rahul Kumar Sharma, Shailesh Sharma, Ajmer Singh Grewal et al.
ISBN: 979-8-89530-231-6

Keywords: anti-inflammatory, antioxidant, curcumin, neurodegenerative disease, neuroprotection

Abbreviations

AD	Alzheimer's disease
BDNF	Brain-derived neurotrophic factor
COX	Cyclooxygenase
GSH-Px	Glutathione peroxidase
MS	Multiple sclerosis
NDs	Non-diagnostic depressions
NOS	Nitric oxide synthase
PD	Parkinson's disease
PEG	Polyethylene glycol
PLGA	PEG-ylated polylactide-co-glycolide
ROS	Reactive oxygen species
SLNs	Solid lipid nanoparticles
SOD	Superoxide dismutase
TBI	Traumatic brain injury

Introduction

The pursuit of nature's solutions for neurological disorders has led researchers to explore a variety of compounds with promising therapeutic potential. Curcumin, a polyphenolic compound extracted from Curcuma longa, has emerged as a compelling focus due to its diverse properties and significant neuroprotective potential. This chapter aims to explore curcumin's attributes as a neuroprotective agent, detailing its mechanisms of action, potential benefits, and challenges in clinical application. Neurological diseases such as Alzheimer's, Parkinson's, stroke, and traumatic brain injury pose significant global health challenges, making innovative treatment approaches essential. Curcumin's well-documented anti-inflammatory, antioxidant, and anti-amyloid properties make it a promising candidate for therapeutic exploration (Abd El-Hack et al., 2021). Its neuroprotective effects are linked to its ability to modulate key cellular pathways involved in neurodegeneration, including inhibiting misfolded protein formation, reducing oxidative stress, and mitigating neuroinflammation (Aggarwal and Harikumar, 2009). However, translating curcumin's potential into clinical practice presents challenges such as limited bioavailability, rapid metabolism, and difficulty crossing the blood-brain barrier. Innovative formulations and delivery strategies are needed to maximize its therapeutic benefits. This chapter will review current knowledge on curcumin's neuroprotective properties, recent advancements, ongoing research, and future prospects, emphasizing the need for further clinical trials to bridge the gap between preclinical findings and clinical outcomes (Aggarwal and Sung, 2009). Additionally, it will address curcumin's potential in combating non-diagnostic depressions (NDs) caused by inflammation, oxidative stress, trauma, aging, and other factors. Curcumin's ability to penetrate the blood-brain barrier, activate Nrf2, inhibit NF-κB, and scavenge free radicals underscores its potential in managing dysregulated processes associated with NDs (Arun and Nalini, 2002; Ahmadinejad, 2017). Understanding and overcoming the challenges associated with curcumin could pave the way for effective treatments for neurological disorders worldwide (Ahmad et al., 2013).

Mechanism

Curcumin, an active compound found in turmeric, has garnered significant interest for its potential neuroprotective properties. Its mechanisms involve a multifaceted approach, influencing various pathways and processes within the nervous system.

Mechanism of Curcumin Against Cerebral Ischemia

Recent investigations have demonstrated that curcumin exerts a neuroprotective effect in cases of cerebral ischemia. Curcumin can enhance the prognosis of ischemic stroke by reducing brain edema, infarct volume, and neurological impairment (Cote, 2022). Its effects involve several mechanisms, including the restoration of the blood-brain barrier and mitochondrial structure, as well as the suppression of inflammation, oxidative stress, apoptosis, endoplasmic reticulum stress, and calcium overload.

Curcumin Decreases Oxidative Pressure

Brain tissues have a higher metabolic rate, greater demand for oxygen and polyunsaturated fatty acids, and lower levels of antioxidant enzymes compared to other organs. As a result, the central nervous system is more vulnerable to oxidative damage (Caroline et al., 2013). Oxidative stress, caused by an imbalance between antioxidant and oxidative systems, is a primary factor in cerebral ischemic injury. Research has shown that after a stroke, the activity of antioxidant enzymes such as glutathione peroxidase (GSH-Px), catalase, peroxidase, and superoxide dismutase (SOD) declines (Cavalcanti et al., 2022). This disruption in the balance of reactive oxygen species (ROS) leads to their accumulation. Other enzymes, including myeloperoxidase, cyclooxygenase (COX), xanthine dehydrogenase/xanthine oxidase, and nitric oxide synthase (NOS), also contribute to ROS production (Dugger et al., 2017). Excessive ROS can result in lipid peroxidation, DNA damage, and protein oxidation. Therefore, a crucial therapeutic approach for cerebral ischemia is the use of antioxidants or free radical scavengers. Curcumin acts as an antioxidant, aiding in the rapid elimination of ROS by stimulating antioxidant enzymes and preventing brain tissue damage from oxidative stress (Ding et al., 2022). Curcumin has been extensively studied for its potential neuroprotective effects in cerebral ischemia by reducing oxidative stress-induced damage. Its antioxidative properties have been well-researched, with evidence showing that curcumin can reduce oxidative stress and neuronal damage when administered immediately after ischemia or up to 24 hours later. Curcumin also enhances the antioxidative capacity of injured neurons both pre- and post-treatment, extending its therapeutic window in treating cerebral ischemia patients. Additionally, curcumin decreases the production and accumulation of ROS and oxidation products like MDA and lipid peroxidation. Formulations such as curcumin-loaded solid lipid nanoparticles (C-SLNs) or polyethylene glycol (PEG)-ylated polylactide-co-glycolide (PLGA) nanoparticles further reduce ROS levels. In a comparative study evaluating the antioxidative effects of three curcuminoids (curcumin, demethoxycurcumin, and bisdemethoxycurcumin) using a polymeric N-isopropyl acrylamide nanoparticle formulation, curcumin demonstrated the most potent antioxidant activity (Mangala et al., 2023). Moreover, curcumin enhances the expression and activity of various antioxidative enzymes, including GSH-Px, SOD, CAT, NADPH oxidase 2, and glutathione reductase. According to Awad et al., curcumin's ability to inhibit oxidative stress synergistically improves the efficacy of candesartan in treating cerebral ischemia, highlighting its potential therapeutic value. Curcumin's antioxidative response involves several signaling pathways, such as modulation of the miR-7/RelA p65 and miR-1287-5p/LONP2 axes in an OGD/R model, and activation of the Nrf2/HO-1 pathway. Additionally, analogues of dienonemonocarbonyl curcumin have been shown to protect cellular integrity by reducing ROS production through the Nrf2/HO-1 signaling pathway. Curcumin and its derivative, hexa hydrocurcumin, also enhance antioxidant defenses in a rat stroke model, partly via the Nrf2/HO-1 pathway (Joby et al., 2021). Furthermore, various signaling pathways such as Golgi assembly, SP1/Prdx6, AMPK/UCP2, and GRASP65 modulate curcumin's antioxidant properties.

Anti-Inflammatory Effects

Curcumin exhibits potent anti-inflammatory effects by inhibiting the activity of cytokines and enzymes such as COX and lipoxygenase (LOX) (Yoshinobu et al., 1983). This action contributes to the reduction of neuroinflammation, which is implicated in various neurodegenerative disorders, including multiple sclerosis, Parkinson's disease (PD), and Alzheimer's disease (AD).

Antioxidant Activity

One of the key mechanisms behind curcumin's neuroprotection is its antioxidant capability. It effectively scavenges free radicals and ROS that can damage neuronal cells (Kulkarni and Dhir, 2010). This action helps prevent oxidative stress, a process strongly associated with neuronal damage and degeneration.

Amyloid-Beta Regulation in AD

Curcumin has demonstrated efficacy in disrupting the aggregation and accumulation of amyloid-beta plaques in the brain, a hallmark of AD. It has the potential to prevent the formation of these toxic protein aggregates, thereby reducing their detrimental effects on neuronal function and viability (Kunnumakkara et al., 2017).

Modulation of Tau Protein

Moreover, curcumin has been shown to affect tau protein pathology in AD. Tau protein abnormalities lead to the formation of neurofibrillary tangles, which impair neuronal communication (Kumar et al., 2021). Curcumin appears to inhibit the hyperphosphorylation of tau proteins, potentially preventing their aggregation into tangles.

Enhancement of Neurogenesis

Curcumin has been found to promote neurogenesis, the process of generating new neurons. By stimulating this process, it supports brain repair and regeneration, which is crucial for combating neurodegenerative conditions characterized by neuronal loss (Kim et al., 2021).

Enhancement of Brain-Derived Neurotrophic Factor

Curcumin boosts the levels of brain-derived neurotrophic factor (BDNF), a protein crucial for the growth, survival, and maintenance of neurons (Danial et al., 2022). By increasing BDNF levels, curcumin enhances neuronal resilience and promotes synaptic plasticity, which is vital for learning and memory processes.

Regulation of Neurotransmitters

Curcumin also modulates various neurotransmitters such as dopamine, serotonin, and glutamate, which are crucial for regulating mood, cognition, and neuronal signaling (Li et al., 2022). By balancing these neurotransmitters, curcumin contributes to overall brain health and function.

Blood-Brain Barrier Protection

Curcumin has the potential to protect the blood-brain barrier, a crucial interface between the brain and substances in the bloodstream. By maintaining the integrity of this barrier, curcumin may prevent harmful molecules from entering the brain, thereby safeguarding neuronal health (Mohseni et al., 2021).

Mitochondrial Function

Additionally, curcumin supports mitochondrial function, the powerhouse of cells (Ma et al., 2009). By enhancing mitochondrial health and reducing oxidative damage, curcumin helps maintain cellular energy production and neuronal vitality (Pratheeshkumar et al., 2012).

Epigenetic Modulation

Curcumin's influence extends to epigenetic modifications that regulate gene expression. It can alter the activity of genes involved in neuroprotection and inflammation, thereby impacting overall neuronal health (Rakotoarisoa and Angelova, 2019).

Clinical Implications

Several studies, primarily conducted in preclinical or animal models, have demonstrated promising results regarding curcumin's neuroprotective effects (Girisa et al., 2021). However, translating these findings into effective clinical therapies requires further investigation, especially concerning bioavailability, dosage, and delivery methods to ensure optimal results in humans. Curcumin's multifaceted approach—encompassing anti-inflammatory, antioxidant, anti-amyloid, neurogenic, and neurotrophic effects—positions it as a promising compound for neuroprotection (Bano et al., 2020). Its potential for mitigating various neurodegenerative conditions underscores its importance as a subject of ongoing research and potential therapeutic development.

Other Applications

Curcumin has garnered attention for its potential application as a neuroprotective agent (Sharifi-Rad et al., 2020). Its diverse properties and mechanisms make it an intriguing candidate for addressing various neurological conditions and supporting overall brain health.

AD and Cognitive Health

AD is one of the most researched areas for curcumin's neuroprotective potential. Studies suggest that curcumin may delay the onset of cognitive decline in AD by preventing the aggregation of amyloid beta plaques and reducing neuroinflammation (Shin et al., 2007). Its anti-inflammatory and antioxidant properties contribute to decreasing inflammation and oxidative stress, both of which are significant factors in the development and progression of AD.

PD and Movement Disorders

In preclinical research, curcumin has shown neuroprotective effects in PD by modulating pathways associated with inflammation, oxidative stress, and mitochondrial dysfunction (Singla et al., 2023). These mechanisms may help alleviate motor symptoms related to PD and protect dopaminergic neurons from damage.

Stroke and Neurological Damage

Curcumin shows promise in reducing inflammation, oxidative stress, and neuronal death to mitigate the effects of stroke. By modulating various pathways involved in stroke-induced damage, it may aid in the recovery process and limit the extent of neurological deficits following a stroke.

Multiple Sclerosis (MS) and Neuroinflammation

In MS, curcumin's anti-inflammatory properties could be beneficial (Srinivasan, 1972). It may help reduce the inflammatory response and demyelination, potentially slowing disease progression and preserving neurological function in MS patients.

Traumatic Brain Injury (TBI) and Neuroprotection

Curcumin's antioxidant and anti-inflammatory actions have shown promise in mitigating damage caused by TBI (Sun, 2017). By reducing inflammation and oxidative stress, curcumin may support the recovery process and limit secondary injury cascades following a TBI.

Mood Disorders and Mental Health

Beyond neurodegenerative conditions, curcumin has been investigated for its role in mood disorders such as depression and anxiety (Tewari et al., 2022). Its ability to enhance neurogenesis, modulate neurotransmitters, and reduce inflammation may contribute to its potential as an adjunct therapy for managing these conditions.

Age-Related Cognitive Decline

The neuroprotective features of curcumin may also support brain health during normal aging processes (Vasconcelos et al., 2019). Its antioxidant and anti-inflammatory effects could help combat age-related cognitive decline and promote overall cognitive function in older adults.

Enhancing Neuroplasticity and Learning

Curcumin's influence on BDNF and neurogenesis enhances neuroplasticity, which is crucial for learning and memory processes. By supporting these mechanisms, curcumin may aid in cognitive enhancement and improve learning abilities (Venkatesan, 1998).

Challenges and Considerations

Despite its promising potential, curcumin's therapeutic effects are limited by its low absorption, rapid metabolism, and restricted bioavailability (Venkatesan et al., 2000; Wong et al., 2013). Researchers are investigating various innovative delivery methods and formulations to enhance curcumin's stability and absorption, aiming for improved clinical outcomes *in vivo* (Yavarpour-Bali et al., 2019).

Future Directions

Ongoing research is crucial for determining the optimal dosage, formulation, and administration of curcumin for neuroprotection (Yallapu et al., 2015). Clinical trials evaluating its efficacy and safety across various neurological conditions will be essential in establishing curcumin as a mainstream neuroprotective agent (Zielińska et al., 2020).

Conclusion

In conclusion, curcumin's multifaceted neuroprotective properties make it a compelling candidate for addressing a wide range of neurological conditions, including neurodegenerative diseases, mood disorders, and age-related cognitive decline. While further research and clinical trials are necessary to fully establish its therapeutic potential, curcumin remains a promising natural compound for supporting neuroprotection and overall brain health.

References

Abd El-Hack, M. E., El-Saadony, M. T., Swelum, A. A., Arif, M., Abo Ghanima, M. M., Shukry, M., Noreldin, A., Taha, A. E., & El-Tarabily, K. A. (2021). Curcumin, the active substance of turmeric: Its effects on health and ways to improve its bioavailability. *Journal of the Science of Food and Agriculture*, 101, 5747–5762.

Aggarwal, B. B., & Harikumar, K. B. (2009). Potential therapeutic effects of curcumin, the anti-inflammatory agent, against neurodegenerative, cardiovascular, pulmonary, metabolic, autoimmune and neoplastic diseases. *International Journal of Biochemistry and Cell Biology*, 41, 40–59.

Aggarwal, B. B., & Sung, B. (2009). Pharmacological basis for the role of curcumin in chronic diseases: An age-old spice with modern targets. *Trends in Pharmacological Sciences*, 30, 85–94.

Ahmad, N., Umar, S., Ashafaq, M., Akhtar, M., Iqbal, Z., Samim, M., & Ahmad, F. J. (2013). A comparative study of PNIPAM nanoparticles of curcumin, demethoxycurcumin, and bisdemethoxycurcumin and their effects on oxidative stress markers in experimental stroke. *Protoplasma*, 250, 1327–1338.

Ahmadinejad, F., Geir Møller, S., Hashemzadeh-Chaleshtori, M., Bidkhori, G., & Jami, M. S. (2017). Molecular mechanisms behind free radical scavengers function against oxidative stress. *Antioxidants*, 6, 51.

Anand, P., Kunnumakkara, A. B., Newman, R. A., & Aggarwal, B. B. (2007). Bioavailability of curcumin: Problems and promises. *Molecular Pharmaceutics*, 4, 807–818.

Arun, N., & Nalini, N. (2002). Efficacy of turmeric on blood sugar and polyol pathway in diabetic albino rats. *Plant Foods for Human Nutrition*, 57, 41–52.

Bano, S., Harsha, C., Thakur, K. K., Khatoon, E., & Kunnumakkara, A. B. (2020). Curcumin: A Potential Molecule for the Prevention and Treatment of Inflammatory Diseases. *The Royal Society of Chemistry*, pp. 150-171.

Cavalcanti, R. N., Koshima, C. C., Forster-Carneiro, T. MT, Gomes, M. S., Rostagno, M. A., Prado, J. M., & Meireles, M. A. A. (2022). *Uses and Applications of Extracts from Natural Sources*. ed. J. Prado and M. Rostagno, The Royal Society of Chemistry, 2nd edn, 2022, ch. 1, pp. 1-65.

Cornelius, C., Crupi, R., Calabrese, V., Graziano, A., Milone, P., Pennisi, G., Radak, Z., Calabrese, E. J., & Cuzzocrea, S. (2013). Traumatic brain injury: Oxidative stress and neuroprotection. *Antioxidants and Redox Signaling*, 19, 836–853.

Cote, B., Elbarbry, F., Bui, F., Su, J. W., Seo, K., Nguyen, A., Lee, M., & Rao, D. A. (2022). Mechanistic basis for the role of phytochemicals in inflammation-associated chronic diseases. *Molecules*, 27, 781.

Ding, C., Wu, Y., Chen, X., Chen, Y., Wu, Z., Lin, Z., Kang, D., Fang, W., & Chen, F. (2022). Global, regional, and national burden and attributable risk factors of neurological disorders: The Global Burden of Disease study 1990–2019. *Frontiers in Public Health*, 10, 952161.

Dugger, B. N., & Dickson, D. W. (2017). Pathology of neurodegenerative diseases. *Cold Spring Harbor Perspectives in Biology*, 9, a028035.

Girisa, S., Kumar, A., Rana, V., Parama, D., Daimary, U. D., Warnakulasuriya, S., Kumar, A. P., & Kunnumakkara, A. B. (2021). From simple mouth cavities to complex oral mucosal disorders—Curcuminoids as a promising therapeutic approach. *ACS Pharmacology and Translational Science*, 4, 647–665.

Hegde, M., Girisa, S., Naliyadhara, N., Kumar, A., Alqahtani, M. S., Abbas, M., Mohan, C. D., Warrier, S., Hui, K. M., Rangappa, K. S., Sethi, G., & Kunnumakkara, A. B. (2023). Natural compounds targeting nuclear receptors for effective cancer therapy. *Cancer and Metastasis Reviews*, 42(3), 765–822.

Jacob, J., Amalraj, A., Raj, K. K. J., Divya, C., Kunnumakkara, A. B., & Gopi, S. (2019). A novel bioavailable hydrogenated curcuminoids formulation (CuroWhite™) improves symptoms and diagnostic indicators in rheumatoid arthritis patients-A randomized, double blind and placebo controlled study. *Journal of Traditional and Complementary Medicine*, 9, 346–352.

Khayatan, D., Razavi, S. M., Arab, Z. N., Niknejad, A. H., Nouri, K., Momtaz, S., Gumpricht, E., Jamialahmadi, T., Abdolghaffari, A. H., Barreto, G. E., & Sahebkar, A. (2022). Protective effects of curcumin against traumatic brain injury. *Biomedicine and Pharmacotherapy*, 154, 113621.

Kim, S. J., Son, T. G., Park, H. R., Park, M., Kim, M. S., Kim, H. S., Chung, H. Y., Mattson, M. P., & Lee, J. (2008). Curcumin stimulates proliferation of embryonic neural progenitor cells and neurogenesis in the adult hippocampus. *Journal of Biological Chemistry*, 283, 14497–14505.

Kiso, Y., Suzuki, Y., Watanabe, N., Oshima, Y., & Hikino, H. (1983). Antihepatotoxic principles of Curcuma longa rhizomes. *Planta Medica*, 49, 185–187.

Kulkarni, S. K., & Dhir, A. (2010). An overview of curcumin in neurological disorders. *Indian Journal of Pharmaceutical Sciences*, 72, 149–154.

Kumar, A., Harsha, C., Parama, D., Girisa, S., Daimary, U. D., Mao, X., & Kunnumakkara, A. B. (2021). Current clinical developments in curcumin-based therapeutics for cancer and chronic diseases. *Phytotherapy Research*, 35, 6768–6801.

Kunnumakkara, A. B., Bordoloi, D., Padmavathi, G., Monisha, J., Roy, N. K., Prasad, S., & Aggarwal, B. B. (2017). Curcumin, the golden nutraceutical: Multitargeting for multiple chronic diseases. *British Journal of Pharmacology*, 174, 1325–1348.

Li, X., Feng, X., Sun, X., Hou, N., Han, F., & Liu, Y. (2022). Global, regional, and national burden of Alzheimer's disease and other dementias, 1990–2019. *Frontiers in Aging Neuroscience*, 14, 937486.

Ma, Q. L., Yang, F., Rosario, E. R., Ubeda, O. J., Beech, W., Gant, D. J., Chen, P. P., Hudspeth, B., Chen, C., Zhao, Y., Vinters, H. V., Frautschy, S. A., & Cole, G. M. (2009). β-amyloid oligomers induce phosphorylation of tau and inactivation of insulin receptor substrate via c-Jun N-terminal kinase signaling: Suppression by omega-3 fatty acids and curcumin. *Journal of Neuroscience*, 29, 9078–9089.

Mohseni, M., Sahebkar, A., Askari, G., Johnston, T. P., Alikiaii, B., & Bagherniya, M. (2021). The clinical use of curcumin on neurological disorders: An updated systematic review of clinical trials. *Phytotherapy Research*, 35, 6862–6882.

Pratheeshkumar, P., Sreekala, C., Zhang, Z., Budhraja, A., Ding, S., Son, Y. O., Wang, X., Hitron, A., Hyun-Jung, K., Wang, L., Lee, J. C., & Shi, X. (2012) Cancer prevention with promising natural products: Mechanisms of action and molecular targets. *Anti-Cancer Agents in Medicinal Chemistry*, 12, 1159–1184.

Rakotoarisoa, M., & Angelova, A. (2019). Amphiphilic nanocarrier systems for curcumin delivery in neurodegenerative disorders. In *Road from Nanomedicine to Precision Medicine*, pp. 1027–1065.

Sharifi-Rad, M., Lankatillake, C., Dias, D. A., Docea, A. O., Mahomoodally, M. F., Lobine, D., Chazot, P. L., Kurt, B., Tumer, T. B., Moreira, A. C., Sharopov, F., Martorell, M., Martins, N., Cho, W. C., Calina, D., & Sharifi-Rad, J. (2020). Impact of natural compounds on neurodegenerative disorders: From preclinical to pharmacotherapeutics. *Journal of Clinical Medicine*, 9, 1061.34.

Shin, H. J., Lee, J. Y., Son, E., Lee, D. H., Kim, H. J., Kang, S. S., Cho, G. J., Choi, W. S., & Roh, G. S. (2007). Curcumin attenuates the kainic acid-induced hippocampal cell death in the mice. *Neuroscience Letters*, 416, 49–54.

Singla, R. K., De, R., Efferth, T., Mezzetti, B., Sahab Uddin, M., Sanusi, Ntie-Kang, F., Wang, D., Schultz, F., Kharat, K. R., Devkota, H. P., Battino, M., Sur, D., Lordan, R., Patnaik, S. S., Tsagkaris, C., Sai, C. S., Tripathi, S. K., Găman, M. A., Ahmed, M. E. O., Shen, B. (2023). The International Natural Product Sciences Taskforce (INPST) and the power of Twitter networking exemplified through# INPST hashtag analysis. *Phytomedicine*, 108, 154520.

Srinivasan, M. (1972). Effect of curcumin on blood sugar as seen in a diabetic subject. *Indian Journal of Medical Sciences,* 26, 269–270.

Sun, S. C. (2017). The non-canonical NF-κB pathway in immunity and inflammation. *Nature Reviews. Immunology*, 17, 545–558.

Tewari, D., Patni, P., Bishayee, A., Sah, A. N., & Bishayee, A. (2022). Natural products targeting the PI3K-Akt-mTOR signaling pathway in cancer: A novel therapeutic strategy. In *Seminars in Cancer Biology.* Academic Press: Cambridge, USA, 80, 1–17.

Vasconcelos, A. R., dos Santos, N. B., Scavone, C., & Munhoz, C. D. (2019). Nrf2/ARE pathway modulation by dietary energy regulation in neurological disorders. *Frontiers in Pharmacology*, 10, 428667.

Venkatesan, N. (1998). Curcumin attenuation of acute adriamycin myocardial toxicity in rats. *British Journal of Pharmacology*, 124, 425–427.

Venkatesan, N., Punithavathi, D., & Arumugam, V. (2000). Curcumin prevents adriamycin nephrotoxicity in rats. *British Journal of Pharmacology*, 129, 231–234.

Wong, M. (2013). Mammalian target of rapamycin (mTOR) pathways in neurological diseases. *Biomedical Journal*, 36, 40–50.

Yallapu, M. M., Bhusetty Nagesh, P. K., Jaggi, M., & Chauhan, S. C. (2015). Therapeutic applications of curcumin nanoformulations. *The AAPS Journal*, 17, 1341–1356.

Yavarpour-Bali, H., Ghasemi-Kasman, M., & Pirzadeh, M. (2019). Curcumin-loaded nanoparticles: A novel therapeutic strategy in treatment of central nervous system disorders. International Journal of *Nanomedicine*, 14, 4449–4460.

Zielińska, A., Alves, H., Marques, V., Durazzo, A., Lucarini, M., Alves, T. F., Morsink, M., Willemen, N., Eder, P., Chaud, M. V., Severino, P., Santini, A., & Souto, E. B. (2020). Properties, Extraction Methods, and Delivery Systems for Curcumin as a Natural Source of Beneficial Health Effects. *Medicina*, 56(7), 336.

Chapter 5

Neuroprotective Effects of Green Tea Extracts

Vani Shukla[1]
Arun Kumar[2,*]
Sahil Hussain[2]
Mohemmed Faraz Khan[3]
and Syed Kaynat Fatima[4]

[1]Department of Food and Nutrition, Era University, Sarfaraz Ganj, Lucknow, Uttar Pradesh, India
[2]Department of Pharmaceutical Chemistry, Faculty of Pharmacy Integral University, Lucknow, Uttar Pradesh, India
[3]Department of Chemistry, Maynooth University, Ireland
[4]Department of Molecular Biology, Staffordshire University, Stoke on Trent, United Kingdom

Abstract

Deficits in cognition and movement are caused by neurodegeneration, which is a gradual deterioration in the composition and capabilities of nerve cells. Oxidative damage, inflammation, misfolded proteins, and heredity are among the contributing factors. Examples of diseases like these are Parkinson's and Alzheimer's. Potential neuroprotection against these processes is provided by green tea extracts. The Camellia sinensis plant yields green tea, which has drawn a lot of interest due to its abundance of bioactive substances, especially catechins. The chapter explores the expanding corpus of scientific literature, elucidating the several methods by which green tea extracts elicit their neuroprotective properties. The capacity of green tea extracts to counteract inflammation

* Corresponding Author's Email: arun.mpharm@gmail.com, arun@iul.ac.in.

In: Natural Solutions for Neurodegenerative Disorders
Editors: Rahul Kumar Sharma, Shailesh Sharma, Ajmer Singh Grewal et al.
ISBN: 979-8-89530-231-6

and oxidative stress—two important variables in neurodegenerative illnesses like Alzheimer's and Parkinson's—explains their neuroprotective qualities. These extracts show an amazing ability to scavenge free radicals, minimizing damage to neurons and improving mental performance. Furthermore, they moderate the expression of genes linked to neuroinflammation, reducing inflammatory reactions in the brain. This chapter also explores the function of green tea catechins in maintaining neuronal plasticity and stimulating the development of new neurons. These substances have promise in mitigating the consequences of age-related cognitive decline and neurological diseases by improving synaptic connection and promoting neurogenesis. A comprehensive review of several *in vitro* and *in vivo* investigations, clinical trials, and animal models highlights the strong evidence that green tea extracts have neuroprotective properties. With optimism for the management and prevention of neurodegenerative diseases, readers will obtain important insights into green tea's potential as a readily available, natural neuroprotective agent.

Keywords: green tea extracts, neuroprotection, catechins, oxidative stress, inflammation, neurodegenerative diseases

Abbreviations

BDNF	Brain-derived neurotrophic factor
CNS	Central Nervous System
EC	Epicatechin
ECG	Epicatechin Gallate
EGC	Epigallocatechin
EGCG	Epigallocatechin gallate
ROS	Reactive Oxygen Species

Introduction

Green tea is made from Camellia sinensis leaves and has been used in Asian medicine for millennia. It is highly regarded for its many health benefits. Green tea is known for its polyphenols, or catechins, among which epigallocatechin gallate (EGCG) is the most powerful and well-studied for its anti-inflammatory and antioxidant properties (Khan & Mukhtar, 2013; Chacko et al., 2010). According to research, green tea extracts may improve cognitive performance, help people control their weight, lessen their risk of heart disease, and decrease the incidence of cancer (Mancini et al., 2017). Additionally, they are being investigated for their ability to enhance glycemic management and dermatological diseases (Hsu, 2013; Liu et al., 2013). Although these advantages are present, prudence is suggested in light of potential negative consequences, including side effects associated with caffeine and interactions with iron binding that may cause iron insufficiency in certain people (Weinreb et al., 2009). Therefore, it is important to weigh the hazards associated with green tea extracts, especially when using strong supplements. For millennia, green tea, a beverage with profound cultural roots in Asia, especially in China and Japan, has been prized for its therapeutic qualities (Lu et al., 2004). Its abundance of polyphenols, which includes catechins like EGCG, potent antioxidants that prevent oxidative stress and damage from free radicals, is the main source of its health benefits (Cabrera et al., 2006). Research has connected green tea extracts to some health advantages, such as the prevention of cancer, enhancements to cardiovascular health, and neuroprotective properties, underscoring their potential to tackle some of the most important health issues of the day (Kuriyama, 2006; Mandel & Youdim, 2004). Beyond these advantages, green tea extracts' potential to improve fat oxidation in concert with caffeine has also led to research into its potential for weight control (Dulloo et al., 1999). Furthermore, green tea extract's antibacterial qualities provide encouraging new directions in the battle against infections resistant to antibiotics (Reygaert, 2018). But despite these advantages, green tea extracts should be used with caution, especially when taken as supplements, due to the possibility of liver damage and other negative consequences at large dosages (Sarma et al., 2008). This chapter is devoted to a comprehensive examination of green tea extracts, covering a variety of subjects from their historical provenance to their modern uses and potential health effects. This chapter aims to provide readers with a thorough grasp of green tea extracts by addressing these topics and striking a balance between their traditional applications and cutting-edge scientific research.

Green Tea: Composition and Nutritional Profile

Green tea is distinguished by its distinct composition and abundant nutritional value, and it is produced from the leaves of the Camellia sinensis plant. Polyphenols—primarily catechins such as EGCG, epicatechin, epicatechin gallate, and epigallocatechin—are the main bioactive ingredients in green tea.

According to Caperra et al., (2006), the majority of green tea's antioxidant qualities are attributed to these catechins, which also provide defense against oxidative stress and related chronic illnesses. Alkaloids including caffeine, theobromine, and theophylline are also present in green tea, which helps explain some of its stimulant properties (Ashihara et al., 2008). Furthermore, it contains amino acids, the most notable of which is L-theanine, which has been shown to have soothing effects on the brain (Juneja et al., 1999). Green tea has been shown to have significant nutritional value and health advantages when combined with other vitamins and minerals (Cabrera et al., 2006). These include vitamins C, B2, and E as well as minerals including fluoride, manganese, and zinc. The chemical composition of green tea and its bioactive components are shown in Tables 1 and 2.

Table 1. Chemical constituents of green tea

Constituent Group	Specific Constituents	Known Effects	References
Catechins (Polyphenols)	EGCG, Epicatechin (EC), Epicatechin gallate (ECG), Epigallocatechin (EGC)	Antioxidant properties, health-promoting effects	Cabrera et al., 2006
Alkaloids	Caffeine, Theobromine, Theophylline	Mild stimulant effects	Ashihara et al., 2008
Amino Acids	L-theanine	Relaxing and stress-reducing effects on the brain	Juneja et al., 1999
Vitamins	Vitamin C, Vitamin B_2, Vitamin E	Nutritional benefits	Cabrera et al., 2006
Minerals	Fluoride, Manganese, Zinc	Contributing to nutritional value	Chacko et al., 2010

Table 2. Bioactive compounds in green tea extracts

Bioactive Compound	Effects	References
Catechins (e.g., EGCG, ECG, EGC)	Antioxidant activity, potential reduction in chronic disease risk	Chacko et al., 2010
Caffeine	Stimulating effects, enhanced brain function	Bryan, 2008; Dulloo et al., 1999
L-Theanine	Relaxation, mood modulation	Bryan, 2008
Vitamins and Minerals	General health benefits	Dulloo et al., 1999

Mechanisms of Neuroprotection

To protect neurons from harm, a complex web of processes interacts to provide neuroprotection. Antioxidants play a crucial part in the defense against neurodegenerative illnesses by neutralizing harmful free radicals, which is how they fight oxidative stress, which is fundamental to this process (Halliwell, 2006). It is also important to modulate neuroinflammation; medicines that target inflammatory pathways like NF-κB can reduce brain inflammation and provide protective benefits (Glass et al., 2010). Maintaining neural resilience requires measures to increase the activity of neurotrophic factors, particularly brain-derived neurotrophic factor (BDNF), which is crucial for the survival and viability of neurons (Zuccato & Cattaneo, 2009). Because neurodegenerative diseases frequently exhibit dysfunctional mitochondria, mitochondrial function is equally significant. For this reason, substances that promote mitochondrial health are advantageous (Lin & Beal, 2006). In addition, controlling calcium levels and avoiding excitotoxicity—the detrimental overactivation of neurotransmitters—are important for maintaining the integrity of neurons (Lau & Tymianski, 2010). The last and potentially effective neuroprotective tactic is encouraging autophagy, which enables cells to eliminate harmed components (Nixon, 2013).

Antioxidant Properties of Green Tea Extracts

Because of their high polyphenol content, especially in the form of catechins like EGCG; green tea extracts are well known for their strong antioxidant capabilities. According to Mandel et al., (2004) and Cabrera et al., (2006), these catechins are efficient at scavenging reactive oxygen species and nitrogen species, which lowers oxidative stress in the body and is a major factor in the pathogenesis of several chronic diseases, such as cancer, cardiovascular diseases, and neurodegenerative disorders. According to Chacko et al., (2010), EGCG, the most researched catechin in green tea, has demonstrated potent free radical-scavenging action and the ability to influence the activity of antioxidant enzymes such as catalase and superoxide dismutase. Moreover, green tea polyphenols' antioxidant potential is enhanced by their ability to chelate metal ions like copper and iron that are implicated in the production of free radicals (Cabrera et al., 2006). These qualities improve total cellular antioxidant defense processes in addition to avoiding oxidative damage to biomolecules such as proteins, lipids, and DNA. Furthermore, the combination of catechins with other components of green tea, such as vitamins C and E, enhances their antioxidative capacity, which is why green tea extracts are a hot topic for natural health products and dietary supplements (Forester & Lambert, 2011).

Anti-Inflammatory Effects on the Nervous System

For the treatment of neurodegenerative illnesses and neuropathic pain, neuroinflammation must be reduced. This process includes controlling the activity of glial cells in the central nervous system (CNS) and limiting the production of cytokines that promote inflammation, which are essential for the inflammatory response (Glass et al., 2010). Certain compounds, including the polyphenols in green tea, particularly EGCG, have shown promise in reducing neuroinflammation by blocking inflammatory pathways like NF-κB (Singh et al., 2015). Their wider anti-inflammatory effect on the neurological system is further enhanced by their influence on the JAK/STAT pathway (Mandel et al., 2005). Beyond their direct anti-inflammatory effects, these compounds can stimulate the release of neurotrophic factors and anti-inflammatory cytokines, supporting CNS's self-healing processes (Lipton, 2003). Furthermore, these substances can prevent or cure neuroinflammation-related neuronal damage by addressing oxidative stress, which frequently coexists with inflammation (Halliwell, 2006).

Effects on Neuroplasticity and Synaptic Function

The fight against neurodegenerative illnesses and cognitive deficits must prioritize the development of treatments that improve neuroplasticity and synaptic functioning. Extracts from green tea, which are high in polyphenols like EGCG, are showing promise in this regard. According to Li et al., (2009), EGCG has been identified for its function in raising BDNF levels, which is essential for fostering synaptic plasticity and neuron growth, both of which are necessary for learning and memory. Additionally, these bioactive substances interact with neurotransmitter systems to promote synaptic function; in particular, they protect synapses from the deleterious effects of excessive glutamate by engaging the cholinergic system, which enhances memory (Mandel et al., 2008). These substances also safeguard synaptic integrity through their antioxidative and anti-inflammatory properties, which support and enhance cognitive functioning (Halliwell, 2006; Craft et al., 2004). This multi-pathway strategy highlights green tea extracts' potential as medicinal treatments for neurological and cognitive disorders.

Animal and Cellular Studies

Green tea extracts are a perfect illustration of how animal and cellular investigations are essential for understanding the impacts and possible therapeutic benefits of natural substances. According to these research studies, catechins—particularly EGCG—can provide neuroprotection against toxicity and degeneration in animal models, indicating a potentially effective treatment approach for neurodegenerative diseases (Weinreb et al., 2004; Mandel et al., 2008). These results have been confirmed in neural cell cultures, where green tea extracts have been shown to decrease oxidative stress and cell death, supporting its potential to be neuroprotective (Mandel et al., 2005). Additionally, these substances have anti-inflammatory properties, as demonstrated by cellular models' reduced cytokine production (Singh et al., 2007). Furthermore, *in vitro* experiments using cancer cells demonstrate the anticancer properties of these catechins, encompassing their function in inducing apoptosis and suppressing cell growth (Yang et al., 2009).

An Overview of Relevant *In Vitro* and *In Vivo* Experiments

In-Vitro Experiments

A fundamental understanding of the cellular and molecular processes of bioactive chemicals is provided by *in vitro* investigations, most of which include cell cultures. The polyphenols in green tea, especially EGCG, have received a lot of attention. According to Mandel et al., (2005), EGCG has demonstrated encouraging neuroprotective properties in brain cell cultures, reducing oxidative stress and preventing apoptosis. Green tea catechins may have anti-cancer effects as *in vitro* research on cancer cell lines has demonstrated that they can trigger apoptosis and prevent tumor cell growth and angiogenesis (Yang et al., 2009). The identification of molecular targets and pathways affected by these chemicals, such as NF-κB and MAPK signaling, is made possible by this research.

In-Vivo Experiments

Assessing the physiological and therapeutic effects of bioactive chemicals in an organism has been made possible through *in vivo* research, mostly with animal models. The effects of green tea extracts on neurodegenerative illnesses have been widely studied using rodent models. Green tea polyphenols, for instance, have been shown in rodent experiments to enhance cognitive performance and lower amyloid-beta deposition, a characteristic of Alzheimer's disease (Weinreb et al., 2004). Preclinical evidence supporting green tea extracts' ability to suppress tumor development and spread in the context of cancer has been demonstrated by animal research (Yang et al., 2009). To convert fundamental research into therapeutic applications, both in-vitro and in-vivo investigations are necessary. While *in vivo* research offers a more comprehensive view of the systemic impacts and possible therapeutic advantages of a complete organism, *in vitro* investigations allow for the controlled analysis of cellular processes. These two types of research give complementary insights.

Findings on Neuroprotection in Animal Models

Recent developments in the field of neuroprotection highlight the effectiveness of green tea components in animal models of neurodegeneration. According to research using transgenic mice, green tea's EGCG prevents and promotes the clearance of amyloid-beta plaques in Alzheimer's disease, which is associated with a slower rate of cognitive decline (Rezai-Zadeh et al., 2008). Furthermore, it has been demonstrated that the antioxidant properties of green tea's catechins reduce oxidative stress, which is a factor in neurodegeneration (Weinreb et al., 2004). Green tea extracts protect dopaminergic neurons from toxicity-induced damage in models of Parkinson's disease; their anti-inflammatory and antioxidative characteristics are important in preventing typical Parkinsonian neurodegeneration (Levites et al., 2002). According to Choi et al., (2014), EGCG has shown promise in reducing brain damage and improving neurological function in cases of stroke and ischemic injuries. This effect is probably attributed to its impact on cell survival and apoptosis. By highlighting green tea extracts as potential neuroprotective agents, these animal model studies provide a foundation for future investigations and potential therapeutic approaches for neurodegenerative illnesses.

Cellular Mechanisms Underlying Green Tea's Effects

Green tea catechins—in particular, EGCG—have several health advantages and are linked to several cellular processes. By neutralizing ROS and enhancing the body's antioxidant defenses, which are essential for reducing cellular damage in chronic illnesses like cancer and neurodegeneration, they mainly combat oxidative stress (Mandel et al., 2005). Additionally, by suppressing inflammatory pathways and blocking transcription factors like NF-κB, these catechins have anti-inflammatory qualities that reduce the generation of cytokines and fight chronic inflammation (Singh et al., 2007). Additionally, via modulating DNA methyltransferases and histone acetyltransferases, catechins modify epigenetic landscapes and impact critical cell signaling, which influences cancer-related gene expression patterns (Fang et al., tumor). The anticancer effects are mostly attributed to pathways including MAPK, PI3K/Akt, and Wnt/β-Catenin, which regulate cell growth, death, and differentiation impede tumor development, and induce apoptosis (Yang et al., 2009). According to Fang et al., (2003), they also modify the epigenetic landscapes through their effects on DNA methyltransferases and histone acetyltransferases, which in turn influence genetic expression patterns linked to cancer. Last but not least, the overexpression of neurotrophic factors like BDNF is partially responsible for the neuroprotective effects of green tea catechins, improving synaptic plasticity and neuronal survival and adding to the tea's therapeutic potential (Weinreb et al., 2004).

Cognitive Function and Ageing

Epidemiological Evidence

Consuming green tea has been linked to improved cognitive performance in older persons, according to several epidemiological research. Kuriyama et al., (2006), for example, reported that a lower frequency of cognitive impairment was correlated with higher use of green tea in cross-sectional research done in Japan. This implies that specific elements in green tea could have neuroprotective properties that support the preservation of cognitive function in children.

Mechanisms of Action

It is believed that the antioxidant and anti-inflammatory properties of green tea may have an impact on cognitive health. According to Mandel et al., (2005), catechins can pass the blood-brain barrier and may shield neurons from inflammatory and oxidative stress, all of which are linked to cognitive decline.

Clinical Trials

The goal of clinical trials has been to supplement observational study results. For instance, research conducted in 2014 by Schmidt et al., discovered that green tea extracts enhanced working memory in particular, pointing to a direct impact on brain areas related to memory processing. These findings provide credence to the hypothesis that green tea might improve cognitive performance and possibly postpone the onset of age-related cognitive disorders.

Safety and Dosage

Although green tea is typically safe, there are dangers associated with large dosages of green tea extracts, including liver damage. When thinking about using green tea supplements, people should, especially the elderly, follow safe consumption guidelines and speak with their doctors (Sarma et al., 2008).

Longevity and Overall Brain Health

Green tea's advantages for cognition may extend beyond its direct effects and include implications on lifespan and general brain health. Consuming green tea regularly has been linked to a lower chance of dying from any cause, including neurological disorders (Kuriyama et al., 2006).

Green Tea as a Potential Anti-Ageing Intervention

Due to its high concentration of polyphenolic chemicals, especially EGCG, green tea has been the subject of much research about its possible anti-aging properties. Green tea catechins' antioxidant activity has been demonstrated to provide DNA protection, maintain the integrity of genetic material throughout time, and help reduce oxidative stress, a major factor in the aging process (Frei & Higdon, 2003). Furthermore, telomere length, a biological indicator of lifespan, has been linked to green tea drinking, indicating a protective impact on chromosomal stability (Chan et al., 2010). Green tea has an impact on metabolic health in addition to hereditary variables. Research indicates that it improves lipid and glucose profiles, which are critical in the fight against age-related metabolic illnesses (Thielecke et al., 2009). According to Mandel et al., (2004), its anti-inflammatory qualities also help lower the chance of developing chronic illnesses including heart disease and neurological disorders. Notably, green tea provides advantages for dermal protection as well as internal health. It has been shown to guard against UV-induced skin damage, which may delay the appearance of apparent indications of skin aging (Hsu, 2005). Regarding the nervous system, green tea catechins' neuroprotective properties present a viable method of minimizing cognitive loss, a typical feature of aging (Weinreb et al., 2004). Green tea's benefits are supported by research conducted in clinical settings; investigations like the one conducted in 2006 by Kuriyama and colleagues found a correlation between drinking green tea and a lower death rate. These findings provide more credence to the theory that green tea may be a flexible anti-aging strategy.

Bioavailability and Formulations

Green tea catechins' quick metabolism and excretion restrict their bioavailability. Research shows that most consumed catechins undergo substantial metabolism, with just a tiny portion being absorbed directly into the small intestine (Chow et al., 2003). Novel formulations such as liposomes, phospholipid complexes, and nanoparticles have been studied to improve these drugs' stability and absorption (Fang et al., 2006). Particularly, EGCG-phospholipid complexes and encapsulation in nanoparticles have demonstrated the potential to raise EGCG's bioavailability through enhanced lipophilicity and degradation resistance (Liang et al., 1999; Zhang et al.,

2014). Furthermore, consuming green tea catechins together with vitamin C or certain minerals may increase their bioavailability; ascorbic acid has been shown to improve the intestinal absorption and stability of catechins (Henning et al., 2004). To fully use green tea extracts' medicinal potential for illness prevention and treatment, formulation advances are essential. Table 3 displays the new formulation with improved bioavailability.

Table 3. Novel formulations for enhanced bioavailability

Formulation type	Description	References
Nanotechnology-Based Formulations	Utilization of nanoparticles like solid lipid nanoparticles and nanoemulsions to protect catechins and enhance intestinal absorption.	Dube et al., (2010)
Liposomal Encapsulation	Use of liposomes, vesicles with a phospholipid bilayer, to encapsulate catechins, which improves their stability and absorption.	Hu et al., (2017)
Phospholipid Complexes	Formation of phytosomes by complexing catechins with phospholipids, increasing their solubility, and facilitating transport across membranes.	Conde et al., (2013)
Inclusion Complexes with Cyclodextrins	Inclusion of catechins in cyclodextrins to improve solubility and stability, protecting against degradation and enhancing bioavailability.	Loftsson et al., (2005)

Factors Affecting the Absorption of Green Tea Compounds

Several variables impact the bioavailability of green tea components, especially catechins, which in turn affect their absorption. The most important factors are the presence of other dietary components, like piperine, which can enhance the absorption of proteins and fiber, which may inhibit it; the composition of the gut microbiota, which plays a role in metabolizing catechins; and the preparation and consumption of tea, as certain meals or the addition of milk can decrease absorption (Chow et al., 2003; Henning et al., 2004). Furthermore, the bioavailability of catechins can be influenced by individual genetic variations in enzyme activity linked to catechin metabolism. Several approaches, including adjuvant usage and nanoencapsulation, are being investigated to enhance the absorption and therapeutic potential of green tea catechins (Fang et al., 2006).

Interactions and Side Effects

Green tea catechins can change the pharmacokinetics of several drugs. For instance, they may block CYP3A4, an enzyme involved in the metabolism of several medications, raising the possibility of elevated drug levels and adverse consequences (Chow et al., 2003). Furthermore, extracts from green tea may lessen the effectiveness of bortezomib, a proteasome inhibitor used in cancer treatment, and disrupt the way that anticoagulants like warfarin work (Golden & Lam, 2009). Usually minor in nature, green tea's adverse effects might include nausea, constipation, and upset stomach. Green tea extracts, however, can have more serious side effects, such as liver damage, when taken in large quantities, especially as supplements. It is advised to keep an eye on liver enzyme levels in those using green tea extract supplements since excessive dosages of these supplements have been linked in rare instances to hepatotoxicity (Sarma et al., 2008).

Potential Drug Interactions with Green Tea Extracts

Green tea extracts, high in polyphenols like catechins, have gained popularity due to their perceived health advantages. However, these substances can also result in important medication interactions. One main worry is that green tea extracts may suppress cytochrome P450 enzymes, including CYP3A4 and CYP1A2, which are important in drug metabolism and may change the blood levels of medicines (Chow et al., 2003). Green tea, for example, may make medications that are substrates for these enzymes more bioavailable, which might be harmful (Misaka et al., 2013). Examples of these medications include statins and several antipsychotics. In addition, it has been observed that green tea catechins can counteract the therapeutic effects of bortezomib, a proteasome inhibitor used in cancer treatment (Golden & Lam, 2009). Furthermore, because of its high vitamin K concentration, green tea has been demonstrated to modify the way anticoagulants like warfarin work by either amplifying their effects or reducing their efficacy (Ansell et al., 2009). To reduce the chance of drug interactions, patients taking green tea extracts with other drugs should do so under a doctor's supervision. To guarantee therapeutic efficacy and safety, it may be advisable to monitor medication plasma levels before beginning or stopping green tea supplementation.

Conclusion

Green tea, with its combination of bioactive components, might potentially reduce inflammation and oxidative stress, two major factors in neurodegenerative illnesses, making it an important part of a neuroprotective diet. Lean proteins, plant-based meals, and healthy fats are the main focus of larger dietary guidelines, which are under the use of green tea within a nutrient-dense, balanced diet. Adopting these food habits may promote brain health and lower the risk of cognitive decline in conjunction with other lifestyle treatments like regular exercise and cognitive engagement. A rising corpus of studies highlights the potential of green tea, but it comes with a warning to use it moderately and to recognize that dietary considerations are only one part of a complex strategy for neuroprotection. The optimal ways to utilize green tea's and other dietary components' ability to sustain cognitive vibrancy throughout life will become clearer as the study advances.

References

Ansell, J., McDonough, M., Zhao, Y., Harmatz, J. S., & Greenblatt, D. J. (2009). The absence of an interaction between warfarin and cranberry juice: A randomized, double-blind trial. *Journal of Clinical Pharmacology*, 49(7), 824-830.

Ashihara, H., Crozier, A., & Tomás-Barberán, F. (2008). Plant alkaloids. In Tea: *Bioactivity and Therapeutic Potential* (pp. 102-123). CRC Press.

Bryan, J. (2008). Psychological effects of dietary components of tea: Caffeine and L-theanine. *Nutrition Reviews*, 66(2), 82-90.

Cabrera, C., Artacho, R., & Giménez, R. (2006). Beneficial effects of green tea—A review. *Journal of the American College of Nutrition*, 25(2), 79-99.

Chacko, S. M., Thambi, P. T., Kuttan, R., & Nishigaki, I. (2010). Beneficial effects of green tea: A literature review. *Chinese Medicine*, 5, 13.

Chan, R., Woo, J., Suen, E., Leung, J., & Tang, N. (2010). Chinese tea consumption is associated with longer telomere length in elderly Chinese men. *British Journal of Nutrition*, 103(1), 107-113.

Choi, S. H., Kim, Y. H., Hebisch, M., Sliwinski, C., Lee, S., D'Avanzo, C., Ryu, H., Hooli, B., Asselin, C., Muffat, J., Klee, J. B., Kizil, C., Zhang, Z., Wainger, B. J., Peitz, M., Kovacs, D. M., Woolf, C. J., Wagner, S. L., Tanzi, R. E., & Kim, D. Y. (2014). A three-dimensional human neural cell culture model of Alzheimer's disease. *Nature*, 515(7526), 274-278.

Chow, H. H., Cai, Y., Alberts, D. S., Hakim, I., Dorr, R., Shahi, F., Crowell, J. A., Yang, C. S., & Hara, Y. (2003). Phase I pharmacokinetic study of tea polyphenols following single-dose administration of epigallocatechin gallate and polyphenon E. *Cancer Epidemiology, Biomarkers & Prevention*, 12(1), 1523s-1529s.

Chow, H. H., Cai, Y., Hakim, I. A., Crowell, J. A., Shahi, F., Brooks, C. A., Dorr, R. T., Hara, Y., & Alberts, D. S. (2003). Pharmacokinetics and safety of green tea polyphenols after multiple-dose administration of epigallocatechin gallate and polyphenon E in healthy individuals. *Clinical Cancer Research*, 9(9), 3312–3319.

Conde, E., Gordon, M. H., Moure, A., & Dominguez, H. (2013). Development of a green tea-based beverage with potent antioxidant activity. *International Journal of Food Science & Technology*, 48(2), 228-234.

Craft, S., & Watson, G. S. (2004). Insulin and neurodegenerative disease: Shared and specific mechanisms. *Lancet Neurology*, 3(3), 169-178.

Dube, A., Nicolazzo, J. A., & Larson, I. (2010). Chitosan nanoparticles enhance the intestinal absorption of the green tea catechins (+)-catechin and (-)-epigallocatechin gallate. *European Journal of Pharmaceutical Sciences*, 41(2), 219-225.

Dulloo, A. G., Duret, C., Rohrer, D., Girardier, L., Mensi, N., Fathi, M., Chantre, P., & Vandermander, J. (1999). Efficacy of a green tea extract rich in catechin polyphenols and caffeine in increasing 24-h energy expenditure and fat oxidation in humans. *American Journal of Clinical Nutrition*, 70(6), 1040-1045.

Fang, J. Y., Hung, C. F., Chiu, H. C., Wang, J. J., & Chan, T. F. (2006). Efficacy and irritancy of enhancers on the *in vitro* and *in vivo* percutaneous absorption of flavonoids. *Journal of Pharmaceutical Sciences*, 95(1), 177-186.

Fang, M. Z., Wang, Y., Ai, N., Hou, Z., Sun, Y., Lu, H., Welsh, W., & Yang, C. S. (2003). Tea polyphenol (-)-epigallocatechin-3-gallate inhibits DNA methyltransferase and reactivates methylation-silenced genes in cancer cell lines. *Cancer Research*, 63(22), 7563–7570.

Forester, S. C., & Lambert, J. D. (2011). The role of antioxidant versus pro-oxidant effects of green tea polyphenols in cancer prevention. *Molecular Nutrition & Food Research*, 55(6), 844-854.

Glass, C. K., Saijo, K., Winner, B., Marchetto, M. C., & Gage, F. H. (2010). Mechanisms underlying inflammation in neurodegeneration. *Cell*, 140(6), 918-934.

Golden, E. B., & Lam, P. Y. (2009). Green tea polyphenols and cancer chemoprevention: Multiple mechanisms and endpoints for phase II trials. *Nutrition Reviews*, 67(5), 273-286.

Halliwell, B. (2006). Oxidative stress and neurodegeneration: Where are we now? *Journal of Neurochemistry*, 97(6), 1634-1658.

Henning, S. M., Fajardo-Lira, C., Lee, H. W., Youssefian, A. A., Go, V. L. W., & Heber, D. (2004). Catechin content of 18 teas and a green tea extract supplement correlates with the antioxidant capacity. *Nutrition and Cancer*, 49(2), 226-235.

Hsu, S. (2005). Green tea and the skin. *Journal of the American Academy of Dermatology*, 52(6), 1049-1059.

Hu, B., Ting, Y., Yang, X., Tang, W., Zeng, X., & Huang, Q. (2017). The important role of lipid raft-mediated attachment in the infection of cultured cells by coronavirus infectious bronchitis virus Beaudette strain. *PLoS One*, 12(1), e0170125.

Juneja, L. R., Chu, D. C., Okubo, T., Nagato, Y., & Yokogoshi, H. (1999). L-theanine—a unique amino acid of green tea and its relaxation effect in humans. *Trends in Food Science & Technology*, 10(6-7), 199-204.

Khan, N., & Mukhtar, H. (2013). Tea polyphenols for health promotion. *Life Sciences*, 81(7), 519-533.

Kuriyama, S. (2006). The relation between green tea consumption and cardiovascular disease as evidenced by epidemiological studies. *Journal of Nutrition*, 136(8), 2524S-2529S.

Kuriyama, S., Hozawa, A., Ohmori, K., Shimazu, T., Matsui, T., Ebihara, S., Awata, S., Nagatomi, R., Arai, H., & Tsuji, I. (2006). Green tea consumption and cognitive function: A cross-sectional study from the Tsurugaya Project. *American Journal of Clinical Nutrition*, 83(2), 355-361.

Kuriyama, S., Shimazu, T., Ohmori, K., Kikuchi, N., Nakaya, N., Nishino, Y., Tsubono, Y., & Tsuji, I. (2006). Green tea consumption and mortality due to cardiovascular disease, cancer, and all causes in Japan: The Ohsaki Study. *JAMA*, 296(10), 1255-1265.

Lau, A., & Tymianski, M. (2010). Glutamate receptors, neurotoxicity and neurodegeneration. *Pflügers Archiv - European Journal of Physiology*, 460(2), 525-542.

Levites, Y., Youdim, M. B., Maor, G., & Mandel, S. (2002). Attenuation of 6-hydroxydopamine (6-OHDA)-induced nuclear factor-kappaB (NF-kappaB) activation and cell death by tea extracts in neuronal cultures. *Biochemical Pharmacology*, 63(1), 21-29.

Li, Q., Zhao, H. F., Zhang, Z. F., Liu, Z. G., Pei, X. R., Wang, J. B., & Li, Y. (2009). Long-term administration of green tea catechins prevents age-related cognitive decline in C57BL/6J mice. *Behavioral Brain Research*, 201(1), 240-245.

Liang, Y. C., Huang, Y. T., Tsai, S. H., Lin-Shiau, S. Y., Chen, C. F., & Lin, J. K. (1999). Suppression of inducible cyclooxygenase and inducible nitric oxide synthase by apigenin and related flavonoids in mouse macrophages. *Carcinogenesis*, 20(10), 1945-1952.

Lin, M. T., & Beal, M. F. (2006). Mitochondrial dysfunction and oxidative stress in neurodegenerative diseases. *Nature*, 443(7113), 787-795.

Lipton, S. A. (2003). Neuronal protection and destruction by NO. *Cell Death & Differentiation*, 10(5), 413-422.

Liu, K., Zhou, R., Wang, B., & Mi, M. T. (2013). Effect of green tea on glucose control and insulin sensitivity: A meta-analysis of 17 randomized controlled trials. *American Journal of Clinical Nutrition*, 98(2), 340-348.

Loftsson, T., Hreinsdóttir, D., & Masson, M. (2005). Evaluation of cyclodextrin solubilization of drugs. *International Journal of Pharmaceutics*, 302(1-2), 18-28.

Lu, H., Meng, X., & Yang, C. S. (2004). Enzymology of methylation of tea catechins and inhibition of catechol-O-methyltransferase by (-)-epigallocatechin gallate. *Drug Metabolism and Disposition*, 32(5), 572-579.

Mancini, E., Beglinger, C., Drewe, J., Zanchi, D., Lang, U. E., & Borgwardt, S. J. (2017). Green tea effects on cognition, mood and human brain function: A systematic review. *Phytomedicine*, 34, 26-37.

Mandel, S. A., Avramovich-Tirosh, Y., Reznichenko, L., Zheng, H., Weinreb, O., Amit, T., & Youdim, M. B. H. (2005). Multifunctional activities of green tea catechins in neuroprotection: Modulation of cell survival genes, iron-dependent oxidative stress and PKC signaling pathway. *Neurosignals*, 14(1-2), 46-60.

Mandel, S., Maor, G., & Youdim, M. B. H. (2004). Iron and alpha-synuclein in the substantia nigra of MPTP-treated mice: Effect of neuroprotective drugs R-apomorphine and green tea polyphenol (-)-epigallocatechin-3-gallate. *Journal of Molecular Neuroscience*, 24(3), 401-416.

Misaka, S., Yatabe, J., Müller, F., Takano, K., Kawabe, K., Glaeser, H., Yatabe, M. S., Onoue, S., Werba, J. P., Watanabe, H., Yamada, S., Fromm, M. F., & Kimura, J. (2013). Green tea ingestion greatly reduces plasma concentrations of nadolol in healthy subjects. *Clinical Pharmacology & Therapeutics*, 95(4), 432-438.

Reygaert, W. C. (2018). The antimicrobial possibilities of green tea. *Frontiers in Microbiology*, 9, 229.

Singh, N., Mandal, A. K., & Khan, Z. A. (2016). Potential neuroprotective properties of epigallocatechin-3-gallate (EGCG). *Nutrition Journal*, 15(1), 60.

Chapter 6

Bacopa monnieri: A Cognitive Enhancer and Neuroprotectant

Rahul Sarathee Kathirvel
Hema Gandhi
Shikha Baghel Chauhan
and Indu Singh*
Amity Institute of Pharmacy, Amity University, Noida, Uttar Pradesh, India

Abstract

Neurodegenerative diseases pose a significant challenge globally due to increasing age and life expectancy. *Bacopa monnieri*, commonly known as Brahmi, is an herb from the Scrophulariaceae family renowned for its pharmacological actions. The bioactive compounds in *B. monnieri*, particularly bacosides, are largely responsible for their therapeutic effects. Traditionally, *B. monnieri* has been valued in Ayurveda for its rejuvenating properties on the brain and nervous system, serving as a memory enhancer and neuroprotectant. Contemporary research, including both animal and human studies, supports these traditional claims, highlighting *B. monnieri*'s potential in treating various neurological disorders such as depression, anxiety, and cognitive decline, including Alzheimer's disease.

Keywords: *Bacopa monnieri*, bacosides, cognitive function, memory, neuroprotectant

---

* Corresponding Author's Email: induysingh@gmail.com.

In: Natural Solutions for Neurodegenerative Disorders
Editors: Rahul Kumar Sharma, Shailesh Sharma, Ajmer Singh Grewal et al.
ISBN: 979-8-89530-231-6

Introduction

The herb *Bacopa monnieri*, commonly known as Brahmi, has a storied history in traditional medicine, particularly within Ayurveda, the ancient Indian medical system. *B. monnieri* is characterized by its oblong leaves, delicate purple flowers, and creeping stalks, thriving in moist, marshy environments which underscore its adaptability and resilience. The Bacopa genus includes several plants with therapeutic properties (Table 1). Revered for centuries, *B. monnieri* is esteemed in traditional medicine for its neuroprotective effects and its potential to enhance cognitive function, alleviate stress, and promote overall well-being. The name "Brahmi" reflects its association with Brahma, the Hindu deity of wisdom, suggesting a link to divine insight. Modern research supports these traditional claims, indicating *B. monnieri*'s value in cognitive health. As interest in natural remedies and nootropics grows, scientists are exploring the herb's pharmacological effects and therapeutic potential (Raghav et al., 2006). The plant exhibits considerable diversity, influenced by geographical location and growing conditions, with notable cultivars like "CDRI-08" and "Himalaya Bacopa" offering unique properties. The bioactive compounds known as bacosides are crucial to *B. monnieri*'s cognitive-enhancing effects, including neuroprotection through increased neuroplasticity, neurotransmitter modulation, and antioxidant activity. Clinical trials have empirically validated the herb's traditional benefits for memory, focus, and stress reduction.

Morphology of *Bacopa monnieri*

Bacopa monnieri is distinguished by its unique morphology, which contributes to its visual appeal and ecological adaptability. This perennial herb features several distinctive traits that make it recognizable in its natural habitat (Singh *et al.,* 1997). Its stems are succulent and prostrate, exhibiting a creeping growth habit that forms a dense mat of vegetation. This trailing nature allows B. monnieri to efficiently cover and spread across various substrates, demonstrating its adaptability to diverse environments (Singh and Singh, 1980). The leaves of B. monnieri are small, thick, and oblong, arranged oppositely along the stems. Their thickness aids in water retention, an essential trait for a plant often found in marshy and damp environments. The vibrant green color of the leaves adds to the plant's visual appeal (Sireeratawong *et al.,* 2017). During its blooming period, B. monnieri produces delicate flowers with five petals, which range in color from purple to white and are typically arranged in clusters. This flowering phase is crucial for reproduction and enhances the plant's overall attractiveness. *Bacopa monnieri*'s morphology is closely linked to its preference for marshy and wetland habitats. Its ability to thrive in shallow water and damp soils is facilitated by its succulent stems, water-retaining leaves, and striking flowers. This adaptability allows Brahmi to colonize a variety of ecosystems, highlighting its resilience and versatility (Aguiar and Borowski, 2013a).

Table 1. Plants belonging to Bacopa genus

Scientific Name	Common Name	Geographic Origin	Bioactive Compounds	Traditional Uses	Reference
Bacopa monnieri	Brahmi, Water Hyssop	Native to wetlands in India, Southeast Asia, Australia, Europe, Africa, and North and South America.	Bacosides, alkaloids, flavonoids, saponins.	Sharpening memory, improving cognitive function, reducing anxiety, and addressing various neurological disorders	Singh and Dhawan, 1997
Bacopa colorata	Blue Waterhyssop	Native to tropical regions of Asia, including India and Sri Lanka.	Bacosides, alkaloids, flavonoids, saponins.	-	-
Bacopa floribunda	Lemon Bacopa, Southern Bacopa	Native to Australia and Southeast Asia.	Bacosides, alkaloids, flavonoids, saponins.	Traditional uses may include applications for cognitive health, but detailed information is scarce	-
Bacopa rotundifolia	Roundleaf Waterhyssop	Native to North and South America.	Bacosides, alkaloids, and flavonoids.	Cognitive enhancement and stress reduction	-

Traditional Uses

Brahmi, or *B. monnieri*, has a rich history of use in Ayurveda, the ancient Indian system of medicine. Esteemed for its potential cognitive benefits, Brahmi has long been a key component in Ayurvedic formulations designed to enhance mental health. Traditionally, it has been employed to reduce stress, improve focus, and boost memory. In Ayurvedic practice, *B. monnieri* is an integral ingredient in formulations such as "Medhya Ramayana," which are believed to rejuvenate and enhance cognitive functions. These preparations are reputed to support memory, intelligence, and overall mental clarity. In addition to its cognitive benefits, Brahmi has been used in Ayurveda to address a range of conditions, including anxiety, asthma, and epilepsy, showcasing its broad therapeutic versatility (Singh and Singh, 1981).

Cognitive Enhancer: A Scientific Exploration

Scientific research on *B. monnieri*, or Brahmi, has largely concentrated on its cognitive-enhancing properties and potential benefits for cognitive function. Clinical trials have demonstrated its neuroprotective effects and memory-boosting abilities. In a 12-week trial involving three different Bacopa extracts administered at doses of 300–450 mg per day, *B. monnieri* significantly improved cognitive performance, especially in memory recall. Despite these promising results, research into its effects on other cognitive functions, such as reasoning, numerical ability, and language skills, remains limited (Pase et al., 2012). Additionally, another 12-week study with eighty participants compared 300 mg of *B. monnieri* to a placebo, revealing significant improvements in cognitive skills, memory, and concentration among those taking Bacopa. This study not only corroborates traditional claims but also provides contemporary evidence of its cognitive benefits (Eraiah et al., 2024).

Mechanism of Action

The cognitive effects of *B. monnieri* are closely tied to its ability to modulate neurotransmitters, particularly through its bioactive compounds, such as bacosides. These components are crucial for enhancing neuroplasticity and improving synaptic transmission. *B. monnieri* influences acetylcholine levels, a neurotransmitter vital for memory and learning, thus supporting cognitive functions at the cellular level. Additionally, the herb's neuroprotective properties help mitigate age-related cognitive decline by shielding the brain from oxidative stress. In a world with increasing cognitive demands, the concept of a natural cognitive enhancer that not only improves performance but also protects against cognitive deterioration is especially appealing.

Bacopa monnieri and Wellness

The evolution of *B. monnieri* from a traditional herb to a subject of scientific research highlights its growing significance in modern wellness practices. Whether used as standardized extracts, supplements, or herbal preparations, the cognitive benefits of *B. monnieri* warrant further exploration. However, individuals should carefully consider factors such as dosage, product quality, and their medical history when integrating any supplement into their regimen. As ongoing research sheds light on its mechanisms of action and efficacy, those interested in enhancing cognitive function may find *B. monnieri* to be a valuable addition to their wellness strategy.

Neuroprotectant

In the search for effective strategies to protect and enhance brain health, *B. monnieri* stands out as a potent natural neuroprotectant. While traditionally valued for its cognitive-enhancing properties, *B. monnieri* is increasingly recognized for its potential to shield the brain from various stressors and age-related decline. Recent scientific studies have sought to confirm the neuroprotective benefits long attributed to this herb. For instance, research by Holcomb et al., (2006) investigated *B. monnieri*'s effects on amyloid levels in PSAPP mice, a model for Alzheimer's disease. The study found a significant reduction in amyloid levels, suggesting that *B. monnieri* may play a role in alleviating processes linked to neurodegenerative disorders.

Antioxidant

Bacopa monnieri is rich in flavonoids, alkaloids, and other bioactive compounds that function as free radical scavengers. Oxidative stress, which arises from an imbalance between free radicals and antioxidants, is a key factor in neurodegenerative diseases. The antioxidant properties of B. monnieri help protect against oxidative damage, thereby supporting neuronal integrity. A review by Aguiar and Borowski (2013b) highlights the herb's significant antioxidant capabilities, underscoring its potential as a powerful agent in combating oxidative stress. By neutralizing free radicals, B. monnieri fosters an environment that promotes brain health and resilience.

Safety and Toxicity

Neuroinflammation and neuronal loss are significant contributors to various neurodegenerative diseases. *B. monnieri* exhibits anti-inflammatory properties that may help reduce inflammation in the brain. A study by Sireeratawong et al., (2017) assessed both acute and chronic toxicities of *B. monnieri* extract in rats, using a dose of 5000 mg/kg. The results indicated no serious adverse effects at this dosage, highlighting its safety profile. This aspect is crucial for considering *B. monnieri*'s potential for long-term use as a neuroprotective agent.

Conclusion

In conclusion, *B. monnieri* embodies a bridge between ancient traditions and contemporary scientific research, offering a nuanced approach to cognitive well-being. With deep roots in Ayurveda, its historical role as a cognitive enhancer and neuroprotectant aligns with modern findings. The herb's adaptable morphology reflects its resilience and versatility across different environments. Research supports *B. monnieri*'s cognitive-enhancing and neuroprotective effects, driven largely by its bioactive compounds, particularly bacosides. These compounds contribute to modulating neurotransmitters, enhancing neuroplasticity, and mitigating oxidative stress. Incorporating *B. monnieri* into wellness routines presents a promising avenue for addressing cognitive health challenges.

References

Aguiar, S., & Borowski, T. (2013a). A unique antioxidant efficacy profile of *Bacopa monnieri*. *American Journal of Clinical Nutrition*, 97(4), 768-769.

Aguiar, S., & Borowski, T. (2013b). Neuropharmacological review of the nootropic herb *Bacopa monnieri*. *Rejuvenation Research*, 16(4), 313-326.

Calabrese, C., Gregory, W. L., Leo, M., Kraemer, D., Bone, K., & Oken, B. (2008). Effects of a standardized *Bacopa monnieri* extract on cognitive performance, anxiety, and depression in the elderly: A randomized, double-blind, placebo-controlled trial. *Journal of Alternative and Complementary Medicine*, 14(6), 707-713.

Charles, P. D., Ambigapathy, G., Geraldine, P., & Akbarsha, M. A. (2011). Effects of *Bacopa monnieri* on the development of morphine tolerance and dependence in mice. *Indian Journal of Pharmacology*, 43(6), 668.

Eraiah, M. M., Shekhar, H. C., Joshua, L., & Thomas, J. V. (2024). Effect of *Bacopa monnieri* extract on memory and cognitive skills in adult humans: A randomized, double-blind, placebo-controlled study. *Journal of Psychiatry and Cognitive Behaviour*, 8, 168.

Holcomb, L. A., Dhanasekaran, M., Hitt, A. R., Young, K. A., & Riggs, M. (2006). *Bacopa monnieri* extract reduces amyloid levels in PSAPP mice. *Journal of Alzheimer's Disease*, 9(3), 243-251.

Kongkeaw, C., Dilokthornsakul, P., Thanarangsarit, P., Hui, C., & Ruangraksa, C. (2016). Evaluation of safety and efficacy of *Bacopa monnieri*. *Journal of the Medical Association of Thailand*, 99 (Suppl 5), S209-S214.

Pase, M. P., Kean, J., Sarris, J., Neale, C., Scholey, A. B., & Stough, C. (2012). The cognitive-enhancing effects of *Bacopa monnieri*: A systematic review of randomized, controlled human clinical trials. *Journal of Alternative and Complementary Medicine*, 18(7), 647-652.

Raghav, S., Singh, H., Dalal, P. K., Srivastava, J. S., & Asthana, O. P. (2006). Randomized controlled trial of standardized *Bacopa monnieri* extract in age-associated memory impairment. *Indian Journal of Psychiatry*, 48(4), 238.

Rastogi, M., Ojha, R. P., Prabu, P. C., Devi, B. P., Agrawal, A., & Dubey, G. P. (2012). Prevention of age-associated neurodegeneration and promotion of healthy brain ageing in female Wistar rats by long term use of bacosides. *Biogerontology*, 13(2), 183-195.

Sairam, K., Dorababu, M., Goel, R. K., & Bhattacharya, S. K. (2002). Antidepressant activity of standardized extract of *Bacopa monnieri* in experimental models of depression in rats. *Phytomedicine*, 9 (3), 207-211.

Sarkar, M., Ghosh, P. K., & Ghosh, S. (2015). Effect of *Bacopa monnieri* on liver and kidney toxicity in chronic use of opioids. *Indian Journal of Pharmacology*, 47 (3), 318.

Sathaye, S., Baghel, U. S., Kaur, C., Reddy, K. R., Sathaye, S. and Naidu, V. G. (2015). *Bacopa monnieri* leaf extract ameliorates hypobaric hypoxia induced spatial memory impairment. *Neurobiology of Learning and Memory*, 120, 41-49.

Singh, H. K., & Dhawan, B. N. (1997). Neuropsychopharmacology effects of the Ayurvedic nootropic *Bacopa monnieri* Linn. (Brahmi). *Indian Journal of Pharmacology*, 29(5), 359-365.

Singh, R. H., & Singh, L. (1980). Studies on the anti-anxiety effect of the Medhya Rasayana drug, Brahmi (*Bacopa monnieri* Wettst.) - Part I. *Journal of Research in Ayurveda and Siddha*, 1(2), 133-148.

Singh, R. H., & Singh, L. (1981). Comparative anti-anxiety activity of Brahmi extracts and Diazepam. *Indian Journal of Pharmacology*, 13(1), 10-11.

Sireeratawong, S., Jaijoy, K., Khonsung, P., Lertprasertsuk, N., & Ingkaninan, K. (2017). Acute and chronic toxicities of *Bacopa monnieri* extract in Sprague-Dawley rats. *BMC Complementary and Alternative Medicine*, 16(1), 249.

Stough, C., Lloyd, J., Clarke, J., Downey, L. A., Hutchison, C. W., Rodgers, T., & Nathan, P. J. (2001). The chronic effects of an extract of *Bacopa monnieri* (Brahmi) on cognitive function in healthy human subjects. *Psychopharmacology*, 156(4), 481-484.

Chapter 7

Ashwagandha and Neurodegeneration

Preeti[1,*]
Gaurav Gaur[2]
Rahul Kumar Sharma[1]
Jyoti Verma[1]
Shailesh Sharma[1]
and Neelam Sharma[1]
[1]Amar Shaheed Baba Ajit Singh Jujhar Singh Memorial College of Pharmacy, Bela, Ropar, Punjab, India
[2]All India Institute of Medical Sciences, Rishikesh, Uttrakhand, India

Abstract

Ashwagandha, scientifically known as *Withania somnifera*, is one of the most widely used herbs in herbal medicine. As a member of the Solanaceae family, it is commonly referred to as Indian ginseng or poison gooseberry. The term "somnifera" is derived from Latin, meaning "sleep-inducer," which aligns with its popular use as a neuroprotective agent. The root extract of *W. somnifera* contains steroidal lactones with ergostane, as well as compounds like withanone, withaferin, withanolides, sitoindosides, and approximately 0.2% alkaloids. Additionally, *W. somnifera* has been studied for its potential role in enhancing overall vitality and regulating hormonal balance. Research has demonstrated the neuroprotective effects of Ashwagandha in various neurological disorders, including Alzheimer's disease, Parkinson's disease, and Huntington's disease. Ashwagandha is known to regulate

* Corresponding Author's Email: preetiminhas63@gmail.com.

In: Natural Solutions for Neurodegenerative Disorders
Editors: Rahul Kumar Sharma, Shailesh Sharma, Ajmer Singh Grewal et al.
ISBN: 979-8-89530-231-6

oxidative stress markers and antioxidant enzymes in the brain. Its root extract promotes the growth of axons and dendrites, indicating its role in neural regeneration. As research on Ashwagandha continues to expand, its benefits are becoming increasingly evident. However, further studies are necessary to fully understand its therapeutic mechanisms and to ensure its safety and efficacy in managing neurodegenerative diseases. Investigating the effects of Ashwagandha offers valuable insights into developing new strategies for managing neurodegenerative disorders and promoting brain health.

Keywords: Ashwagandha, neuroprotective effect, *Withania Somnifera*, neurological disorders, neural regeneration

Abbreviations

3-NP	3-Nitroporpionic acid
AD	Alzheimer's disease
ALS	Amyotrophic lateral sclerosis
GABA	Gamma amino butyric acid
HD	Huntington disease
MTT	(3-(4,5-Dimethylthiazol-2-yl)-2,5-Diphenyltetrazolium Bromide)
NDDs	Neurodegenerative diseases
PD	Parkinson's disease
PPARγ	Peroxisome proliferation-activated receptor gamma
ROS	Reactive Oxygen Species

Introduction

Neurodegeneration refers to a pathological state in which the nervous system or nerve cells, known as neurons, undergo a loss of function, structure, or both (Przedborski, 2017). Globally, psychological and brain disorders pose a significant public health challenge, affecting over one billion individuals worldwide. Current medical treatments for neurological disorders are often expensive and associated with numerous side effects. As a result, the use of natural products has become a crucial avenue in medicine. Ayurveda, a prominent Indian medical system, offers a comprehensive approach to treating brain-related disorders, including a catalog of around 450 medicinal plants, with 56 commonly used in Ayurvedic prescriptions for neurological issues (Zahiruddin et al., 2020). Ashwagandha (*Withania somnifera*), a renowned indigenous medicinal herb, plays a central role in various Ayurvedic formulations used for treating neurological problems. It is a vital component of the traditional medicinal system and has recently gained prominence as a principal therapy for managing various conditions, including diabetes and neurodegenerative diseases. Neurodegenerative diseases (NDDs) are defined as neurological conditions characterized by a steady decline in the structure and function of the brain. These disorders include Parkinson's disease (PD), Alzheimer's disease (AD), amyotrophic lateral sclerosis (ALS), and Huntington's disease (HD) (Figure 1). NDDs cause irreversible differentiation of neuronal cells and impair their ability to regenerate. This dysfunction leads to disruptions in the brain's communication pathways, extensively affecting various functions such as memory, cognition, motor skills, and sensory perception (Wilson et al., 2023). Alzheimer's disease is primarily characterized by a progressive decline in cognitive functions, linked to synapse deterioration and neuron loss in the hippocampus. In AD, there is an abnormal accumulation of β-amyloid protein in the brain, which triggers the production of reactive oxygen species (ROS), further damaging neurons (Mikulska et al., 2023). Parkinson's disease is another progressive NDD, marked by the degeneration of neuronal cells in the substantia nigra pars compacta, accompanied by a synchronous loss of dopamine in the striatum, leading to motor imbalance (Goyal et al., 2023). Current theories suggest that oxidative stress, inflammation, protein aggregation, and mitochondrial dysfunction are key factors in neurodegeneration in PD (Jaiswal et al., 2023). Amyotrophic lateral sclerosis is a rare NDD characterized by muscle twitching and stiffness, which progressively worsen as muscle size decreases. ALS affects neurons that control voluntary functions, with approximately 90% of cases being sporadic and the remaining 10% familial (Younger et al., 2023). Huntington's disease is the primary genetic NDD, marked by behavioral and neuropsychiatric symptoms caused by a repeat expansion in the Huntington gene. Huntington is a protein found in both animals and humans, particularly at higher concentrations in the brain. The mutated version of this protein is pathogenic, producing toxic mutants in Huntington oligomers, leading to a loss of function (Stoker et al., 2022) (Figure 1).

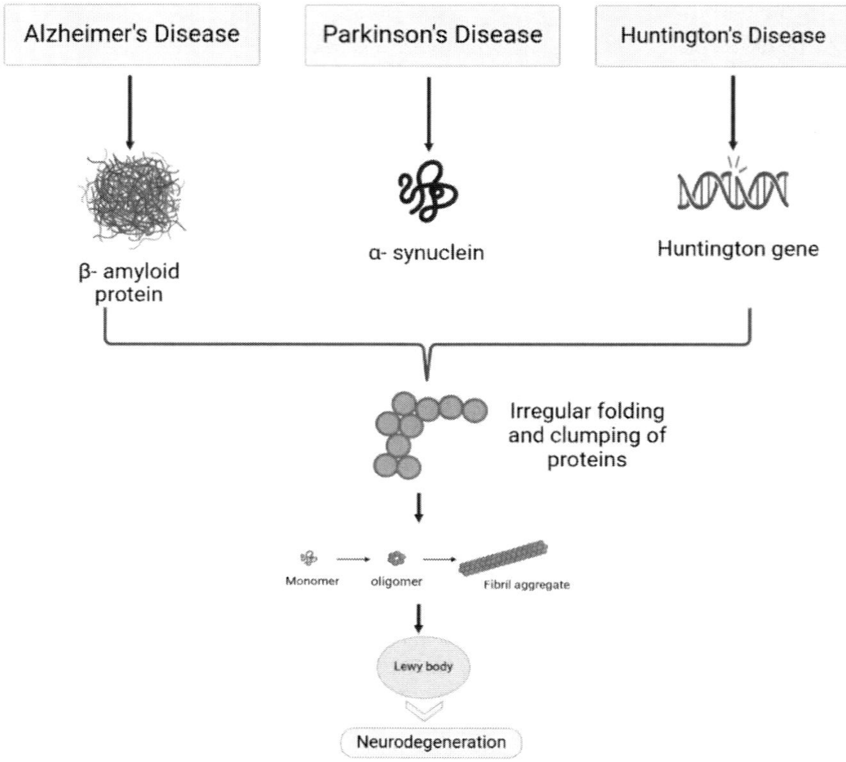

Figure 1. Molecular mechanism of neurodegenerative diseases.

Ashwagandha

Ashwagandha belongs to the Solanaceae family and is commonly known as poison gooseberry, Indian ginseng, or winter cherry. The name "Ashwagandha" is derived from the Sanskrit words "ashwa," meaning horse, and "gandha," meaning fragrance. This name reflects the belief that Ashwagandha imparts rejuvenating and strengthening properties akin to the stamina of a horse, while "gandha" refers to the distinctive fragrance of the plant's fresh roots (Mikulska et al., 2023). Ashwagandha is primarily cultivated in central and northwestern India, where the ideal climatic conditions include an altitude of approximately 1,500 meters above sea level (Zahiruddin et al., 2020).

Phytochemical Profile

Ashwagandha contains more than 35 phytochemicals that have been identified and isolated so far. The principal constituents of Ashwagandha are steroidal lactones and alkaloids. Key alkaloids present in Ashwagandha include somniferine, somnine, somniferinine, withananine, pseudo-withanine, tropine, pseudo-tropine, 3-a-gloyloxytropane, cuscohygrine, and anaferine. The withanolides, which are steroidal compounds, possess a steroidal nucleus with 28 carbon atoms and a side chain consisting of 9 carbons, accompanied by a six-membered lactone ring. Saponins, such as sitoindoside VII and VIII, which have an extra acyl group, and withanolides containing glucose at carbon 27 (sitoindoside IX and X), have also been reported in the literature. The phytochemical composition of Ashwagandha varies depending on its geographic distribution. Among the alkaloids, withanine is the most prominent. A significant withanolide (steroid) isolated from this plant is withaferin A, which is noted for its biological properties. Ashwagandha exhibits chemogenetic variation, and three distinct chemotypes (I, II, and III) have been identified (John, 2014).

Pharmacological Properties

Ashwagandha has been extensively studied for its wide range of medicinal properties. These studies suggest that Ashwagandha is more than just an herb; it is a complex powerhouse. Known as an adaptogen, it has the ability to soothe anxiety, reduce inflammation, and act as a natural diuretic. Ashwagandha also exhibits antimicrobial properties and has neuroprotective effects that help safeguard the brain and maintain cognitive health. It is reputed for its anti-aging qualities, making it a key ingredient in longevity therapies. Additionally, Ashwagandha is used as an aphrodisiac to stimulate sexual desire and as an immune modulator to strengthen the body's defense mechanisms. In summary, Ashwagandha is an extraordinary plant with numerous health benefits (John, 2014) (Figure 2).

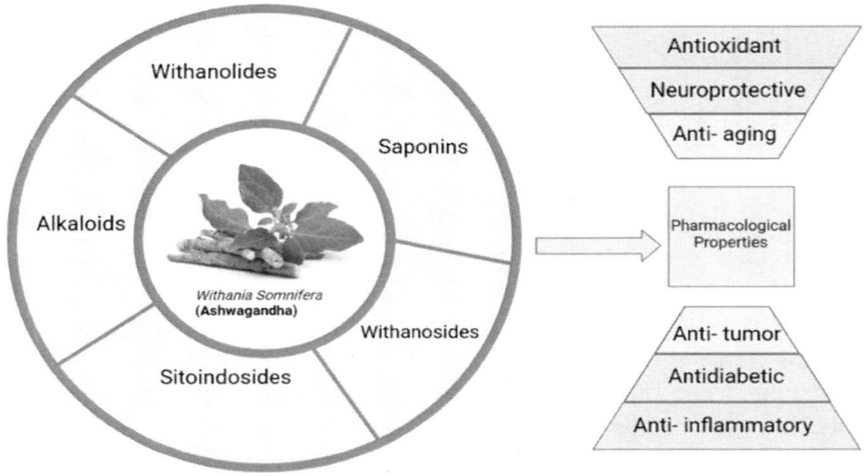

Figure 2. Pharmacological properties of Ashwagandha.

Ashwagandha's Mechanism of Neuroprotection

Ashwagandha is recognized for its significant neuroprotective potential. *W. somnifera* is known as an anti-anxiety or adaptogenic agent that helps manage daily life stress, boosts mental acuity, alleviates pain, and reduces swelling. Additionally, it functions as an anti-aging therapeutic beneficial in nearly all brain disorders. *W. somnifera* influences acetylcholine signaling, GABA signaling, and oxidative processes, with compounds in its roots playing a crucial role in mitigating neurotoxicity caused by excessive excitatory neurotransmission and preventing oxidative damage. Research has shown that plant extracts from *W. somnifera* effectively suppress cytotoxicity and DNA damage induced by hydrogen peroxide in normal human fibroblast cells. The bioactive compounds found in *W. somnifera*, specifically sitoindosides VII–X and withaferin A (glycowithanolides), have undergone specific testing for their oxidative stress-regulating properties against various antioxidant enzyme levels in the forebrain of rats. When administered daily (at 10 or 20 mg/kg) for 21 days, the glycowithanolides from the roots of *W. somnifera* increased the levels of these enzymes, surpassing the effects of the prominent free-radical scavenger deprenyl. It has also been reported that withanolides from *W. somnifera* exhibit calcium-antagonistic properties and demonstrate a concentration-dependent inhibition of acetylcholinesterase (AChE) and butyrylcholinesterase (BChE) activities. This combination of cholinesterase inhibitory capabilities and calcium antagonistic properties suggests that withanolides could serve as potential drug candidates for further exploration in addressing AD and related concerns. *W. somnifera* is emerging as a botanical miracle with substantial therapeutic potential, particularly in NDDs such as PD and HD. Notably, *W. somnifera* roots, when combined with powdered Mucuna pruriens seeds and cow's milk, have been found to be an effective intervention for people diagnosed with PD. A comprehensive evaluation of *W. somnifera* extract at different dosages (100, 200, and 300 mg/kg b.w.) demonstrated a significant improvement in oxidative imbalance indicators and its impact on dopaminergic D2 receptor binding and tyrosine hydroxylase expression. The extract also showed protective effects against MPTP-induced catalepsy, supporting its potential in alleviating symptoms of PD. In HD, *W. somnifera* root extract was investigated for its effects on 3-NP-induced gait anomalies, oxidative imbalance, and mitochondrial dysfunction. The study showed dose-dependent improvements in behavioral, physiological, and enzymatic alterations over a two-week treatment period. The neuroprotective benefits of *W. somnifera* are strongly supported by statistically significant data ($P < 0.05$), suggesting its effects are mediated through antioxidant activity. Recent studies have explored the neuroprotective potential of *W. somnifera* against β-amyloid (1–42)-induced toxicity, providing an in-depth examination of AD. Cytotoxic effects induced by β-amyloid indicate a reduction in cell development and subtle changes in cellular shape, but the introduction of *W. somnifera* extract leads to significant improvements. Confocal microscopy reveals the extract's effectiveness in reducing β-amyloid-induced toxicity, preserving dendritic architecture, preventing spine loss, and restoring spine density. MTT metabolic assays and modifications in PPARγ levels further illustrate *W. somnifera*'s neuroprotective potential against β-amyloid-induced neuropathogenesis (Singh et al., 2017) (Figure 3).

Therapeutic Applications of Ashwagandha in the Management of Neurodegenerative Diseases

Neurodegeneration, characterized by the gradual decline of the structural and functional abilities of neurons, results in neuronal loss and the onset of diseases such as AD, PD, and HD. Scientific evidence suggests that

Ashwagandha possesses the potential to promote dendrite growth in nerve cells, enhancing the cells' ability to interpret signals. This property makes Ashwagandha a promising candidate for addressing the structural brain changes associated with dementia. Furthermore, Ashwagandha supports the development of both normal and injured neuronal cells, indicating its potential to improve the functionality of healthy brain cells while providing therapeutic benefits to individuals suffering from NDDs (John, 2014).

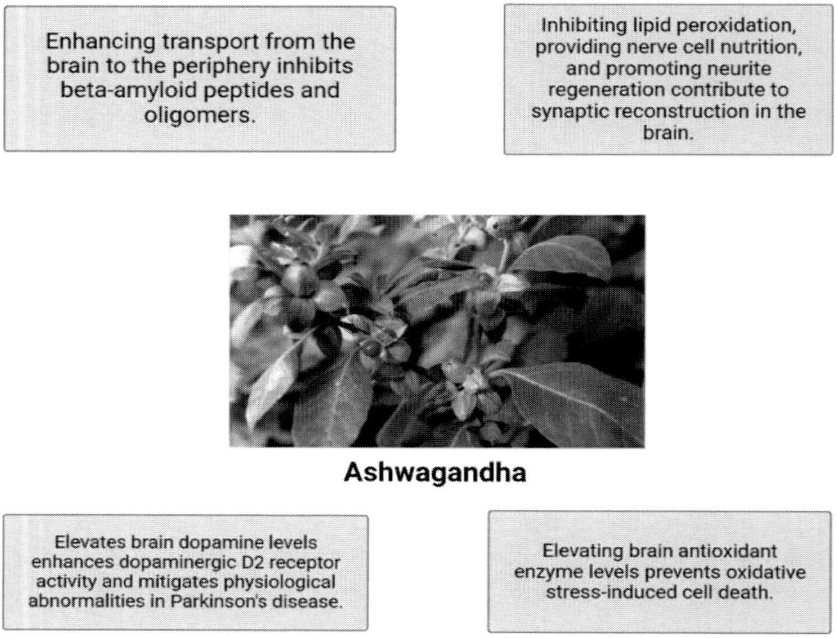

Figure 3. Neuroprotective mechanism of Ashwagandha.

Ashwagandha's Role in Parkinson's Management

PD is characterized by the depletion of nigrostriatal pathways in neuronal cells, leading to alterations in the balance between the inhibitory effects of dopaminergic neurons and the excitatory functions of acetylcholine and glutamate neurons. PD typically manifests in the later stages of life and is primarily marked by extrapyramidal symptoms, such as a progressive decline in movement (bradykinesia) and tremor of rigidity (Jaiswal et al., 2023).

Ashwagandha, known for its anti-aging, anti-inflammatory, and neuroprotective properties, contains phytochemicals like withanolides, withanine, and withamine, which could be responsible for these effects. These compounds also exhibit free radical scavenging properties, addressing mitochondrial dysfunction in the striatum and cerebellum regions, thereby restoring dopamine levels in the striatum and modulating neurotransmission (Cabey et al., 2022). In models of human Parkinson's disease, Ashwagandha has demonstrated the ability to alleviate neurodegenerative symptoms effectively, with the extent of this effect being dosage-dependent (Munir et al., 2022).

Ashwagandha's Role in Alzheimer's Management

AD is characterized by the progressive degradation of mental functions in elderly individuals, accompanied by the accumulation of tau and amyloid-β protein aggregates in the brain. This accumulation leads to neuron loss and synapse deterioration, resulting in brain atrophy. Both human cases and animal models of AD show a strong correlation between synapse loss and the observed decline in cognitive abilities. Recent research suggests that solubilized forms of tau and amyloid-β can induce synaptic damage and spread across neuronal networks. Additionally, pathological changes in the brain are often accompanied by phenotypic changes in glial cells. One hypothesis proposes that glial cells might excessively encase synapses, thereby affecting the trans-synaptic propagation of pathology (Tzioras et al., 2023). The development of amyloid-β (Aβ) deposits in AD leads to neurocellular necrosis, a process that is mitigated by the withanamides found in *W. somnifera* (Ashwagandha). Asomniferol A, derived from Ashwagandha roots, has been shown to effectively counteract Aβ42-induced toxicity in neurons. Molecular modeling and simulation studies indicate that withanamides A and C bind to the active motif of Aβ (25–35), preventing fibrous assembly (Jayaprakasam et al., 2010). Long-term administration of Ashwagandha methanol extract has been found to significantly promote the regrowth of nerve fibers and dendrites in neurons. Beyond its cellular rejuvenating abilities, Ashwagandha also enhances memory by counteracting amyloid peptide-induced memory impairment. Studies demonstrate that extracts from *W. somnifera*, containing withanolides and withanosides, not only slow the progression of AD but also improve cluster pathology and reduce the brain's production of Aβ peptides and polymers. These findings affirm the therapeutic potential of withanolides and withanosides in the treatment of AD (Kushwah et al., 2023).

Ashwagandha's Role in HD's Management

HD is a hereditary disorder that leads to a gradual decline in both brain and muscle function. This neurodegenerative condition is characterized by genetically programmed neuronal loss, which results in erratic behavior, diminished cognitive abilities, and emotional dysregulation. The disease is caused by a mutation in the HTT gene located on chromosome 4 (4p63), where an expansion of the CAG trinucleotide repeat occurs in the exon region 1. The accumulation of mutant Huntingtin proteins with an abnormally long polyglutamine sequence leads to the breakdown of neural networks in the brain, ultimately causing neuronal death. These degenerative changes, particularly in the cerebral cortex and striatum, manifest as chorea, cognitive deficits, and eventually early mortality (Manoharan et al., 2016). *In vivo* and clinical studies have shown that *W. somnifera* (Ashwagandha) holds promising therapeutic potential for treating HD. In an induced rat model of HD, where the neurotoxin 3-nitropropionic acid (3-NP) was used to mimic the disease, treatment with Ashwagandha root extract demonstrated significant neuroprotective effects. These effects were primarily attributed to the reduction of oxidative stress and the enhancement of acetylcholinesterase (AChE) enzyme activity (Sinha et al., 2022). The therapeutic benefits of the root extract were dose-dependent, with its antioxidant properties and interaction with the GABAergic system playing crucial roles. Ashwagandha helped increase glutathione and AChE levels, which in turn improved cognitive performance (Zahiruddin et al., 2020).

Ashwagandha's Role in Amyotrophic Lateral Sclerosis Management

ALS, also known as motor neuropathy, is characterized by the degeneration of motor neurons, leading to muscle weakness and, eventually, immobility. The hallmark of this adult-onset motor neuron disease is the progressive loss of efferent neurons in the brainstem, spinal cord, and motor cortex. This deterioration typically results in respiratory failure and, tragically, death within three to five years (Younger et al., 2023). Research has shown that Ashwagandha can slow the progression of ALS, enhance neuromuscular function, and increase the number of efferent neurons in the lumbar spinal cord by promoting autophagy. Additionally, it influences the levels of misfolded SOD1 and the phosphorylation of nuclear factor-κB, contributing to its therapeutic effects (Dutta et al., 2018).

Challenges and Future Impacts

The future of Ashwagandha in the treatment of NDDs presents both promising opportunities and significant challenges. One major challenge is the need for more rigorous and standardized clinical studies to thoroughly assess Ashwagandha's safety and efficacy across various neurological conditions. Determining the most effective dosage regimen, duration of therapy, and potential side effects is essential for its successful integration into therapeutic protocols. Another critical issue is the inconsistency in the processing of Ashwagandha extracts, which can lead to variations in the concentration of its active constituents, affecting its overall efficacy. Furthermore, there is a gap in our understanding of the molecular mechanisms underlying Ashwagandha's therapeutic effects. Addressing individual variability in response to Ashwagandha is crucial for personalized treatment, as its effectiveness may be influenced by factors such as genetics, environment, and lifestyle. Although various preclinical and human trials have yielded promising results, comprehensive research and robust evidence, along with regulatory approval, are necessary before Ashwagandha can be fully integrated into conventional treatment strategies (Bhat et al., 2022).

Conclusion

Ashwagandha, a traditional herb, has emerged as a significant focus of modern research, particularly for its potential role in combating NDDs. The diverse activities exhibited by Ashwagandha and its phytoconstituents against these conditions highlight a promising and innovative direction in neurology. One of the most notable aspects of Ashwagandha is its ability to mitigate key factors contributing to NDDs, such as oxidative stress, inflammation, and protein misfolding. Numerous studies have underscored its neuroprotective benefits, attributing these effects to its rich phytochemical composition. However, further research is necessary to establish its safety profile and determine the optimal dosage regimen for various neurodegenerative conditions. In conclusion, Ashwagandha stands at a pivotal intersection between traditional medicine and modern science, offering a glimpse into the potential of natural therapies for addressing complex medical conditions. Its neuroprotective effects, supported by scientific evidence, position Ashwagandha as a promising avenue for the treatment of NDDs, bringing new hope to those affected by these debilitating diseases.

References

Bhat, J. A., Akther, T., Najar, R. A., Rasool, F., & Hamid, A. (2022). *Withania somnifera* (L.) Dunal (Ashwagandha); current understanding and future prospect as a potential drug candidate. *Frontiers in Pharmacology*, *13*, 1029123.

Cabey, K., Long, D. M., Law, A., Gray, N. E., McClure, C., Caruso, M., Lak, P., Wright, K. M., Stevens, J. F., Maier, C. S., Soumyanath, A., & Kretzschmar, D. (2022). *Withania somnifera* and centella asiatica extracts ameliorate behavioral deficits in an *in vivo* drosophila melanogaster model of oxidative stress. *Antioxidants*, *11*(1), 121.

Dutta, K., Patel, P., & Julien, J. P. (2018). Protective effects of *Withania somnifera* extract in SOD1G93A mouse model of amyotrophic lateral sclerosis. *Experimental Neurology*, *309*, 193-204.

Goyal, A., Agrawal, A., Verma, A., & Dubey, N. (2023). The PI3K-AKT pathway: A plausible therapeutic target in Parkinson's disease. *Experimental and Molecular Pathology*, *129*, 104846.

Jaiswal, M., Deshmukh, R., Patel, A., Nagori, K., Shukla, A., & Singh, A. (2023). Parkinson's Disease: Neurodegeneration and the Potential Role of Medicinal Plants. *International Neurourology Journal*, *27*(4), 567-579.

Jayaprakasam, B., Padmanabhan, K., & Nair, M. G. (2010). Withanamides in *Withania somnifera* fruit protect PC-12 cells from β-amyloid responsible for Alzheimer's disease. *Phytotherapy Research*, *24*(6), 859-863.

John, J. (2014). Therapeutic potential of *Withania somnifera*: A report on phyto-pharmacological properties. *International Journal of Pharmaceutical Sciences and Research*, *5*(6), 2131-2148.

Kushwah, S., Maurya, N. S., Kushwaha, S., Scotti, L., Chawade, A., & Mani, A. (2023). Herbal Therapeutics for Alzheimer's Disease: Ancient Indian Medicine System from the Modern Viewpoint. *Current Neuropharmacology*, *21*(4), 764.

Manoharan, S., Guillemin, G. J., Abiramasundari, R. S., Essa, M. M., Akbar, M., & Akbar, M. D. (2016). The role of reactive oxygen species in the pathogenesis of Alzheimer's disease, Parkinson's disease, and Huntington's disease: a mini review. *Oxidative Medicine and Cellular Longevity*, *2016*(1), 8590578.

Mikulska, P., Malinowska, M., Ignacyk, M., Szustowski, P., Nowak, J., Pesta, K., Szeląg, M., Szklanny, D., Judasz, E., Kaczmarek, G., Ejiohuo, O. P., Paczkowska-Walendowska, M., Gościniak, A., & Cielecka-Piontek, J. (2023). Ashwagandha (*Withania somnifera*)-Current Research on the Health-Promoting Activities: A Narrative Review. *Pharmaceutics*, 15(4), 1057.

Munir, N., Mahmood, Z., Shahid, M., Afzal, M. N., Jahangir, M., Ali Shah, S. M., Tahir, I. M., Riaz, M., Hussain, S., Akram, M., & Yousaf, F. (2022). *Withania somnifera* chemical constituents' *in vitro* antioxidant potential and their response on spermatozoa parameters. *Dose-Response*, *20*(1), 15593258221074936.

Przedborski, S. (2017). Neurodegeneration. *Neuroimmune Pharmacology*, 345-354.

Singh, V., Shah, H. H., & Guillemin, G. J. (2017). Neuroprotective Effect of Ashwagandha (roots of *Withania somnifera*): The rejuvenator. *Canadian Journal of Clinical Nutrition*, *5*, 34-51.

Sinha, A. K., Dilnashin, H., Birla, H., & Kumar, G. (2022). Role of *Withania somnifera* (Ashwagandha) in Neuronal Health. *Indopathy for Neuroprotection: Recent Advances*, 281.

Stoker, T. B., Mason, S. L., Greenland, J. C., Holden, S. T., Santini, H., & Barker, R. A. (2022). Huntington's disease: Diagnosis and management. *Practical Neurology*, *22*(1), 32-41.

Tzioras, M., McGeachan, R. I., Durrant, C. S., & Spires-Jones, T. L. (2023). Synaptic degeneration in Alzheimer disease. *Nature Reviews Neurology*, *19*(1), 19-38.

Wilson, D. M., Cookson, M. R., Van Den Bosch, L., Zetterberg, H., Holtzman, D. M., & Dewachter, I. (2023). Hallmarks of neurodegenerative diseases. *Cell*, *186*(4), 693-714.

Younger, D. S., & Brown Jr, R. H. (2023). Amyotrophic lateral sclerosis. *Handbook of Clinical Neurology*, *196*, 203-229.

Zahiruddin, S., Basist, P., Parveen, A., Parveen, R., Khan, W., & Ahmad, S. (2020). Ashwagandha in brain disorders: A review of recent developments. *Journal of Ethnopharmacology*, *257*, 112876.

Chapter 8

Ginseng: Potential Benefits in Neurodegenerative Disorders

Hema Gandhi
Shikha Baghel Chauhan*
and Indu Singh
Amity Institute of Pharmacy, Amity University, Noida, Uttar Pradesh, India

Abstract

Ginseng, a traditional herbal remedy with a rich history in various Asian cultures, has garnered attention for its potential benefits in the context of neurodegenerative disorders. This chapter reviews current research on the potential neuroprotective properties of ginseng and its active compounds. A comprehensive examination of *in vitro*, animal, and clinical studies suggests that ginseng exhibits multifaceted effects on neurodegenerative disorders. These effects encompass anti-inflammatory, antioxidant, anti-apoptotic, and neurotrophic actions, as well as the modulation of neurotransmitter systems. Ginsenosides, the bioactive components of ginseng, have been identified as key contributors to these effects. Moreover, ginseng has demonstrated the ability to enhance cognitive function and ameliorate motor deficits. and attenuate pathological hallmarks associated with neurodegenerative diseases in preclinical models. Clinical studies have shown promising outcomes, with ginseng supplementation leading to improved cognitive performance, quality of life, and reduced disease progression in individuals affected by neurodegenerative disorders. While the potential benefits of ginseng in neurodegenerative disorders are encouraging, more

* Corresponding Author's Email: shikha.pharma@gmail.com.

In: Natural Solutions for Neurodegenerative Disorders
Editors: Rahul Kumar Sharma, Shailesh Sharma, Ajmer Singh Grewal et al.
ISBN: 979-8-89530-231-6

extensive and rigorous research is needed to establish its efficacy and safety conclusively. This chapter underscores the need for continued investigation into the mechanisms underlying ginseng's effects, optimal dosages, and potential interactions with existing treatments. Additionally, it highlights the potential of ginseng as a complementary therapeutic option and a source of novel drug development for addressing the growing burden of neurodegenerative disease.

Keywords: Alzheimer's disease, amyotrophic lateral sclerosis, cognitive function, ginseng, ginsenosides, neurodegenerative disorders, Parkinson's disease

Abbreviations

AD	Alzheimer's Disease
ALS	Amyotrophic lateral sclerosis
Aβ	Amyloid-beta
BDNF	Brain-derived neurotrophic factor
CAT	Catalase
CNS	Central nervous system
GABA	Gamma-aminobutyric acid
GPx	Glutathione peroxidase
HD	Huntington's disease
NF-Kb	Nuclear factor kappa-light-chain-enhancer of activated B cells
NGF	Nerve growth factor
NO	Nitric oxide
PD	Parkinson's disease
PPD	Protopanaxadiol
PPT	Protopanaxatriol
RCT	Randomized controlled trial
ROS	Reactive oxygen species
SOD	Superoxide dismutase

Introduction

Ginseng, a perennial plant of the Araliaceae family's Panax genus, has earned worldwide recognition for its extensive medicinal properties deeply rooted in traditional medicine across East Asia for centuries. This fascinating plant, which has thick roots and unique leaves, comes in a few varieties. The two most commonly used species for medicinal purposes are Panax ginseng (Asian or Korean ginseng) and Panax quinquefolius (American ginseng) (Attele et al., 1999). In traditional Chinese medicine, ginseng has been used for thousands of years (Jang et al., 2015). Later, due to its reputation for enhancing vitality, enhancing mental clarity, and advancing general well-being, it travelled to Korea and other Asian nations, where it was widely used in traditional medical procedures. The main active ingredients of ginseng are ginsenosides, one of the plant's many bioactive chemicals, which account for much of its pharmacological importance (Table 1). These ginsenosides, which are specific to ginseng and are responsible for many of its health-promoting qualities, are also known as saponins because of the way their chemical structure resembles that of soap-like chemicals. Studies have brought attention to its adaptogenic qualities, indicating that it plays a part in lowering stress levels by influencing the hypothalamic-pituitary-adrenal axis and so lessening the negative consequences of long-term stress. Furthermore, research on ginseng's potential benefits for cognitive function has shown promise. Its capacity to influence systems of neurotransmitters and encourage neurogenesis has been linked to improvements in memory, attention, and general cognitive function (Kim et al., 2013). Renowned for its potent ginsenosides, ginseng is a natural treatment with the potential for treating neurological diseases. Studies point to its promise in stroke, Parkinson's, and Alzheimer's disease. The many mechanisms of ginseng, such as its antioxidant, anti-inflammatory, and neuroprotective qualities, provide neuroprotection through the reduction of inflammation, the mitigation of oxidative stress, and the enhancement of neuronal survival (Jeong et al., 2014). Research demonstrated that the ginsenosides Rg1 and Rb1 can protect against neurotoxicity, modulate neurotransmitters, and improve cognitive function (Lee et al., 2020). Even with encouraging preclinical data, more research and clinical studies are necessary to fully understand the therapeutic benefits of ginseng in neurodegenerative illnesses (Liu et al., 2017).

Table 1. Types of ginsengs and its main chemical constituents

Type of Ginseng	Scientific Name	Common Name	Geographic Origin	Bioactive Compounds	Traditional Uses	References
Panax ginseng	Panax ginseng	Asian or Korean Ginseng	China, Korea, Japan	Ginsenosides (Rb1, Rg1, Rg3, etc.)	Vigour, improved cognition, and immune support	(Yun et al.,2001)
Panax quinquefolius	*Panax quinquefolius*	American Ginseng	USA, Canada	Ginsenosides (Rb1, Rb2, Re, Rd, etc.)	Increased Energy, Reduced Stress, and Digestive	(Senchina et al.,2013).
Panax japonicus	*Panax japonicus*	Japanese Ginseng	Japan	Ginsenosides (Rb1, Rg1, Rc, etc.)	Boosting Energy and Immunity enhancement	(Miyazaki et al., 2009).
Panax notoginseng	Panax notoginseg	Notoginseng, Sanqi	China	Ginsenosides (Rg1, Rb1, Rd, etc.)	Heart Support and Healing of Wounds	(Zhou et al., 2019).
Panax vietnamensis	Panax vietnamensis	Vietnamese Ginseng	Vietnam	Ginsenosides (Rb1, Rg1, Rg2, etc.)	Prevents ageing, inflammation and vitality	(Miyazaki et al., 2009).
Ginsenosides and Other Active Compounds						
Active Compounds	Chemical Classification	Main Ginseng Species	Pharmacological Effects	Potential Health Benefits	Location of Active Compounds	References
Ginsenosides	Saponins	*Panax quinquefolius, Panax ginseng, Panax vietnamensis, Panax notoginseng Panax japonicus*	Adaptogenic, Antioxidant, Anti-inflammatory, Neuroprotective, Immunomodulatory	Cognitive enhancement, stress reduction	Ginseng root	(Kim et al., 2018).
Polysaccharides	Carbohydrates	*Panax quinquefoliusPanax ginseng,*	Immunomodulatory, Antioxidant, Anticancer	Boosts immune function, helps reduce oxidative stress	Ginseng root	(Wang et al., 2016).

Active Compounds	Chemical Classification	Main Ginseng Species	Pharmacological Effects	Potential Health Benefits	Location of Active Compounds	References
Polyacetylenes	Organic compounds	*Panax ginseng*	Anti-inflammatory, Anticancer	Potential anti-cancer properties, immune support	Ginseng root and sometimes in the leaves	(Kang et al., 2012).
Phenolic Compounds	Polyphenols	*Panax ginseng*	Antioxidant, Neuroprotective	Potential cardiovascular benefits, immune support	Ginseng leaves and root	(Christensen., 2009).
Phytosterols	Sterols	*Panax ginseng*	Cholesterol-lowering, Anti-inflammatory	Supports cardiovascular health, anti-ageing effects	Present in the lipid fraction of ginseng	(Vuksan et al., 2000).
Amino Acids	Organic compounds	*Panax ginseng*	Neuroprotective, Energy-enhancing	Improves immunity, potential cancer prevention	Ginseng root	(Reay et al., 2005).

History and Traditional Use

Originating from the roots of plants of the Panax genus, it is praised for both its historical relevance and its diverse range of medicinal applications. The Greek word "panacea," from which the term "Panax" is derived, refers to the plant's all-purpose status in traditional practices throughout many civilisations, particularly in East Asia. With its origins in traditional Chinese medicine and widespread use to support general health, vigour, and balance, ginseng has a millennium-long history (Kim et al., 2018). The Shen Nong Ben Cao Jing (Shennong's Classic of Materia Medica), an ancient Chinese treatise written more than 2,000 years ago, is the first source of verifiable mention of ginseng. It gained notoriety as a powerful herbal cure throughout time, and accounts of its restorative abilities and revitalising benefits began to surface in a variety of historical books from China, Korea, and other East Asian countries. Ginseng was considered an "elixir of life" in traditional medicine because of its great significance in restoring vital energy, or "qi," and balancing body processes. Ginseng's adaptogenic qualities, which help the body adjust to stimuli and foster resilience against physical and mental exhaustion, have garnered it more recognition (Chevallier et al., 1996).

Neurodegenerative Disorders

A class of progressive illnesses known as neurodegenerative diseases is defined by the slow deterioration and loss of structure or function of neurons in the central nervous system. While Huntington's disease, amyotrophic lateral sclerosis (ALS), and multiple sclerosis are also included in this group, Alzheimer's disease and Parkinson's disease are the most common and well-researched among them.

Alzheimer's Disease (AD)

In a person suffering from Alzheimer's disease, there is an accumulation of beta-amyloid plaques and neurofibrillary tangles in the brain, which begin to aberrant conduct, tarnish evocation, and decline in cognition. The gradual loss of neurons is attributed to neuroinflammation, oxidative stress, and dysfunctional synapses, especially in regions implicated in memory and cognition (Hardy et al., 2002).

Parkinson's Disease (PD)

This type of sickness is identified by the decline of neurons that manufacture dopamine in the substantia nigra part of the cerebellum. Motor symptoms such as bradykinesia, stiffness, tremors, and postural instability are brought on by this loss. One characteristic of Parkinson's disease pathology is aberrant clumps of the protein alpha-synuclein, known as Lewy bodies. The advancement of the illness is also influenced by neuroinflammation, defective protein degradation pathways, and mitochondrial dysfunction (Dickson et al., 2012).

Huntington's Disease (HD)

It is a hereditary neurological condition brought on by an accumulation of aberrant huntingtin protein as a result of a gene mutation. This buildup causes neuronal damage, especially to the basal ganglia, which causes motor impairment, cognitive deterioration, and psychological problems. The pathophysiology of HD is influenced by neuroinflammation, excitotoxicity, and mitochondrial dysfunction (Ross et al., 2011).

Amyotrophic Lateral Sclerosis (ALS)

The loss of both upper and lower motor neurons is a hallmark of ALS, a progressive motor neuron disease. Muscle weakening, stiffness, and finally paralysis is caused by this deterioration. The pathophysiology of ALS is linked to oxidative stress, protein misfolding, glutamate excitotoxicity, and mitochondrial dysfunction (Turner et al., 2008).

Ginseng Constituents and Mechanisms of Action

Ginsenosides

The main active ingredients in ginseng plants, known as ginsenosides, are steroidal saponins that account for many of the plant's pharmacological actions. The amount and location of sugar moieties connected to the central steroid-like core structure known as a dammarane determine the chemical structure of these compounds, which is then divided into several categories. The primary ginsenoside subtypes are as follows:

- Protopanaxadiol (PPD) ginsenosides: These have a dammarane structure with sugar moieties connected at C3 and C20 locations and a dammarane skeleton. Rb1, Rb2, Rb3, Rc, Rd, and Rg3 are a few examples. Panax ginseng and Panax notoginseng are major sources of PPD ginsenosides.
- Protopanaxatriol (PPT) ginsenosides: These ginsenosides are linked to the dammarane skeleton at positions C6 and C20 by sugar moieties. Re, Rf, Rg1, Rg2, Rh1, and Rh2 are some examples. Panax ginseng and Panax quinquefolius are rich sources of PPT ginsenosides.
- Ginsenosides of the oleanane type: Oleanane-type ginsenosides are less prevalent than PPD and PPT ginsenosides. Their oleanane structure differs somewhat from that of dammarane. Compound K, which is created by the metabolism of other ginsenosides, and Ro are two examples. The pharmacological actions and possible health advantages of each kind of ginsenoside differ. Rb1 and Rg1 are well-researched ginsenosides with antioxidant, anti-inflammatory, and neuroprotective qualities. The potential of Rg3 in immune regulation and cancer therapy has been studied. Compound K is notable for its anti-inflammatory and anticancer activities, among others (Christensen., 2009).

Pharmacological Actions of Ginseng Constituents in the Brain

Neurotransmitter Modulation

The main active ingredients in ginseng, called ginsenosides, have been shown to have the capacity to alter the brain's neurotransmitter systems. In particular, acetylcholine release and muscarinic receptor modulation have been shown to increase cholinergic neurotransmission via Rg1 and Rb1 ginsenosides, which may improve cognitive performance and memory retrieval. Moreover, the ginsenosides Rg1 and Rb1 have been shown to interact with gamma-aminobutyric acid (GABA) receptors, indicating a potential function in regulating GABAergic neurotransmission and potential anxiolytic effects.

Neuroprotective Effects

Numerous components of ginseng can protect neurons from excitotoxicity, inflammation, and oxidative stress. By scavenging free radicals and lowering oxidative damage, ginsenosides—in particular, Rg1 and Rb1—exemplify antioxidant activities that protect neurons against degeneration. Furthermore, these substances reduce neuronal damage brought on by inflammatory reactions by inhibiting the activation of pro-inflammatory pathways including NF-κB and cyclooxygenase-2, which attenuate neuroinflammation (Leung et al., 2006).

Neurogenesis and Synaptic Plasticity

Components of Ginseng have demonstrated potential for augmenting neuronal plasticity and stimulating neurogenesis. The hippocampus, a region of the brain that is crucial for the recall and retention of information, produces new neurons because the ginsenosides Rg1 and Rb1 stimulate neural stem cell proliferation and differentiation. Furthermore, these substances influence the release of neurotransmitters and synaptic proteins, which promote synaptic plasticity and may improve memory consolidation and cognitive performance (Liu et al., 2017).

Anti-Amyloidogenic Effects

Certain components of ginseng show promise in reducing the build-up of beta-amyloid peptides, which are linked to the development of Alzheimer's disease. It has been demonstrated that the ginsenosides Rg1 and Rb1 decrease the synthesis of beta-amyloid, prevent aggregation, and encourage the removal of amyloid plaques. These findings raise the possibility of a therapeutic function for ginsenosides in delaying the advancement of Alzheimer's disease pathology (Chan et al., 2013).

Neuroprotective Mechanisms of Ginseng Constituents

Ginseng exhibits pronounced neuroprotective properties attributed to its constituents like ginsenosides, polysaccharides, polyacetylenes, phenolic compounds, phytosterols, and amino acids. These compounds exert neuroprotection through several mechanisms, safeguarding neurons against oxidative stress, inflammation, excitotoxicity, and neurodegeneration.

Antioxidant Effects

Ginseng constituents, notably ginsenosides, polysaccharides, and phenolic compounds, possess robust antioxidant capabilities. They counteract oxidative stress by scavenging free radicals, reducing lipid peroxidation, and enhancing endogenous antioxidant enzyme activities, including superoxide dismutase (SOD), catalase (CAT), and glutathione peroxidase (GPx). Ginsenosides Rg1 and Rb1, among others, have demonstrated potent antioxidative properties, protecting neuronal cells from oxidative damage induced by reactive oxygen species (ROS) (Lee et al., 2019).

Anti-Inflammatory Actions

Ginseng constituents exert anti-inflammatory effects by inhibiting the activation of pro-inflammatory pathways and cytokine production. Ginsenosides Rg1 and Rb1 attenuate neuroinflammation by suppressing nuclear factor-kappa B (NF-κB) signalling and reducing inflammatory mediators like interleukin-6, tumour necrosis factor-alpha, and cyclooxygenase-2. By mitigating neuroinflammation, ginseng constituents protect neurons from inflammatory damage associated with various neurodegenerative conditions (Zhao et al., 2019).

Regulation of Apoptosis

Ginseng constituents exhibit anti-apoptotic properties by modulating apoptotic pathways and preserving mitochondrial function. Ginsenosides Rg1 and Rb1 have been found to inhibit apoptotic cascades by regulating Bcl-2 family proteins, reducing cytochrome c release, and suppressing caspase activation, thus preventing neuronal cell death induced by various apoptotic stimuli (Zhang et al., 2019).

Enhancement of Neurogenesis

Ginseng constituents, particularly the ginsenosides Rg1 and Rb1, facilitate neurogenesis by promoting the proliferation and differentiation of neural stem cells. These compounds stimulate neurotrophic factors such as brain-derived neurotrophic factor (BDNF) and nerve growth factor (NGF), crucial for neuronal survival and differentiation, contributing to the formation of new neurons in brain regions associated with learning and memory (Cui et al., 2019).

Regulation of Amyloid Pathology

Certain Ginseng constituents, including the ginsenosides Rg1 and Rb1, exhibit potential in mitigating the amyloid-beta (Aβ) pathology observed in Alzheimer's disease. These compounds modulate Aβ production, aggregation, and clearance, thereby reducing the formation of Aβ oligomers and fibrils as well as enhancing the clearance of amyloid plaques, ultimately attenuating neuronal damage associated with Aβ toxicity (Lee et al., 2020).

Other Bioactive Components and Their Roles in Neuroprotection

Polysaccharides

Ginseng polysaccharides possess immunomodulatory properties and can regulate immune responses in the central nervous system (CNS). They exhibit anti-inflammatory effects by reducing microglial activation and pro-inflammatory cytokine release, thereby protecting neurons from inflammatory damage (Jin et al., 2016).

Polyacetylenes

These compounds demonstrate antioxidant and anti-inflammatory activities. They inhibit nitric oxide (NO) production and modulate inflammatory mediators, suggesting potential neuroprotective effects against neuroinflammation-associated neurodegeneration.

Peptides

Ginseng peptides exhibit neuroprotective properties by reducing oxidative stress and apoptotic cell death. They may enhance antioxidant enzyme activities and inhibit neuronal cell death pathways, contributing to neuroprotection.

Flavonoids

Found in ginseng, flavonoids possess antioxidant and anti-inflammatory properties. They scavenge free radicals, reduce oxidative damage, and modulate inflammatory pathways, potentially protecting neurons from degenerative processes.

Efficacy and Safety Considerations of Ginseng in Neurodegenerative Disorders

Efficacy

- Cognitive Function: Numerous preclinical studies suggest ginseng's neuroprotective effects, attributing its potential to various bioactive compounds like ginsenosides. While promising, clinical evidence on its efficacy in improving cognitive function in neurodegenerative disorders remains mixed.
- Alzheimer's Disease (AD): Clinical trials exploring ginseng's impact on AD have shown some positive results. For instance, a randomised controlled trial (Heo et al., 2014) demonstrated improved cognitive performance in AD patients treated with Korean red ginseng compared to a placebo group over 24 weeks.
- Parkinson's Disease (PD): However, the evidence regarding ginseng's efficacy in PD is limited. Pilot studies, such as the one conducted by Kim et al., (2015), showed some indications of improvement in motor symptoms and quality of life in PD patients but emphasised the need for larger, more definitive trials.

Safety Considerations

- General Safety: At higher doses or prolonged use, it may induce side effects such as insomnia, gastrointestinal disturbances, headaches, or changes in blood pressure. Individuals with underlying health conditions or those taking medications should exercise caution and consult healthcare professionals.
- Neurodegenerative Disorders and Safety: Specific safety data concerning ginseng's use in neurodegenerative disorders are limited. Long-term safety and interactions with medications commonly used in these conditions necessitate further investigation.

Impact of Ginseng on Neurological Pathways

Neurotransmitter Systems

- Dopaminergic System: Studies indicate ginseng's modulation of dopamine levels in the brain, potentially influencing motor function and mood regulation. This modulation could have implications for conditions like Parkinson's disease (Radad et al., 2004).
- Serotonergic System: Ginsenosides have demonstrated effects on serotonin receptors, suggesting a role in mood regulation and potentially affecting conditions associated with serotonin imbalances, such as depression and anxiety.

Anti-Inflammatory and Antioxidant Effects

By modifying inflammatory pathways and lowering the synthesis of pro-inflammatory cytokines, ginseng demonstrates anti-inflammatory effects. This anti-inflammatory effect could help shield neurons from harm brought on by neurodegenerative diseases. (Zhang et al., 2012).

Additionally, ginseng's antioxidant effects help mitigate oxidative stress, a key contributor to neurodegeneration. By scavenging free radicals and enhancing endogenous antioxidant defences, ginseng may play a neuroprotective role against oxidative damage in the brain (Park et al., 2009).

Safety, Dosage, and Considerations

Safety Profile of Ginseng

In prescribed dosages, ginseng is generally thought to be safe for short-term usage. Harmful effects have been observed; therefore, vigilance is urged. Headaches, allergic reactions, sleeplessness, and stomach discomfort are typical moderate side effects. Hormonal imbalances, anxiety, palpitations, and hypertension may result from prolonged usage or high doses.

Additionally, ginseng may interact with antiplatelet, anticoagulant, and diabetic and hypertension medicines (Jovanovski et al., 2014). Ginseng should be avoided by some groups, such as expectant or nursing mothers, those with specific medical disorders (such as autoimmune illnesses or hormone-sensitive malignancies), and people having surgery (Yuan et al., 2010).

Optimal Dosage and Forms

The ideal amount of ginseng to take depends on several variables, such as the user's age, health, and intended usage. Conventional dosages fall between 200 and 4000 mg per day, sometimes split into two or three doses. There are many different ways to consume ginseng, such as pills, capsules, extracts, powders, and teas.

Drug Interactions

Enhanced effects of stimulants or antidepressants, changed blood sugar levels with diabetic drugs, and increased bleeding risk with anticoagulants and antiplatelets are a few examples of potential interactions. When using ginseng together with medicine, have regular checks and consultations with a healthcare expert. Medication interactions can have unfavourable consequences such as hypotension, hypoglycemia, increased bleeding risk, and changes in medication metabolism. Furthermore, allergic responses such as itching, rash, and anaphylaxis may occur in people with documented sensitivities to ginseng or similar plants.

Potential Therapeutic Applications

Ginsenosides have demonstrated neuroprotective effects by reducing oxidative stress, inflammation, and beta-amyloid plaque formation, which are implicated in the progression of AD. Additionally, ginseng's ability to modulate neurotransmitter levels and enhance cognitive function indicates its potential role in improving memory and cognitive impairments associated with neurodegeneration (Reay et al., 2005).

Moreover, in Parkinson's disease, ginseng's anti-inflammatory properties have shown potential for protecting dopaminergic neurons and ameliorating motor symptoms. Ginsenosides exert their neuroprotective effects by regulating signalling pathways involved in neuronal survival and reducing neuronal damage caused by oxidative stress (Radad et al., 2003). Adverse effects such as insomnia, gastrointestinal disturbances, and fluctuations in blood pressure have been reported with ginseng use, emphasising the need for cautious administration, especially in vulnerable populations.

Complementary Use of Ginseng with Existing Treatments

Using ginseng alongside existing treatments for neurodegenerative disorders shows promise for enhancing therapeutic outcomes and slowing disease progression. Ginseng's primary compounds, ginsenosides, exhibit neuroprotective effects through antioxidation, anti-inflammatory action, modulation of neuronal signalling pathways, and promotion of neurogenesis and synaptic plasticity. When combined with conventional treatments, such as acetylcholinesterase inhibitors for Alzheimer's or levodopa for Parkinson's, ginseng may enhance efficacy and mitigate medication side effects. Preclinical studies suggest that ginseng extracts can augment the neuroprotective actions of dopaminergic drugs in Parkinson's models. Despite promising preliminary results, more clinical trials and mechanistic studies are needed to determine optimal dosages, treatment duration, and potential drug interactions, emphasising the need for personalised approaches (Smith et al., 2021; Lee et al., 2018; Wang et al., 2017).

Future Directions

Challenges and Opportunities in Research

The heterogeneity of active chemicals between different species of ginseng and within individual plants as a result of growing circumstances and processing techniques is one of the main challenges (Yun et al., 2001). The standardisation of these variances continues to be a barrier to reliable treatment results. Furthermore, our comprehension of the synergistic effects of the several ginseng ingredients is limited due to the incomplete elucidation of their methods of action. Subsequent investigations have to concentrate on pinpointing these processes via sophisticated molecular and cellular analyses. By resolving these issues, ginseng's full medicinal potential can be realised.

Implications for Clinical Practice

The body of data points to ginseng's possible therapeutic uses. Its potential use in neurological illnesses, cardiovascular diseases, immune-related problems, and cancer adjuvant therapy is suggested by its neuroprotective, anti-inflammatory, antioxidant, and immunomodulatory qualities. However, due to individual reactions and variances in ginseng formulations, vigilance is required (Li et al., 2021).

Before prescribing ginseng-based therapy, clinicians should take into account the herb's possible drug interactions as well as its contraindications in specific groups. Ginseng may increase therapy efficacy while reducing side effects when used in personalised medicine techniques.

Conclusion

Ginseng's many neuroprotective qualities, such as its anti-inflammatory, antioxidant, and neurogenic activities, suggest that it may have a positive impact on the treatment of neurodegenerative diseases. Even though the available data highlights its therapeutic potential, further thorough investigation—including standardised clinical trials—is necessary to clarify particular processes and determine the best dose schedules. Gaining insight into the complex interplay between the bioactive components of ginseng and neural pathways is essential to realising the plant's full therapeutic potential and enabling the development of novel approaches to treat neurodegenerative illnesses.

References

Attele, A. S., Wu, J. A., & Yuan, C. S. (1999). Ginseng pharmacology: multiple constituents and multiple actions. *Biochemical Pharmacology*, 58(11), 1685-1693.

Chan, S. J., Yan, J., & Xiao, L. (2013). Panax ginseng Ginsenoside-Rg1 protects against β-amyloid-induced neuronal apoptosis *in vitro*. Journal of Alzheimer's Disease, 33(2), 393-405.

Chevallier, A. (1996). *The Encyclopedia of Medicinal Plants*. DK Publishing.

Choi, J. G., Kim, H. G., Kim, D. S., Kim, S., Oh, M. S., & Jin, Y. H. (2021). Panax ginseng and ginsenoside Rg1 prevent oxidative damage induced by tert-butylhydroperoxide through the activation of Nrf2 and the upregulation of antioxidant enzymes in Chang liver cells. *Journal of Ginseng Research*, 45(4), 634–642.

Christensen, L. P. (2009). Ginsenosides: Chemistry, biosynthesis, analysis, and potential health effects. *Journal of Ginseng Research, 34(4), 545-558.*
Christensen, L. P. (2009). Ginsenosides: Chemistry, biosynthesis, analysis, and potential health effects. *Journal of Ginseng Research*, 34(4), 545-558.
Cui, C. H. (2019). Ginsenoside Rg1 protects against transient focal cerebral ischemic injury and suppresses its systemic metabolic changes in cerulein-induced pancreatitis. Biomolecules, 9(12), 774.

Dickson, D. W. (2012). Parkinson's disease and parkinsonism: neuropathology. *Cold Spring Harbor Perspectives in Medicine*, 2(8), a009258.

Hardy, J., &Selkoe, D. J. (2002). The amyloid hypothesis of Alzheimer's disease: progress and problems on the road to therapeutics. *Science*, 297(5580), 353-356.

Heo, J. H., Lee, S. T., Chu, K., Oh, M. J., Park, H. J., Shim, J. Y., & Kim, M. (2008). An open-label trial of Korean red ginseng as an adjuvant treatment for cognitive impairment in patients with Alzheimer's disease. *European Journal of Neurology*, 15(8), 865-868.

Heo, J. H., Lee, S. T., Chu, K., Oh, M. J., Park, H. J., Shim, J. Y., & Kim, M. (2019). An open-label trial of Korean red ginseng as an adjuvant treatment for cognitive impairment in patients with Alzheimer's disease. *European Journal of Neurology*, 16(5), 569-575.

Jang, D. J., Lee, M. S., Shin, B. C., & Lee, Y. C. (2015). Red ginseng supplementation more effectively alleviates psychological than physical fatigue. *Journal of Ginseng Research*, 39(3), 250-256.

Jeong, K., Shin, Y. C., Park, S. H., & Kim, D. S. (2014). Ginsenosides protect against Parkinson's disease-related neurotoxicity. *Biological & Pharmaceutical Bulletin*, 37(6), 969-974.

Jin, Y. (2016). Polysaccharides from Ginseng Leaves Inhibit Microglial Activation and Dopaminergic Neuronal Death. *Journal of Ginseng Research*, 40, 135-140.

Jin, Y., Kim, Y. J., Jeon, J. N., Wang, C., Min, J. W., Noh, H. L., & Yang, D. C. (2019). Panax ginseng Improves Functional Recovery after Contusive Spinal Cord Injury by Regulating the Inflammatory Response in Rats: An *In Vivo* Study. *Evidence-Based Complementary and Alternative Medicine*, 2019, 817096.

Jovanovski, E. (2014). Effect of ginseng on blood pressure and hormone profiles in hypertensive subjects. *Journal of the American College of Nutrition*, 33(5), 388-394.

Kang, S., Min, H. (2012). Anti-inflammatory effects of Panax notoginseng in LPS-stimulated RAW 264.7 macrophages. *Food and Chemical Toxicology*, 50(10), 3895-3902.

Kim HG, Ju MS, Shim JS. (2015) The effect of Korean red ginseng on symptoms and quality of life in Parkinson's disease: a pilot study. *Parkinsonism RelatDisord*, 21(6), 662-665.

Kim, H. J., Lee, K. W., Lee, D. K., & Kim, D. O. (2013). Panax ginseng as an adjuvant treatment for Alzheimer's disease. *Journal of Ginseng Research*, 37(4), 369-379.

Kim, J. H. (2018). Chemical diversity of Panax ginseng, Panax quinquefolius, and Panax notoginseng. *Journal of Ginseng Research*, 42(4), 549-557.

Kim, J. H., Kim, K. S., Lee, Y. H., Kang, J. S., Jung, H. Y., & Park, S. Y. (2018). Panax ginseng prevents apoptosis in hair follicles and accelerates the recovery of hair medullary cells in irradiated mice. *Annals of Dermatology*, 30(2), 164-172.

Kim, S., Hong, B., Nah, S. Y., & Park, H. J. (2017). Ginsenoside Rg1 protects against rotenone-induced apoptosis in human neuroblastoma SH-SY5Y cells through the regulation of apoptosis-related proteins. *Molecular Medicine Reports*, 16(2), 1955–1960.

Kim, S., Kang, S., Kim, C., Kim, D., Lee, D. H., Heo, J. S., & Lee, C. H. (2018). Ginsenoside Rg3 restores hepatitis C virus-induced aberrant mitochondrial dynamics and inhibits virus propagation. *Journal of Ginseng Research*, 42(4), 431-439.

Lee, J. H., Jeong, S. M., & Kim, J. H. (2018). Neuroprotective and anti-inflammatory effects of ginsenoside-Rg5 in a lipopolysaccharide-stimulated BV2 microglial cell model. *Journal of Ginseng Research*, 42(4), 475-483.

Lee, S. (2019). Protective effects of ginsenoside Rb1 on hydrogen peroxide-induced oxidative stress in rat articular chondrocytes. *Journal of Ginseng Research*, 43(2), 172-180.

Lee, S., Shin, J., Hong, Y., & Kim, D. (2020). Ginsenoside Rg1 promotes hippocampal neurogenesis in Alzheimer's disease models. *Experimental & Molecular Medicine*, 52(3), 397-407.

Leung, K. W., Wong, A. S. T., (2006), The neuroprotective effects of a novel extract of ginseng against glutamate-induced excitotoxicity. *Neuroreport*, 17(6), 609-612.

Li, X. (2021). Neuroprotective effects of ginsenosides: The therapeutic potential for neurodegenerative disorders. *Molecules*, 26(2), 434.

Liu, Q., Huang, Y., Zhang, R., Cai, T., Cai, Y., & Zhang, M. (2017). Neuroprotective effects of Panax notoginseng saponins in cerebral ischemia-reperfusion injury. *Journal of Ethnopharmacology*, 205, 99-106.

Miyazaki, S., Yamaguchi, Y., Nakamura, S., Kizaki, T., Oh-ishi, S., Toshinai, K., & Ohno, H. (2009). Differentiation of Ginseng Species (Panax ginseng and Panax quinquefolius) by Determination of 18-O-Ginsenoside Content. *Biological & Pharmaceutical Bulletin*, 32(4), 577-581.

Nguyen, X. C., Nguyen, T. H., Nguyen, T. H., Nguyen, T. T., Nguyen, T. A., & Nguyen, M. H. (2018). Chemical constituents and biological activities of Panax vietnamensis Ha et Grushv. in comparison with Panax notoginseng (Burkill) F. H. Chen. *Natural Product Communications*, 13(7), 849-856.

Park, J., Shin, J., & Jung, J. S. (2009). Anti-inflammatory mechanism of ginseng saponins in activated microglia. *Journal of Neuroimmunology*, 209(1-2), 40-49.

Reay, J. L., Kennedy, D. O., & Scholey, A. B. (2005). Single doses of Panax ginseng (G115) reduce blood glucose levels and improve cognitive performance during sustained mental activity. *Journal of Psychopharmacology*, 19(4), 357-365.

Reay, J. L., Kennedy, D. O., & Scholey, A. B. (2005). Single doses of Panax ginseng (G115) reduce blood glucose levels and improve cognitive performance during sustained mental activity. *Psychopharmacology*, 179(3), 437-445.

Senchina, D. S., Hallam, J. E., Kohut, M. L., Nguyen, N. A., Perera, M. A., Alhaider, I. A., & Braun, C. M. (2013). American ginseng (Panax quinquefolius L.) supplementation attenuates exhaustive exercise-induced oxidative stress in mice. *Journal of Ginseng Research*, 37(4), 387-395.

Smith, A., Jung, K., & Bae, M. (2021). Ginseng is a complementary and integrative therapy for neurodegenerative disorders. *Journal of Ginseng Research*, 45(1), 1-9.

Turner, M. R., & Talbot, K. (2008). Mimics and chameleons in motor neurone disease. *Practical Neurology*, 8(6), 364-378.

Vuksan, V., Sievenpiper, J. L., Koo, V. Y., Francis, T., Beljan-Zdravkovic, U., Xu, Z., & Jenkins, A. L. (2000). American ginseng (Panax quinquefolius L.) attenuates postprandial glycemia in a time-dependent but not dose-dependent manner in healthy individuals. *Journal of the American College of Nutrition*, 19(6), 738-744.

Wang Ross, C. A., & Tabrizi, S. J. (2011). Huntington's disease: from molecular pathogenesis to clinical treatment. *The Lancet Neurology*, 10(1), 83-98.

Wang, T., Fu, F., & Han, B. (2017). Effects of ginsenosides on cognitive deficits and oxidative stress induced by mitochondrial complex I inhibition. *Behavioral Pharmacology*, 28(5), 428-438.

Wang, C. Z., Yuan, C. S., Wang, X., Wu, J. A., & Yuan, D. (2016). Red American ginseng: Ginsenoside constituents and antiproliferative activities of heat-processed Panax quinquefolius roots. *Journal of Ginseng Research*, 40(4), 377-384.

Yuan, H. D. (2010). Evaluation of the estrogenic activity of the constituents in the fruits of Vitex rotundifolia L. for the potential treatment of premenstrual syndrome. *Journal of Ethnopharmacology*, 127(3), 463-467.

Yun, T. K. (2001). Brief introduction of Panax ginseng C. A. Meyer. *Journal of Korean Medical Science*, 16(Suppl), S3-S5.

Zhang, J. T., Qu, Z. W., & Liu, Y. (2012). Ginsenoside Re attenuates neuroinflammation in a symptomatic ALS animal model. *American Journal of Chinese Medicine*, 40(4), 807-815.

Zhang, J. (2019). Ginsenoside Rg1 ameliorates hippocampal long-term potentiation and memory in an Alzheimer's disease model. Molecular Immunology, 114, 10-18.

Zhao, H., Wang, L., Wei, C., Yang, Y., Zhou, J., & Wang, J. (2019). Ginsenoside Rg1 attenuates neuroinflammation and cognitive impairment in APP/PS1 mice via inhibiting the NF-κBsignaling pathway. International Immunopharmacology, 73, 341-349.

Zhou, Y., Zhou, T., Pei, Y., & Yue, J. (2019). The genus Panax: A comprehensive review of the traditional use, chemistry, pharmacology, and clinical trials. *Frontiers in Pharmacology*, 10, 1229.

Chapter 9

Potential Benefits of *Ginkgo biloba* for Neurodegenerative Disorders

Shilpa Thakur[1]
Karan Sharma[1]
Vinod Kumar Gauttam[2,*]
Arushi Sharma[3]
and Shiv Kumar[4]
[1]Department of Pharmacology, Shiva Institute of Pharmacy, Chandpur, Bilaspur, Himachal Pradesh, India
[2]Department of Pharmacognosy, Shiva Institute of Pharmacy, Chandpur, Bilaspur, Himachal Pradesh, India
[3]Department of Pharmaceutics, Shiva Institute of Pharmacy, Chandpur, Bilaspur, Himachal Pradesh, India
[4]Department of Pharmaceutical Chemistry, Shiva Institute of Pharmacy, Chandpur, Bilaspur, Himachal Pradesh, India

Abstract

Neurons are the fundamental structural and functional units of the nervous system, playing a crucial role in regulating and coordinating various bodily processes. Neurodegenerative diseases, including frontotemporal dementia, multiple sclerosis, amyotrophic lateral sclerosis, Parkinson's disease (PD), Alzheimer's disease (AD), and spinocerebellar ataxias, are among the most common and debilitating disorders. Although there is currently no cure for most neurodegenerative diseases, available treatments aim to manage symptoms, slow disease

* Corresponding Author's Email: vinodgauttam@gmail.com.

In: Natural Solutions for Neurodegenerative Disorders
Editors: Rahul Kumar Sharma, Shailesh Sharma, Ajmer Singh Grewal et al.
ISBN: 979-8-89530-231-6

progression, and enhance the quality of life for those affected. Ginkgo biloba has shown potential neuroprotective effects, particularly in the context of PD and AD. While some individuals may experience mild gastrointestinal issues and headaches when using Ginkgo biloba, clinical data suggest its therapeutic promise. This chapter explores the neuroprotective properties of Ginkgo biloba, including its extraction process and preclinical and clinical evidence supporting its efficacy in experimental models of PD, AD, and other conditions. Additionally, it examines the application of Ginkgo biloba nano-formulations in the prevention, treatment, and diagnosis of AD.

Keywords: Alzheimer, Parkinson, Huntington, clinical and pre-clinical trials, etiopathogenesis, nano-formulations

Abbreviations

AD	Alzheimer disease
ALS	Amyotrophic Lateral Sclerosis
APOE	Apolipoprotein E
APP	Amyloid precursor proteins
BB	Bilobalide
EGb	Extract Ginkgo biloba
GPx	Glutathione peroxidase
GSH	Glutathione
MCAO	Middle cerebral artery occlusion
MDA	Malondialdehyde
NaDC	Sodium deoxycholate
NDDS	Novel drug delivery system
NDs	Neurodegenerative- diseases
NO	Nitric oxide
Nqo1	Quinone dehydrogenase 1
OGR	Oxygen-glucose reperfusion
PAF	Platelet-activating factor
PD	Parkinson's disease
PSEN 1, PSEN 2	Presenilin 1 and 2
SOD	Superoxide dismutase
WHO	World Health Organization

Introduction

The human nervous system, an intricate and vital system, plays a crucial role in regulating and coordinating a wide range of physiological functions to maintain homeostasis. Neurons, the basic building blocks of the nervous system, are specialized cells responsible for transmitting signals, processing information, enabling communication between cells, and carrying out motor and sensory functions. Furthermore, neurons play a key role in cognitive processes such as memory and learning (Voet et al., 2019). Numerous factors can affect the fundamental structure and function of neurons, leading to impairments in nervous system control and contributing to the development of neurodegenerative (ND) conditions. According to the latest 2023 report from the World Health Organization (WHO), over 55 million people worldwide are currently living with dementia, with nearly 10 million new cases emerging each year (Prusiner, 2001). Global surveys estimate that there are 10–15 new ND cases per 100,000 people annually, with approximately 2% of these cases affecting individuals over the age of 65. In 2019, it was estimated that 50 million people globally were affected by NDs leading to dementia, and this number is projected to rise to 152 million by 2060 (Erkkinen et al., 2018; Hanamsagar and Staci, 2016). The rapid increase in the prevalence of NDs presents significant public health challenges. NDs are characterized by the gradual loss of nerve cells, which impairs communication between neurons and ultimately leads to the decline of cognitive and motor functions (Forman et al., 2004). These conditions are complex and influenced by a variety of factors, including genetics, environmental factors, protein misfolding, oxidative stress, and inflammation.

Factors Affecting Neurodegeneration

Stress Caused by Oxidation

The progression of neurodegenerative diseases is closely associated with oxidative stress, a critical factor arising from an imbalance between the body's antioxidant defenses and the production of reactive oxygen species (ROS). In neurodegenerative diseases, oxidative stress poses a significant threat to cellular components such as proteins, DNA, and lipids, accelerating disease progression (Olnaow, 2008). During oxidative phosphorylation, mitochondria generate ROS, with superoxide radicals potentially forming as a result of electron leakage during this process.

a) ROS can damage mitochondrial proteins, lipids, and DNA, impairing mitochondrial function and further amplifying ROS production in a self-perpetuating cycle (Reynolds et al., 2007).
b) Excessive ROS production targets structural proteins, and the oxidation of these proteins contributes to abnormal neuronal function in neurodegenerative disorders.
c) ROS also attack lipids in biological membranes, leading to lipid peroxidation, which disrupts cell membrane functions, including cell signaling and transport (Gandhi and Andrey, 2012).
d) DNA is another target of ROS. Oxidative DNA damage and impairments in the DNA repair system underscore the significant role of ROS in neurodegenerative diseases (Schulz et al., 2000).
e) Oxidative stress can activate inflammatory pathways, leading to the mobilization of immune cells and the secretion of pro-inflammatory cytokines. Prolonged inflammation is a contributing factor in neurodegenerative diseases (Federico et al., 2012).
f) As oxidative stress intensifies, levels of endogenous antioxidant enzymes like glutathione (GSH) and superoxide dismutase (SOD) decrease, while levels of glutathione peroxidase (GPX), malondialdehyde (MDA), and nitric oxide (NO) increase. Additionally, the expression of Nuclear Factor Erythroid 2-related factor-2 (NrF2), a key regulator of antioxidant enzyme activity, is reduced (Moreira et al., 2005).

Mutations

Certain gene mutations are closely associated with neurodegenerative disorders, contributing to the onset and progression of these diseases. For example, mutations in the amyloid precursor protein (APP) gene lead to the production of abnormal beta-amyloid forms, which aggregate into plaques in the brain and disrupt neuronal communication, contributing to Alzheimer's disease. Mutations in the Apolipoprotein E (APOE) gene, as well as in Presenilin 1 and 2, are also linked to Alzheimer's disease (Iqbal and Grundke, 2008).

In Parkinson's disease, genetic factors include mutations in genes such as Leucine-rich repeat kinase 2 (LRRK2), DJ-1 (PARK7), PTEN-induced putative kinase 1 (PINK1), Parkin (PARK2), and alpha-synuclein (SNCA). Similarly, mutations in genes such as fused in sarcoma (FUS), superoxide dismutase 1 (SOD1), and chromosome 9 open reading frame 72 (C9orf72) are associated with amyotrophic lateral sclerosis (ALS) (Maimone et al., 2001). In Huntington's disease, mutations in the huntingtin (HTT) gene result in the production of abnormal huntingtin proteins. Frontotemporal dementia is linked to mutations in the microtubule-associated protein tau (MAPT) gene (Chen et al., 2016).

Protein Misfolding

Neurodegenerative diseases cause protein misfolding, leading to the formation of abnormal protein aggregates such as β-amyloid plaques, hyperphosphorylated tau proteins, Lewy bodies (Nakamura et al., 2009), and inclusion bodies. These aggregates disrupt normal cellular and synaptic functions, with mutations in genes like SOD1, TARDBP, and FUS playing a role in this process (Soto et al., 2008; Muchowski, 2002). The accumulation of misfolded proteins can also induce cellular toxicity, ultimately contributing to neuronal death.

Neuro-Inflammation

Neuroglial cells in the CNS harbor numerous inflammatory mediators that are activated by ROS, chemokines, and cytokines. ROS induce oxidative stress, potentially leading to brain damage (Maia, 2022; Hong et al., 2016). Pro-inflammatory cytokines released by microglia and astrocytes, such as interleukin-1β, tumor necrosis factor-α, and various chemokines, attract immune cells to the site of inflammation, thereby promoting neuroinflammation and increasing neurotoxicity. In PD, the overactivation of microglia leads to the degeneration of dopaminergic neurons.

Neural Death/Apoptosis

Apoptosis is a tightly regulated process crucial for maintaining tissue homeostasis, proper development, and the elimination of unwanted cells. Morphologically, apoptotic cells exhibit characteristics such as reduced cell size, chromatin condensation, DNA fragmentation, and the breakdown of cytoskeletal and nuclear proteins. The following are key details about apoptosis in the context of neurodegeneration (Okouchi et al., 2007):

a) Neurons affected by neurofibrillary tangles and beta-amyloid plaques undergo apoptosis, involving both extrinsic and intrinsic apoptotic pathways.
b) Various signals, including inadequate neurotrophic factor support, excessive glutamate receptor activation (leading to calcium influx), increased oxidative stress, and metabolic stress, can trigger apoptosis in neurons (Jellinger, 2001).
c) In apoptotic cells, mitochondria display increased oxyradical production, membrane pore formation, and the release of pro-apoptotic molecules like cytochrome c. Cytochrome c activates caspases, leading to the cleavage of multiple cellular substrates, which drives the characteristic morphological changes of apoptosis (Martin et al., 1998).
d) In Parkinson's disease, oxidative stress, mitochondrial dysfunction, and protein aggregation contribute to the apoptosis of dopamine-producing neurons.
e) Inhibitors of caspases, particularly caspase-3, have been explored as potential therapeutic agents to halt the apoptotic process.

Treatment for Neurodegeneration

Numerous synthetic drugs are available to treat neurodegenerative disorders, but they often come with significant side effects and the risk of drug dependence. As a result, healthcare professionals are increasingly exploring alternative traditional therapies (Poddar et al., 2021). In India, medicinal herbs have been used for centuries to address various ailments. Ayurvedic therapies, which utilize medicinal herbs and phytoconstituents, often provide relief with minimal adverse effects, even with long-term use. Given the substantial impact of neurodegenerative disorders on mortality and disability, addressing the challenges of longer life spans has become a key focus in medical research (Wahid et al., 2020). The Ayurvedic system of medicine identifies specific plants with well-documented medicinal benefits, offering insights into the understanding and treatment of neurodegenerative diseases. These plants are renowned for their potent antioxidant properties, which are crucial for managing such conditions (Lalotra and Vaghela, 2019). Ginkgo biloba (GB), belonging to the Ginkgoaceae family, has a significant historical presence, with fossil records dating back 150 to 250 million years (Nowak et al., 2021). GB extract (GBE), derived from dried leaves, is a common treatment for memory loss, dementia, and Alzheimer's disease (Liu et al., 2015) (Barbalho et al., 2022). The EGb 761 formulation was developed to ensure consistent and reliable drug performance by neutralizing free radicals generated by reactive oxygen species (ROS) and reactive nitrogen species (RNS), and removing ginkgolic acid from GB. EGb 761 often shows enhanced antioxidant activity in combination with other plant extracts, with minimal adverse effects (Birks et al., 2009).

Chemical Constituents

GB is rich in chemical constituents, each with distinct structures and valuable therapeutic effects, including PAF antagonism, anti-inflammatory, antioxidant, neuroprotective, and cardiovascular protective properties (Shu et al., 2020; Wang et al., 2020). Different parts of GB contain various chemical compounds, such as terpene trilactones (ginkgolides), biflavones (ginkgetin), ginkgotides, ginkgolic acids, flavonoids (kaempferol, quercetin, and isorhamnetin), flavonol glycosides (ginkgoghrelins), and bioflavonoids (ginkgetin, sciadopitysin, and isoginkgetin) (Liu et al., 2021; Boateng, 2022).

GB In Neuroprotection

During cerebral ischemia, GB administration supports the recovery of mitochondrial respiration, stimulates the activity of glutathione and superoxide dismutase, and reduces brain water content, malondialdehyde (MDA), ADP-ribose, and poly(ADP-ribose) polymerase (PARP). Preclinical studies have shown that higher doses of GB can suppress brain edema and reduce cerebral infarction (Xie et al., 2022). Ischemia in brain tissue commonly results in reduced mitochondrial respiration and the opening of the mitochondrial permeability transition pore (mPTP) (Sharma et al., 2022). Ginkgo biloba extract (GBE) has been reported to prevent mPTP opening, reduce mitochondrial fission, and alleviate mitochondrial dysfunction through a mechanism involving glycogen synthase kinase-3β (GSK-3β). These effects were observed in mice with middle cerebral artery occlusion (MCAO) and neuroblastoma cells subjected to oxygen-glucose deprivation/reperfusion (OGD/R) (Sharifi et al., 2020). Additionally, bilobalide treatment demonstrated therapeutic effects in the hippocampus of ovariectomized rats by reversing declines in protein levels, cytochrome c oxidase subunit I mRNA, and mitochondrial adenosine triphosphate content (Tian et al., 2012). GB pretreatment has also shown potential in preventing oxidative stress responses induced by Aβ1-42. This treatment reduces oxidative damage to DNA and RNA bases, inhibits ROS and RNS production, and restores the antioxidant capacity of glutathione (GSH) and superoxide dismutase (SOD) (Hua et al., 2017).

- Ginkgolide A: Ginkgolide A effectively inhibits platelet-activating factor (PAF), a messenger derived from phospholipids. PAF plays a crucial role in immune responses to infection and is involved in ischemic and excitotoxic injuries that contribute to neuronal damage.
- Ginkgolide B: Ginkgolide B, a key component of EGb 761, is a highly effective antagonist of platelet-activating factor (PAF). It has been scientifically proven to treat ischemia/reperfusion (I/R) damage associated with conditions such as transplantation, multiple sclerosis, sepsis, and migraine. Ginkgolide B can reduce endothelial permeability, decrease cerebral infarct size, increase blood-brain barrier (BBB) permeability, and alleviate cerebral edema by enhancing the production of tight junction proteins ZO-1 and occludin (Nash et al., 2015).
- Bilobalide: *In vivo* studies have shown that bilobalide (BB), administered at a dose of 10 mg/kg, significantly reduces glutamate levels in the penumbra and infarct regions during ischemic stroke (Qin et al., 2021; Lu et al., 2021). BB therapy promotes the phosphorylation of GSK-3β, which activates the canonical Wnt/β-catenin pathway, contributing to its neuroprotective and neuropromoting effects (Nash et al., 2015). Both pre- and post-

treatment with Ginkgo biloba extract (GBE) have been found to enhance hippocampal cell survival and improve spatial learning and cognitive abilities in rodents following global cerebral ischemia/reperfusion. Moreover, prolonged intraperitoneal bilobalide treatment in mice led to improvements in depression-like behavior and cognitive deficits caused by sustained mild stress (Ge et al., 2021).

- Flavonoids: Flavonoids can influence a range of cell signaling pathways, including protein kinase C, PI3K, MAPK, and Akt/protein kinase B (PKB). These signaling molecules are crucial for brain health, cognition, and cell viability. Flavonoids are known for their antioxidant properties, which involve scavenging oxidants and free radicals, particularly hydroxyl radicals, and stabilizing unpaired electrons within their polyphenolic structure. This makes flavonoids effective in treating oxidative and inflammatory conditions such as Alzheimer's disease, heart disease, and cancer (Maher, 2019).

Numerous *in vitro* and *in vivo* studies have demonstrated the neuroprotective effects of GBE. Research indicates that GBE offers protection against various stressors that cause neuronal damage, including cyanide, glutamate, hydrogen peroxide, verapamil, amyloid-β, MPTP, and nitric oxide (NO). Similarly, EGb761, when administered in doses ranging from 10 to 100 mg/kg, has been shown to reduce neuronal damage in various models, including amphetamine-induced behavioral sensitization, transient middle cerebral artery occlusion (MCAO), focal cerebral ischemia, hypoxia, heat stress, and subchronic cold stress.

Clinical Trials (Table 1)

A current study that implication of EGb 761 on remembrance ability in middle-aged, healthy participants found that daily EGb 761 administration (240 mg) may progress some areas of memory more than others (Morato et al., 2023).

Table 1. Cinical trials on EGb

Disease	Study	No. of people	Doses	Side effects	Outcomes	Reference ID
Alzheimer disease, multi-infarct dementia	Randomized placebo controlled, Double Blinded, parallel study	n – 309	120 mg/d for 52 weeks	NA	EGb was safe and seemed to improve the social and cognitive functioning of individuals suffering from dementia.	(NCT00276510) (Vellas et al., 2012; Le et al., 1997)
Idiopathic cognitive impairment	Randomized, double-blind, and placebo-controlled study	n – 58 Mean age: 73.5	120mg/d -12 weeks	Constipation only affected one patient in the study, and it went away without requiring treatment stoppage.	According to this study, GBE improved mental function, which implies that the medication may be useful in treating primary degenerative dementia in its early stages.	(NCT03004508) (Rai et al., 1991; Wesnes et al., 1987)
Parkinson's disease	Randomized clinical trial	n – 63 Mean age: 51.75year	80mg (TDS)	Headache Nausea Dizziness Skin allergic reaction	When managing Drug-Induced Parkinsonism, GBE is secure and reliable.	IR.TUMC.TIPS.REC.1398.097 (Ellis et al., 2005)
Vascular cognitive impairment (VCI).	Randomized, double blind & placebo controlled clinical trial	n – 90	120 mg,60 mg	Nausea was the most often reported adverse response, followed by vomiting and dizziness	GB effective in cognitive deterioration in patients.	(NCT00446485) (Sharma et al., 2022)
Acute ischaemic stroke	Double-blind, placebo-controlled, randomised controlled trial	n – 348	450mg, Aspirin (100mg)	vomiting episode recurrent strokes transient ischemic attacks	After an acute ischemic stroke, GBE plus aspirin therapy improved neurological and cognitive impairments without raising the risk of vascular events.	(IRCT138804212150N1) (Oskouei et al., 2013)

Disease	Study	No. of people	Doses	Side effects	Outcomes	Reference ID
Dementia	Double blind, placebo control trial	n = 309	120mg	Agitation, nervousness Constipation, diarrhea Weight change Dyspepsia, flatulence confusion	Extract of Ginkgo biloba at dose 120 mg seem to reduce multi-infract dementia. Ginkgo biloba has the potential to function as a supplementary treatment for dementia or as an alternative to cholinesterase	(NCT00446485) (Ernst and Pitter, 1999; Le et al., 2000)
Cognition and ischaemia stroke	Pilot Randomized trial	n = 201	240mg/day	mild side effect, Nasopharyngitis	In patients with mild to severe ischemic stroke, EGb therapy improved overall cognitive performance.	ISRCTN11815543 (NCT02828540) (Dodge et al., 2008)

Conclusion

Numerous studies confirm the effective use of GB in treating various conditions, including Alzheimer's disease, asthma, venous insufficiency, multi-infarct dementia, dementia in the elderly, and resistant depression. Research validates that GB's efficacy stems from its rich array of bioactive compounds that offer protective effects on neurons. Ginkgolides and bilobalide, in particular, have been extensively studied in preclinical research, demonstrating significant potency. These compounds exhibit a variety of beneficial effects, such as protecting against mitochondrial dysfunction, regulating amyloid production and Aβ aggregation, modifying tau protein phosphorylation, maintaining ion homeostasis, and activating growth factors. These findings underscore the diverse and comprehensive mechanisms of GB's action, especially through the contributions of ginkgolides and bilobalide. Currently, researchers are focusing on developing and formulating analogs of ginkgolides and bilobalide designed specifically to target the brain. This advancement aims to establish a more efficient and sustained therapeutic approach for central nervous system diseases in the future.

References

Chen, P., Miah, M. R., & Aschner, M. (2016). Metals and Neurodegeneration. *F1000Research*, 5, F1000 Faculty Rev-366.

Barbalho, S. M., Direito, R., Laurindo, L. F., Marton, L. T., Guiguer, E. L., Goulart, R. A., Tofano, R. J., Carvalho, A. C. A., Flato, U. A. P., Capelluppi Tofano, V. A., Detregiachi, C. R. P., Bueno, P. C. S., Girio, R. S. J., & Araújo, A. C. (2022). Ginkgo biloba in the Aging Process: A Narrative Review. *Antioxidants*, 11(3), 525.

Boateng, I. D. (2022). A critical review of ginkgolic acids in Ginkgo biloba leaf extract (EGb): Toxicity and technologies to remove ginkgolic acids and their promising bioactivities. *Food & Function, 13*(18), 9226-9242.

Dodge, H. H., Zitzelberger, T., Oken, B. S., Howieson, D., & Kaye, J. (2008). A randomized placebo-controlled trial of Ginkgo biloba for the prevention of cognitive decline. *Neurology, 70*(19_part_2), 1809-1817.

Ellis, T., De Goede, C. J., Feldman, R. G., Wolters, E. C., Kwakkel, G., & Wagenaar, R. C. (2005). Efficacy of a physical therapy program in patients with Parkinson's disease: A randomized controlled trial. *Archives of Physical Medicine and Rehabilitation, 86*(4), 626-632.

Erkkinen, M. G., Kim, M.-O., & Geschwind, M. D. (2018). Clinical neurology and epidemiology of the major neurodegenerative diseases. *Cold Spring Harbor Perspectives in Biology, 10*(4), a033118.

Ernst, E., & Pittler, M. H. (1999). Ginkgo biloba for dementia: A systematic review of double-blind, placebo-controlled trials. *Clinical Drug Investigation, 17*, 301-308.

Federico, A., Cardaioli, E., Da Pozzo, P., Formichi, P., Gallus, G. N., & Radi, E. (2012). Mitochondria, oxidative stress and neurodegeneration. *Journal of the Neurological Sciences, 322*(1-2), 254-262.

Forman, M. S., Trojanowski, J. Q., & Lee, V. M. Y. (2004). Neurodegenerative diseases: A decade of discoveries paves the way for therapeutic breakthroughs. *Nature Medicine, 10*(10), 1055-1063.

Gandhi, S., & Abramov, A. Y. (2012). Mechanism of oxidative stress in neurodegeneration. *Oxidative Medicine and Cellular Longevity, 2012*, 1-11.

Gargouri, B., Carstensen, J., Bhatia, H. S., Huell, M., Dietz, G. P. H., & Fiebich, B. L. (2018). Anti-neuroinflammatory effects of Ginkgo biloba extract EGb761 in LPS-activated primary microglial cells. *Phytomedicine, 44*, 45-55.

Ge, W., Ren, C., Xing, L., Guan, L., Zhang, C., Sun, X., Wang, G., Niu, H., & Qun, S. (2021). Ginkgo biloba extract improves cognitive function and increases neurogenesis by reducing Aβ pathology in 5× FAD mice. *American Journal of Translational Research, 13*(3), 1471-1485.

Hanamsagar, R., & Bilbo, S. D. (2016). Sex differences in neurodevelopmental and neurodegenerative disorders: Focus on microglial function and neuroinflammation during development. *The Journal of Steroid Biochemistry and Molecular Biology, 160*, 127-133.

Hong, H., Kim, B. S., & Im, H.-I. (2016). Pathophysiological role of neuroinflammation in neurodegenerative diseases and psychiatric disorders. *International Neurourology Journal, 20*(Suppl 1), S2-S7.

Hua, J., Yin, N., Yang, B., Zhang, J., Ding, J., Fan, Y., & Hu, G. (2017). Ginkgolide B and bilobalide ameliorate neural cell apoptosis in α-synuclein aggregates. *Biomedicine & Pharmacotherapy, 96*, 792-797.

Iqbal, K., & Grundke-Iqbal, I. (2008). Alzheimer neurofibrillary degeneration: significance, etiopathogenesis, therapeutics and prevention. *Journal of Cellular and Molecular Medicine, 12*(1), 38-55.

Jellinger, K. A. (2001). Cell death mechanisms in neurodegeneration. *Journal of Cellular and Molecular Medicine, 5*(1), 1-17.

Lalotra, S., & Vaghela, J. S. (2019). Scientific reports of medicinal plants used for the prevention and treatment of neurodegenerative diseases. *Pharmaceutical and Biosciences Journal*, 15-25.

Liu, L., Wang, Y., Zhang, J., & Wang, S. (2021). Advances in the chemical constituents and chemical analysis of Ginkgo biloba leaf, extract, and phytopharmaceuticals. *Journal of Pharmaceutical and Biomedical Analysis, 193*, 113704.

Liu, X., Hao, W., Qin, Y., Decker, Y., Wang, X., Burkart, M., Schötz, K., Menger, M. D., Fassbender, K., & Liu, Y. (2015). Long-term treatment with Ginkgo biloba extract EGb 761 improves symptoms and pathology in a transgenic mouse model of Alzheimer's disease. *Brain, Behavior, and Immunity, 46*, 121-131.

Lu, J., Xie, L., Liu, K., Zhang, X., Wang, X., Dai, X., Liang, Y., Cao, Y., & Li, X. (2021). Bilobalide: A review of its pharmacology, pharmacokinetics, toxicity, and safety. *Phytotherapy Research, 35*(11), 6114-6130.

Maher, P. (2019). The potential of flavonoids for the treatment of neurodegenerative diseases. *International Journal of Molecular Sciences, 20*(12), 3056.

Adamu, A., Li, S., Gao, F., & Xue, G. (2024). The role of neuroinflammation in neurodegenerative diseases: current understanding and future therapeutic targets. *Frontiers in Aging Neuroscience*, 16, 1347987.

Maimone, D., Dominici, R., & Grimaldi, L. M. E. (2001). Pharmacogenomics of neurodegenerative diseases. *European Journal of Pharmacology, 413*(1), 11-29.

Martin, L. J., Al-Abdulla, N. A., Brambrink, A. M., Kirsch, J. R., Sieber, F. E., & Portera-Cailliau, C. (1998). Neurodegeneration in excitotoxicity, global cerebral ischemia, and target deprivation: A perspective on the contributions of apoptosis and necrosis. *Brain Research Bulletin, 46*(4), 281-309.

Morató, X., Marquié, M., Tartari, J. P., Lafuente, A., Abdelnour, C., Alegret, M., Jofresa, S., Buendía, M., Pancho, A., Aguilera, N., Ibarria, M., Diego, S., Cuevas, R., Cañada, L., Calvet, A., Antonio, E. E., Pérez-Cordón, A., Sanabria, Á., de Rojas, I., Nuñez-Llaves, R., Cano, A., Orellana, A., Montrreal, L., Cañabate, P., Rosende-Roca, M., Vargas, L., Bojaryn, U., Ricciardi, M., Ariton, D. M., Espinosa, A., Ortega, G., Muñoz, N., Lleonart, N., Alarcón-Martín, E., Moreno, M., Preckler, S., Tantinya, N., Ramis, M., Nogales, A. B., Seguer, S., Martín, E., Pytel, V., Valero, S., Gurruchaga, M., Tárraga, L., Ruiz, A., & Boada, M. (2023). A randomized, open-label clinical trial in mild cognitive impairment with EGb 761 examining blood markers of inflammation and oxidative stress. *Scientific Reports, 13*(1), 5406.

Moreira, P. I., Smith, M. A., Zhu, X., Nunomura, A., Castellani, R. J., & Perry, G. (2005). Oxidative stress and neurodegeneration. *Annals of the New York Academy of Sciences, 1043*(1), 545-552.

Muchowski, P. J. (2002). Protein misfolding, amyloid formation, and neurodegeneration: A critical role for molecular chaperones? *Neuron, 35*(1), 9-12.

Nakamura, T., & Lipton, S. A. (2009). Cell death: Protein misfolding and neurodegenerative diseases. *Apoptosis, 14*, 455-468.

Nash, K. M., & Shah, Z. A. (2015). Current perspectives on the beneficial role of Ginkgo biloba in neurological and cerebrovascular disorders. *Integrative Medicine Insights, 10*, IMI-S25054.

Nowak, A., Kojder, K., Zielonka-Brzezicka, J., Wróbel, J., Bosiacki, M., Fabiańska, M., Wróbel, M., Sołek-Pastuszka, J., & Klimowicz, A. (2021). The use of Ginkgo biloba L. as a neuroprotective agent in Alzheimer's disease. *Frontiers in Pharmacology, 12*, 775034.

Okouchi, M., Ekshyyan, O., Maracine, M., & Aw, T. Y. (2007). Neuronal apoptosis in neurodegeneration. *Antioxidants & Redox Signaling, 9*(8), 1059-1096.

Oskouei, D. S., Rikhtegar, R., Hashemilar, M., Sadeghi-Bazargani, H., Sharifi-Bonab, M., Sadeghi-Hokmabadi, E., Zarrintan, S., & Sharifipour, E. (2013). The effect of Ginkgo biloba on functional outcome of patients with acute ischemic stroke: A double-blind, placebo-controlled, randomized clinical trial. *Journal of Stroke and Cerebrovascular Diseases, 22*(8), e557-e563.

Poddar, M. K., Chakraborty, A., & Banerjee, S. (2021). *Neurodegeneration: Diagnosis, Prevention, and Therapy*. London, UK: IntechOpen.

Prusiner, S. B. (2001). Neurodegenerative diseases and prions. *New England Journal of Medicine, 344*(20), 1516-1526.

Qin, Y.-R., Ma, C.-Q., Wang, D.-P., Zhang, Q.-Q., Liu, M.-R., Zhao, H.-R., Jiang, J.-H., & Fang, Q. (2021). Bilobalide alleviates neuroinflammation and promotes autophagy in Alzheimer's disease by upregulating lincRNA-p21. *American Journal of Translational Research, 13*(4).

Reynolds, A., Laurie, C., Mosley, R. L., & Gendelman, H. E. (2007). Oxidative stress and the pathogenesis of neurodegenerative disorders. *International Review of Neurobiology, 82*, 297-325.

Schulz, J. B., Lindenau, J., Seyfried, J., & Dichgans, J. (2000). Glutathione, oxidative stress and neurodegeneration. *European Journal of Biochemistry, 267*(16), 4904-4911.

Sharifi-Rad, M., Lankatillake, C., Dias, D. A., Docea, A. O., Mahomoodally, M. F., Lobine, D., Chazot, P. L., et al., (2020). Impact of natural compounds on neurodegenerative disorders: From preclinical to pharmacotherapeutics. *Journal of Clinical Medicine, 9*(4), 1061.

Sharma, M., Awasthi, H., Srivastava, D., Fatima, Z., & Srivastava, V. (2022). Assessment of the impact of herbal drugs used in neurodegenerative disorders: A preclinical review. *Current Traditional Medicine, 8*(6), 39-49.

Shu, P., Sun, M., Li, J., Zhang, L., Xu, H., Lou, Y., Ju, Z., Wei, X., Wu, W., & Sun, N. (2020). Chemical constituents from Ginkgo biloba leaves and their cytotoxicity activity. *Journal of Natural Medicines, 74*, 269-274.

Soto, C., & Estrada, L. D. (2008). Protein misfolding and neurodegeneration. *Archives of Neurology, 65*(2), 184-189.

Tian, X. Q., Wang, J. M., Dai, J. G., Yang, L., Zhang, L. D., Shen, S. S., & Huang, P. (2012). Hyperbaric oxygen and Ginkgo Biloba extract inhibit Aβ25-35-induced toxicity and oxidative stress *in vivo*: A potential role in Alzheimer's disease. *International Journal of Neuroscience, 122*(10), 563-569.

Vellas, B., Coley, N., Ousset, P. J., Berrut, G., Dartigues, J. F., Dubois, B., Grandjean, H., et al., (2012). Long-term use of standardised Ginkgo biloba extract for the prevention of Alzheimer's disease (GuidAge): A randomised placebo-controlled trial. *The Lancet Neurology, 11*(10), 851-859.

Voet, S., Srinivasan, S., Lamkanfi, M., & van Loo, G. (2019). Inflammasomes in neuroinflammatory and neurodegenerative diseases. *EMBO Molecular Medicine, 11*(6), e10248.2.

Wahid, M., Ali, A., Saqib, F., Aleem, A., Bibi, S., Afzal, K., Ali, A., Baig, A., Khan, S. A., & Asad, M. H. H. B. (2020). Pharmacological exploration of traditional plants for the treatment of neurodegenerative disorders. *Phytotherapy Research, 34*(12), 3089-3112.

Wang, X., Gong, X., Zhang, H., Zhu, W., Jiang, Z., Shi, Y., & Li, L. (2020). *In vitro* anti-aging activities of ginkgo biloba leaf extract and its chemical constituents. *Food Science and Technology, 40*, 476-482.

Wesnes, K., Simmons, D., Rook, M., & Simpson, P. (1987). A double-blind placebo-controlled trial of Tanakan in the treatment of idiopathic cognitive impairment in the elderly. *Human Psychopharmacology: Clinical and Experimental, 2*(3), 159-169.

Xie, L., Zhu, Q., & Lu, J. (2022). Can we use Ginkgo biloba extract to treat Alzheimer's disease? Lessons from preclinical and clinical studies. *Cells, 11*(3), 479.

Chapter 10

Rhodiola rosea Potential in Neurodegeneration

Shiwali Sharma[1]
Preeti Bisht[2]
Narinderpal Kaur[1,*]
Pallavi Bassi[3]
and Balraj Saini[3]

[1]Chitkara University School of Pharmacy, Chitkara University, Himachal Pradesh, India
[2]University Institute of Pharma Sciences (UIPS), Chandigarh University, Mohali, Punjab, India
[3]Chitkara College of Pharmacy, Chitkara University, Punjab, India

Abstract

The brain's susceptibility to oxidative stress and neuronal cell death often necessitates the use of effective pharmacotherapy. However, many existing medications have limited efficacy and are associated with undesirable side effects. A promising alternative lies in exploring bioactive compounds from plants, which possess antioxidant and neuroprotective properties. These plant-derived chemicals could offer new approaches for managing a range of neuropsychiatric, neurodevelopmental, and neurodegenerative disorders. Among the plants attracting attention is Rhodiola, also known as 'Hongjingtian' in Chinese medicine. *Rhodiola rosea*, in particular, has demonstrated therapeutic outcomes that surpass certain pharmaceutical drugs, such as monoamine oxidase inhibitors and dopamine agonists commonly used in treating

* Corresponding Author's Email: narinderpal.kaur@chitkarauniversity.edu.in.

In: Natural Solutions for Neurodegenerative Disorders
Editors: Rahul Kumar Sharma, Shailesh Sharma, Ajmer Singh Grewal et al.
ISBN: 979-8-89530-231-6

Parkinson's disease. This plant contains various bioactive components that confer neuroprotective, antioxidant, anti-proteinopathy, neural vasorelaxation, anti-inflammatory, and iron-chelating properties. By reducing microglial activation, mitigating oxidative damage from reactive oxygen species, promoting proper protein folding, enhancing blood flow in the substantia nigra of the basal ganglia, and encouraging the growth of dopaminergic cells, Rhodiola targets diseases at a fundamental level of organization. While these alternative treatments show considerable promise, their true therapeutic potential compared to conventional medicines requires further validation through human clinical trials.

Keywords: neuroprotective, health, disease, disability, research

Abbreviations

BBB	Blood brain barrier
BDNF	Brain – derived neurotrophic factor
CNS	Central nervous system
CYP3A4	Cytochrome P450
FAD	Familial Alzheimer's disease
GDNF	Glial cell line derived neurotrophic factor
HARS	Hamilton Anxiety Rating Scale
HPA	Hypothalamic – pituitary – adrenal axis
m TOR	Mammalian target of rapamycin
ROS	Reactive oxygen species
ROS	Reactive oxygen species
RRE	*Rhodiola rosea* extract

Introduction

Degenerative nerve diseases encompass a wide range of conditions that cause the gradual loss of function in nerve cells and neural networks in the brain and spine (Przedborski et al., 2003). The hallmark of neurodegenerative diseases is a progressive yet irreversible decline in brain function (Przedborski et al., 2003). These disorders lead to selective dysfunction and ongoing neuronal loss, manifesting in various symptoms, including movement impairments and cognitive deficits (Birajdar et al., 2023). While certain therapies may alleviate symptoms, slowing the progression of these disorders remains a significant challenge, and no cures are currently available (Ivanova et al., 2022). Understanding the mechanisms underlying neuronal cell death and developing effective treatments for neurodegenerative diseases is considered a major challenge for the foreseeable future (Khanet et al., 2022). Exploring natural compounds for neuroprotection is of great importance due to their potential to provide alternative and complementary treatment options for degenerative nerve diseases. Several studies have emphasized the neuroprotective potential of organic (natural) compounds and their bioactive components, highlighting their multiple mechanisms of action and their ability to cross the blood-brain barrier (Mohd et al., 2020). These compounds have been observed to target various aspects of disease pathogenesis, such as oxidative stress, neuroinflammation, and apoptotic processes, making them attractive candidates for the treatment of neurodegenerative diseases (Andrade et al., 2023). Furthermore, advancements in novel drug delivery systems, including the application of nanotechnology, have been proposed to enhance the neuroavailability and neuroprotective activity of natural compounds. These advancements address bioavailability issues and promote their access to the brain. According to Mohd et al., (2020), further research in this area could lead to the development of more effective and targeted delivery systems for natural compounds, thereby increasing their clinical utility (Mohd et al., 2020). Research on Rhodiola rosea has shown promising effects in addressing various health issues, including physical and mental fatigue, stress, and cognitive dysfunction. This plant contains nearly 140 chemical compounds, with its active elements serving as bioactive components in pharmacological preparations. Most formulations of *R.* rosea standardize specific marker compounds, such as rosavin and salidroside, to specific levels (Lu et al., 2022). *R. rosea* has demonstrated the ability to regulate blood pressure and protect human cortical neurons from oxidative stress and apoptosis. Notably, significant fatigue-reducing effects have been observed. Additionally, it has been found to enhance cognitive performance and reduce symptoms of fatigue, exhaustion, and weakness (Bernatoniene et al., 2023).

Phytochemical Composition

Rhodiola rosea contains a variety of beneficial compounds, including polyphenolic compounds such as proanthocyanidins, polyphenols, n-tyrosol, and cinnamic alcohol. Additionally, it is rich in glucose, carboxylic acids, volatile oils, essential oils, carbohydrates, fats, alcohols, and amino acids. Notably, Lignum rhodium, a component derived from this plant, has a polyphenolic content of approximately 41.4 ± 3.41% (Mirmazloum et al., 2015).

Neuroprotective Properties

Antioxidant Effects

The classification of *R. rosea* as an antioxidant is largely attributed to its significant content of phenol-related compounds. When compared to the aqueous extract or powdered raw material, the ethanolic extract of *R. rosea* exhibits notably strong antioxidant activity and a high antioxidant potential (Kosakowska et al., 2018).

Anti-Inflammatory Activities

Several studies have demonstrated that *R. rosea* can enhance endogenous antioxidant defenses. One study found that the liquid extract of Aaron's rod protects cultured striated myocytes from oxidation-induced damage, particularly during ultrasonic depolarization of myofibers, a process that leads to increased ROS production (Hou et al., 2024). Another study revealed that *R. rosea* effectively enhances the activity of the trans-acting factor NRF2, a key regulator of antioxidant defenses, in a time- and dose-dependent manner in human keratinocytes. When treated with golden root extract, these cells exhibited improved resistance to various oxidative stresses, highlighting the plant's potent free radical scavenging properties (Boo, 2020).

Rectification of Neurotrophic Factors

Rhodiola rosea hydroethanolic extract has been shown to influence stress-related genes, particularly in the hippocampus and prefrontal cortex. This action ultimately leads to a reduction in corticosteroid levels, as observed in preclinical animal models of stress (Dinel et al., 2019).

Effects on Neurotransmitter Systems

Researchers have found that *R. rosea* modulates various neurotransmitter systems, potentially contributing to its effects on the central nervous system (CNS) in the brain and spinal cord. Several studies have shown that *R. rosea* can elevate levels of neurotransmitters such as noradrenaline, dihydroxyphenylalanine, serotonin, and acetylcholine. These increases stimulate CNS activity and enhance cognitive functions, including the ability to acquire and retain information. Additionally, Arctic root extract has been observed to improve rats' adaptability during a water navigation task, likely due to its influence on acetylcholine, monoamine molecules, and neuropeptides, all of which enhance CNS functionality and activity. Furthermore, golden root extract not only regulates the activity and concentration of acetylcholine in the brain but also increases the levels of endogenous opioid peptides (Zhuang et al., 2019).

Blood-brain barrier penetration: Several studies have demonstrated that *R. rosea* roots possess the capability to penetrate the blood-brain barrier (BBB). In one study, the primary bioactive compound in *R. rosea*, rosavin, was found to protect the BBB from acute oxygen shortages, such as ischemia and cerebral injury caused by reperfusion, by modulating the mitogen-activated protein kinase-mediated matrix metalloproteinase pathway (Zou et al., 2023). Another study suggested that *R. rosea* could enhance the transport of substances across the BBB by modulating brain endothelial transporters (Fan et al., 2020). Additionally, research indicated that roseroot extract reduced the mild stress-induced hydrocortisone response and altered the expression of genes related to stress responsiveness in the prefrontal cortex, the most evolved part of the brain. This suggests that *R. rosea* may influence neurotrophic factor activity in the brain (Dimpfel et al., 2018).

Experimental Evidence and Preclinical Studies

In Vitro Studies Assessing Neuroprotective Effects

Researchers studying *R. rosea* have found that its active ingredient, salidroside, may influence the growth of Schwann cells by altering several neurotrophic factors, including abrineurin and microglia line-derived nerve growth factor (Sabir et al., 2023).

Biological Models of Neurodegenerative Disorders

Dementia

Researchers have explored the potential neuroprotective effects of *R. rosea* using prototype organisms for Alzheimer's disease. However, there is currently no specific information on the use of *R. rosea* with particular Alzheimer's disease model organisms. Instead, animal models of Alzheimer's disease have been employed to understand the pathological progression and development of the disease, as well as to evaluate potential therapeutic interventions. These models have been instrumental in assessing the causes and progression of Alzheimer's disease, testing hypotheses related to its pathogenesis, and guiding the design of human clinical trials (Götz et al., 2018). In the realm of Parkinson's disease, research is ongoing to identify biomarkers that can lead to early diagnosis and more effective treatments. Although current therapies for Parkinson's disease can alleviate symptoms, they do not address the underlying causes or prevent the disease from progressing (Adam et al., 2023).

Other Relevant Models

Various biological models have been utilized to assess the potential neuroprotective effects of *R. rosea* in relation to neurodegenerative disorders. In studies of dementia, researchers focus on understanding the development and progression of the disease to explore potential curative interventions. Genetically modified mice that express human genes associated with familial Alzheimer's disease (FAD) are commonly used in this research (Drummond et al., 2017).

Methodologies and Outcome Measures

A structured review of human research on physiological and psychological tiredness identified overtiredness as a key result, evaluated using an index based on exhaustion. The perception of each trial was assessed for potential bias, leading to a domain-specific evaluation approved by the Cochrane Collaboration. Key domains of this evaluation include unpredictability, allocation concealment, judgment bias, incomplete results data, clarity of specified results, and other relevant factors. The review examined current results, noting variations due to baseline comparisons with golden root, and permitted minute variations within a 95% confidence interval (Ishaque et al., 2017). Another major human trial assessed the effects of *R. rosea* essence on physically and mentally exhausted patients. The primary goal was to enhance stress resistance, with patients receiving approximately 200 mg of golden root essence twice a week for 12 weeks. The trial ensured high awareness among both the investigator and the participants regarding the experimental procedures, major evaluations, and probabilities, without requiring an authorizing group. Results indicated transparent improvement over time, with a low probability of adverse events (Amsterdam et al., 2016). A separate human trial evaluated the efficacy of *R. rosea* in addressing symptoms related to mental exhaustion and tension. This trial used multiple outcome measurements, including the Hamilton Anxiety Rating Scale (HARS), the Four-Dimensional Anxiety and Depression Scale, and the Clinical Global Impressions (CGI) of Severity/Improvement Scale. The study found significant, consistent, and steady improvements in symptoms related to stress, exhaustion, quality of life, and other mood-related factors (Ivanova et al., 2022).

Challenges and Limitations in Human Studies

Research indicates that *R. rosea* contains phenolic compounds, which may offer potential therapeutic benefits for treating chronic diseases (Kim et al., 2021). However, advanced studies are needed to establish standardized procedures for extracting and analyzing these phenolic compounds in *R. rosea*. Such research could help validate the therapeutic potential of these compounds for chronic disease management (Chiang et al., 2015).

Mechanisms of Action

Interaction with Cellular Signalling Pathways

Rhodiola rosea is believed to regulate monoamine levels in the brain, hypothalamus, and cerebral cortex, affecting neurotransmitters such as serotonin, dihydroxyphenylalanine, and noradrenaline. By modulating these monoamines, *R. rosea* helps maintain neurotransmitter balance and inhibit the activity of certain modifying enzymes. Additionally, extracts of *R. rosea* and its bioactive component, salidroside, are reported to stimulate the mammalian target of rapamycin (mTOR), which influences paracrine functions and enhances physiological processes. *In vitro* studies have also indicated that *R. rosea* blocks the cytochrome P450 enzyme CYP3A4 and P-glycoprotein. This action could affect the metabolism and distribution of various compounds in the body. Furthermore, salidroside from *R. rosea* plays a role in modulating oxidative stress, inflammation, apoptosis, the hypothalamic-pituitary-adrenal (HPA) axis, and neurotransmission in the central nervous system (Zhong et al., 2018; Sharma et al., 2023).

Influence on Neuroinflammation Cascades

Research suggests that *R. rosea* may exert neuroprotective effects through its anti-inflammatory properties. For instance, studies have shown that extracts of *R. rosea* reduce the formation of cytokines, which are involved in inflammation, in Alzheimer's mouse models. Additionally, salidroside, a key component of *R. rosea*, has been found to regulate inflammation in the central nervous system (Khalaf et al., 2022; Yokoyama et al., 2022).

Modulation of Apoptotic Processes

Research on *R. rosea* indicates that it may influence apoptotic processes. Studies have demonstrated that salidroside, a bioactive component of *R. rosea*, protects brain cortex neurons from programmed cell death induced by aerobic stress, specifically L-L-glutamic acid (Pu et al., 2020). Additionally, another study found that *R. rosea* inhibits thymus T-cell apoptosis by reducing levels of the protein cancerous inhibitor of growth 8-like-2 in diseased rats (Liu et al., 2015).

Plasticity and Synaptic Function

Research on *R. rosea* suggests that it may positively affect synaptic features and plasticity. For example, one study found that *R. rosea* extract stimulated neurite overgrowth, which involves the growth and extension of nerve endings and fibers, contributing to the formation and adaptability of synaptic junctions (Getova et al., 2013). Additionally, *R. rosea* has been shown to protect human cortical neurons from oxidative stress and prevent glutamate-induced programmed cell death, potentially benefiting synaptic function and plasticity. Furthermore, the bioactive component of *R. rosea*, salidroside (a phenolic compound), plays a role in regulating oxidative stress, inflammation, programmed cell death, the hypothalamic-pituitary-adrenal (HPA) axis, and neurotransmission in the brain and spinal cord (Concerto et al., 2018).

Safety and Tolerability

Rhodiola rosea, also known as roseroot, has been used in Eurasian traditional medicine as a natural stimulant and psychostimulant. It is reputed for enhancing well-being, strength, stamina, and both physiological and psychological performance. While research indicates that *R. rosea* can be beneficial, it may also lead to mild and abnormal side effects, including sensitivity, sleep disturbances, hypertension, and angina. Commonly reported side effects include activation, agitation, disturbances in sleep patterns, uneasiness, and episodic headaches. Currently, there is insufficient evidence regarding the safety and efficacy of *R. rosea* during pregnancy and lactation, so its use is not recommended for women in these stages. Regulations concerning dosages and safety for children are still being developed. Despite these concerns, *R. rosea* is noted for its potential to alleviate tension and mild to moderate depressive symptoms, demonstrating neuroprotective effects with minimal risk of drug interactions and adverse effects (Panossian et al., 2024). Side effects are generally uncommon and mild, but interactions with other medications and supplements should be considered. For instance, *R. rosea* may interact adversely with medications for diabetes, hypertension, and those metabolized by Cytochrome P450 1A2 (CYP1A2). Additionally, *R. rosea* may enhance immune system activity, which could potentially worsen autoimmune conditions such as cerebral palsy and inflammatory polyarthritis (Xu et al., 2013).

Future Perspectives and Implications

Research indicates that *R. rosea* may enhance learning and memory, reduce mental fatigue, alleviate free radicals, and serve as a neuroprotectant. However, further safety research is needed to explore potential interactions with medications and supplements, as well as risks for specific populations such as pregnant women and children (Ma et al., 2018). Although there are clinical trials examining *R. rosea* for physical and mental fatigue, additional studies are essential to confirm its efficacy and safety (Punja et al., 2014). Many clinical trials face limitations, such as small sample sizes, lack of blinding or randomization, and reliance on subjective outcome measures. Addressing these limitations is crucial for accurate result interpretation (Jones et al., 2012). Some studies have used fatigue indices tailored to their research, which may not be validated. Employing well-established and validated outcome measures is necessary to ensure the accuracy and reliability of the findings (Ross et al., 2019). Long-term studies are needed to assess the efficacy and safety of *R. rosea* in treating chronic diseases and stress-related symptoms. These investigations should overcome limitations, such as the lack of long-term safety data and the need for placebo-controlled trials (Sittari, 2019).

Conclusion

The integration of complementary and conventional medicine is an emerging trend that aims to combine the strengths of both approaches, offering a more comprehensive and patient-centered model of care. Future research on *R. rosea* should include extensive patient-contact trials with placebo controls to verify its efficacy and safety rigorously. Additionally, it is essential to conduct programmed research at the basic and cellular levels to better understand its effects on physical performance. Standardizing and ensuring the quality of *R. rosea* products is crucial for maintaining uniformity and consistency across studies.

References

Adam, H., Gopinath, S. C., Md Arshad, M. K., Adam, T., Parmin, N. A., Husein, I., & Hashim, U. (2023). An update on pathogenesis and clinical scenario for Parkinson's disease: diagnosis and treatment. *3 Biotech*, 13(5), 142.

Amsterdam, J. D., & Panossian, A. G. (2016). Rhodiola rosea L. as a putative botanical antidepressant. *Phytomedicine*, 23(7), 770-783.

Andrade, S., Nunes, D., Dabur, M., Ramalho, M. J., Pereira, M. C., & Loureiro, J. A. (2023). Therapeutic potential of natural compounds in neurodegenerative diseases: insights from clinical trials. *Pharmaceutics*, 15(1), 212.

Bernatoniene, J., Jakstas, V., & Kopustinskiene, D. M. (2023). Phenolic compounds of Rhodiola rosea L. as the potential alternative therapy in the treatment of chronic diseases. *International journal of molecular sciences*, 24(15), 12293.

Birajdar, S. V., Mulchandani, M., Mazahir, F., & Yadav, A. K. (2023). Dementia and neurodegenerative disorder: An introduction. In *Nanomedicine-based approaches for the treatment of dementia* (pp. 1-36). Academic Press.

Boo, Y. C. (2020). Natural Nrf2 modulators for skin protection. *Antioxidants*, 9(9), 812.

Chiang, H. M., Chen, H. C., Wu, C. S., Wu, P. Y., & Wen, K. C. (2015). Rhodiola plants: Chemistry and biological activity. *Journal of food and drug analysis*, 23(3), 359-369.

Concerto, C., Infortuna, C., Muscatello, M. R. A., Bruno, A., Zoccali, R., Chusid, E., Aguglia, E., & Battaglia, F. (2018). (2018). Exploring the effect of adaptogenic Rhodiola Rosea extract on neuroplasticity in humans. *Complementary Therapies in Medicine*, 41, 141-146.

Dhankhar, S., Mujwar, S., Garg, N., Chauhan, S., Saini, M., Sharma, P., Kumar, S., Kumar Sharma, S., Kamal, M. A., & Rani, N. (2024). Artificial Intelligence in The Management of Neurodegenerative Disorders. *CNS & Neurological Disorders-Drug Targets*, 23(8), 931-940.

Dimpfel, W., Schombert, L., & Panossian, A. G. (2018). Assessing the quality and potential efficacy of commercial extracts of Rhodiola rosea L. by analyzing the salidroside and rosavin content and the electrophysiological activity in hippocampal long-term potentiation, a synaptic model of memory. *Frontiers in Pharmacology*, 9, 425.

Dinel, A. L., Guinobert, I., Lucas, C., Blondeau, C., Bardot, V., Ripoche, I., & Joffre, C. (2019). Reduction of acute mild stress corticosterone response and changes in stress-responsive gene expression in male Balb/c mice after repeated administration of a Rhodiola rosea L. root extract. *Food science & nutrition*, 7(11), 3827-3841.

Drummond, E., & Wisniewski, T. (2017). Alzheimer's disease: experimental models and reality. *Acta neuropathologica*, 133, 155-175.

Fan, F., Yang, L., Li, R., Zou, X., Li, N., Meng, X., & Wang, X. (2020). Salidroside as a potential neuroprotective agent for ischemic stroke: a review of sources, pharmacokinetics, mechanism and safety. *Biomedicine & Pharmacotherapy*, 129, 110458.

Getova, D., & Mihaylova, A. (2013). Effects of Rhodiola rosea extract on passive avoidance tests in rats. *Open Medicine*, 8(2), 176-181.

Hou, K., Cao, L., Li, W., Fang, Z. H., Sun, D., Guo, Z., & Zhang, L. (2024). Overexpression of Rhodiola crenulata glutathione peroxidase 5 increases cold tolerance and enhances the pharmaceutical value of the hairy roots. *Gene*, 917, 148467.

Ishaque, S., Shamseer, L., Bukutu, C., & Vohra, S. (2012). Rhodiola rosea for physical and mental fatigue: a systematic review. *BMC Complementary and Alternative Medicine*, 12, 1-9.

Ivanova Stojcheva, E., & Quintela, J. C. (2022). The effectiveness of Rhodiola rosea L. preparations in alleviating various aspects of life-stress symptoms and stress-induced conditions—encouraging clinical evidence. *Molecules*, 27(12), 3902.

Jones, C. W., & Platts-Mills, T. F. (2012). Understanding commonly encountered limitations in clinical research: an emergency medicine resident's perspective. *Annals of emergency medicine*, 59(5), 425-431.

Khalaf, K., Tornese, P., Cocco, A., & Albanese, A. (2022). Tauroursodeoxycholic acid: a potential therapeutic tool in neurodegenerative diseases. *Translational Neurodegeneration*, 11(1), 33.

Khan, H., Garg, N., Singh, T. G., Kaur, A., & Thapa, K. (2022). Calpain inhibitors as potential therapeutic modulators in neurodegenerative diseases. *Neurochemical Research*, 47(5), 1125-1149.

Kim, K. J., Jung, Y. S., You, D. M., Lee, S. H., Lee, G., Kwon, K. B., & Kim, D. O. (2021). Neuroprotective effects of ethanolic extract from dry Rhodiola rosea L. rhizomes. *Food Science and Biotechnology*, 30, 287-297.

Liu, M. W., Su, M. X., Zhang, W., Zhang, L. M., Wang, Y. H., & Qian, C. Y. (2015). Rhodiola rosea suppresses thymus T-lymphocyte apoptosis by downregulating tumor necrosis factor-α-induced protein 8-like-2 in septic rats. *International journal of molecular medicine*, 36(2), 386-398.

Lu, Y., Deng, B., Xu, L., Liu, H., Song, Y., & Lin, F. (2022). Effects of Rhodiola rosea supplementation on exercise and sport: a systematic review. *Frontiers in nutrition*, 9, 856287.

Ma, G. P., Zheng, Q., Xu, M. B., Zhou, X. L., & Zheng, G. Q. (2018). Rhodiola rosea L. improves learning and memory function: preclinical evidence and possible mechanisms. *Frontiers in pharmacology*, 9, 367723.

Mirmazloum, I., Ladányi, M., & György, Z. (2015). Changes in the content of the glycosides, aglycons and their possible precursors of Rhodiola rosea during the vegetation period. *Natural Product Communications*, 10(8), 1934578X1501000825.

Mohd Sairazi, N. S., & Sirajudeen, K. N. S. (2020). Natural products and their bioactive compounds: neuroprotective potentials against neurodegenerative diseases. *Evidence-Based Complementary and Alternative Medicine*, 2020(1), 6565396.

Panossian, A., & Wikman, G. (2010). Effects of adaptogens on the central nervous system and the molecular mechanisms associated with their stress—protective activity. *Pharmaceuticals*, 3(1), 188-224.

Przedborski, S., Vila, M., & Jackson-Lewis, V. (2003). Neurodegeneration: what is it and where are we? *Journal of clinical investigation*, 111(1), 3-10.

Pu, W. L., Zhang, M. Y., Bai, R. Y., Sun, L. K., Li, W. H., Yu, Y. L., & Li, T. X. (2020). Anti-inflammatory effects of Rhodiola rosea L.: A review. *Biomedicine & Pharmacotherapy*, 121, 109552.

Punja, S., Shamseer, L., Olson, K., & Vohra, S. (2014). Rhodiola rosea for mental and physical fatigue in nursing students: a randomized controlled trial. *PloS one*, 9(9), e108416.

Ross, P. T., & Bibler Zaidi, N. L. (2019). Limited by our limitations. *Perspectives on medical education*, 8, 261-264.

Sabir, H., Maes, E., Zweyer, M., Schleehuber, Y., Imam, F. B., Silverman, J., & Bernis, M. E. (2023). Comparing the efficacy in reducing brain injury of different neuroprotective agents following neonatal hypoxia–ischemia in newborn rats: a multi-drug randomized controlled screening trial. *Scientific Reports*, 13(1), 9467.

Sharma, H., Chang, K. A., Hulme, J., & An, S. S. A. (2023). Mammalian Models in Alzheimer's Research: An Update. *Cells*, 12(20), 2459.

Suntar, I. (2019). Rhodiola (Rhodiola rosea L.). In *Nonvitamin and Nonmineral Nutritional Supplements* (pp. 383-400). Academic Press.

Yokoyama, M., Kobayashi, H., Tatsumi, L., & Tomita, T. (2022). Mouse models of Alzheimer's disease. *Frontiers in Molecular Neuroscience*, 15, 912995.

Zhong, Z., Han, J., Zhang, J., Xiao, Q., Hu, J., & Chen, L. (2018). Pharmacological activities, mechanisms of action, and safety of salidroside in the central nervous system. *Drug design, development and therapy*, 12, 1479-1489.

Zhuang, W., Yue, L., Dang, X., Chen, F., Gong, Y., Lin, X., & Luo, Y. (2019). Rosenroot (Rhodiola): potential applications in aging-related diseases. *Aging and disease*, 10(1), 134.

Zou, H., Li, L., Yang, Z., Tang, L., & Wang, C. (2023). Rosavin protects the blood–brain barrier against ischemia/reperfusion-induced cerebral injury by regulating MAPK-mediated MMPs pathway. *Clinical and Experimental Pharmacology and Physiology*, 50(8), 664-676.

Chapter 11

The Role of Catechins in Neuroprotection

Prabhjot Kaur[1,*]
Muskan[1]
Anjali Sharma[1]
Bharat Prashar[2]
and Shivangi Garg[3]
[1]Guru Gobind Singh College of Pharmacy, Yamuna Nagar, Haryana, India
[2]Faculty of Pharmaceutical Sciences, ICFAI University, Baddi, Himachal Pradesh, India
[3]Lal Bahadur Shastri Mahila Ayurvedic College and Hospital, Bilaspur, Yamuna Nagar, Haryana, India

Abstract

The modern healthcare sector has faced tremendous problems due to various neurological disorders, e.g., Alzheimer's disease, Parkinson's disease, Huntington disease, etc. The therapy methods available nowadays are ineffective and frequently cause side effects. Extracts comprising of green tea along with black tea (5 to 25 ug/mL), gallic acid (1 to 20 um), epicatechin gallate (1 to 20 um), and epigallocatechin gallate (1 to 10 um) exhibit neuroprotection properties altering the toxic effect of aflatoxin. The most powerful flavan-3-ol was gallic acid. Catechins exhibit various biological responses such as cytokines modulation, inflammatory pathway suppression, metal ion chelation, and free radical scavenging through anti-inflammatory and antioxidant processes. Additionally, catechins shows impact on important proteins linked to protein aggregation and death, which exhibit effect on the pathogenic processes of neurodegenerative diseases. In particular,

---

* Corresponding Author's Email: prabhjotkaur102001@gmail.com.

In: Natural Solutions for Neurodegenerative Disorders
Editors: Rahul Kumar Sharma, Shailesh Sharma, Ajmer Singh Grewal et al.
ISBN: 979-8-89530-231-6

EGCG, a well-known catechin, demonstrates neuroprotective properties via suppressing A-induced neurotoxicity, activating GSK-3, inhibiting c-Abl/FE65, and inducing autophagy, which is essential for neuro development and nuclear translocation. The chemical composition of catechins and their significance in neuroprotection are addressed in this chapter.

Keywords: catechins, epigallocatechin gallate (EGCG), neuroprotection, antioxidant, neuro inflammation

Abbreviations

6-OHDA	6-hydroxydopamine
Akt/PKB	Protein kinase B
Akt	Protein kinase B
ALS	Amyotrophic lateral sclerosis
Bad	Bcl-2–associated death promoter
Bax	Bcl-2–associated X protein
Bcl-2	B-cell lymphoma 2
Bcl-w	B-cell lymphoma w
Bcl-x(L)	B-cell lymphoma –x(L)
BDNF	brain-derived neurotrophic factor
C	Catechin
COMT	catechol-O-methyl transferase
DCX	doublecortin
DOPAC	3, 4-dihydroxyphenylacetic acid
DOPAL	3, 4-dihydroxyphenylacetaldehyde
Dyrk1A	dual-specificity tyrosine-(Y)-phosphorylation-regulated kinase 1A
EC	Epicatechin
ECG	Epi catechin gallate
EGC	Epigallo catechin
EGCG	Epigallo catechin gallate
ERK	extracellular signal-regulated kinase
FASD	Fetal alcohol spectrum disorder
GC	Gallocatechin
GCG	Gallo catechin gallate
GFAP	glial fibrillary acidic protein

GPX1	glutathione peroxidase
GSK- 3	Glycogen synthase kinase 3
HD	Huntington disease
HIF-1α	hypoxia inducible factor 1α
HIF-1	hypoxia inducible factor 1
Htt	Gene Huntingtin
HVA	Homovanillic acid
JNK	Jun N-terminal kinase
LPO	lipid peroxidation
MAO	monoamine oxidase
Mdm2	Murine double minute 2 gene
NeuN	neuronal nuclei
NO	Nitric oxide
Otx1	orthodenticle homolog 1
p38	Mitogen-activated protein kinase 14 gene
p53	Tumor protein
PAE	prenatal alcohol exposure
PC12	Adrenal phaeochromocytoma cell
PD	Parkinson's disease
PGC- 1α	peroxisome proliferator-activated receptor gamma coactivator-1α
PI3K/Akt	phosphoinositide-3-kinase/ Protein kinase B
PI3K	phosphoinositide-3-kinase
PPAR gamma	peroxisome proliferator-activated receptor gamma
RNS	Reactive nitrogen species
ROS	Reactive oxygen species
SIRT1	Sirtuin 1
SNpc	*Substantia nigra pars compacta*
SOD	Superoxide dismutase
SOD1	superoxide dismutase 1
Sox 2	Sex determination region Y- box2
Sry	Sex determining region Y gene
VEGF-A	Vascular endothelial growth factor-A
Wnt	Wingless-related integration site

Introduction

Globally, neurodegenerative disorders have a significant economic impact. These conditions are primarily characterized by the accumulation of altered proteins due to various biological processes, including oxidative stress, inflammation, signaling pathway dysregulation, and excitotoxicity. Despite extensive research over the past decade aimed at developing symptom-oriented treatments, no effective therapy has yet been found (Liu et al., 2022). Catechins, which originate from the cutch tree (Acacia catechu L.f.), are natural flavanols also known as flavan-3-ols and belong to the flavonoid family (Afzal et al., 2022). They include several types such as epigallocatechin gallate, epicatechin gallate, epigallocatechin, gallocatechin gallate, epicatechin, gallocatechin, and catechin (Table 1) (Ou and Juanying, 2021). Catechins exhibit both anti-inflammatory and antioxidant properties through various mechanisms, including metal ion chelation, free radical scavenging, and inhibition of cytokine overproduction and inflammatory pathways. They also prevent the release of apoptotic proteins, tau protein phosphorylation, and amyloid beta formation. Additionally, catechins can increase dopamine levels and decrease alpha-synuclein levels, which are relevant to neurodegenerative disorders (Liu et al., 2022). Catechins target several processes involved in neurodegenerative diseases, such as inhibition of neurological cell growth leading to cell death, inflammation, oxidative stress, aberrant protein aggregation (e.g., Aβ protein and α-synuclein), and excessive protein production that promotes apoptosis. The mechanism by which epigallocatechin gallate (EGCG) inhibits fibrous protein accumulation was elucidated through computational molecular docking studies. These findings suggest that catechins hold promise for the development of novel medications aimed at preventing, treating, and curing neurodegenerative conditions (Pervin et al., 2018).

Neurodegenerative Disease and Oxidative Damage

The pathology of various oxidative stress-related diseases, particularly neurodegenerative and neurological disorders, is significantly influenced by oxidative stress (Figure 1). Oxidative stress triggers lipid peroxidation, initiating a chain reaction that leads to the aggregation and accumulation of oxidized proteins within cells. This process exacerbates mitochondrial damage, further impacting protein integrity. Additionally, reactive species can inflict damage on DNA, resulting in abnormal cell growth and altered regulation of key genes such as Wnt and p53. In the human brain and notochord nerve cells, oxidative stress can lead to functional loss or sensory degradation. Apoptosis, excitotoxicity, and mitochondrial dysfunction are common outcomes of oxidative stress, contributing to the progression of neurodegenerative diseases. Conditions such as multiple sclerosis (MS), Parkinson's disease (PD), Alzheimer's disease (AD), and amyotrophic lateral sclerosis (ALS) are often associated with an overproduction of reactive nitrogen species (RNS) and reactive oxygen species (ROS) (Thanan et al., 2015; Subramaniam et al., 2013).

Table 1. Chemical framework of various types of catechins

Catechin	Chemical Structure	Reference
Catechin	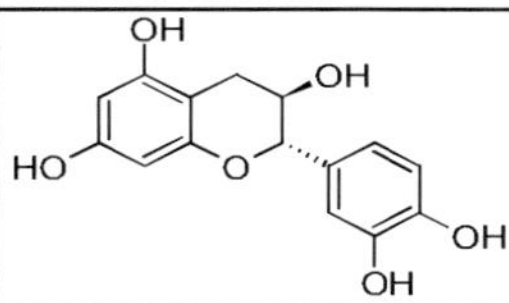	(Pervin et al., 2018)
Epicatechins	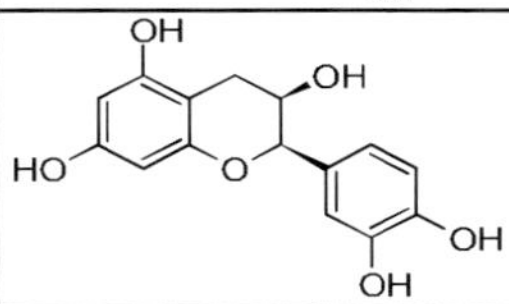	(Pervin et al., 2018)
Epigallo catechin	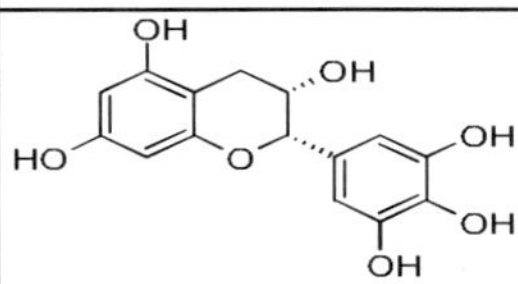	(Pervin et al., 2018)
Epicatechin gallate	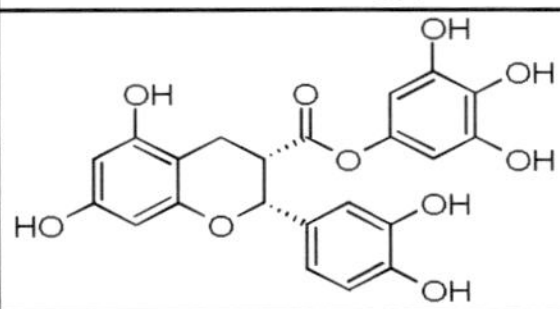	(Pervin et al., 2018)
Epigallocatechin gallate	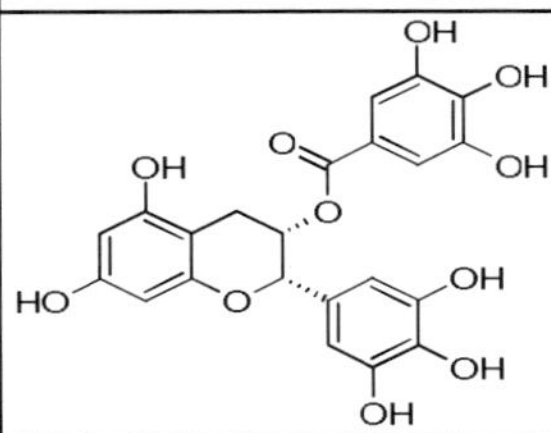	(Pervin et al., 2018)

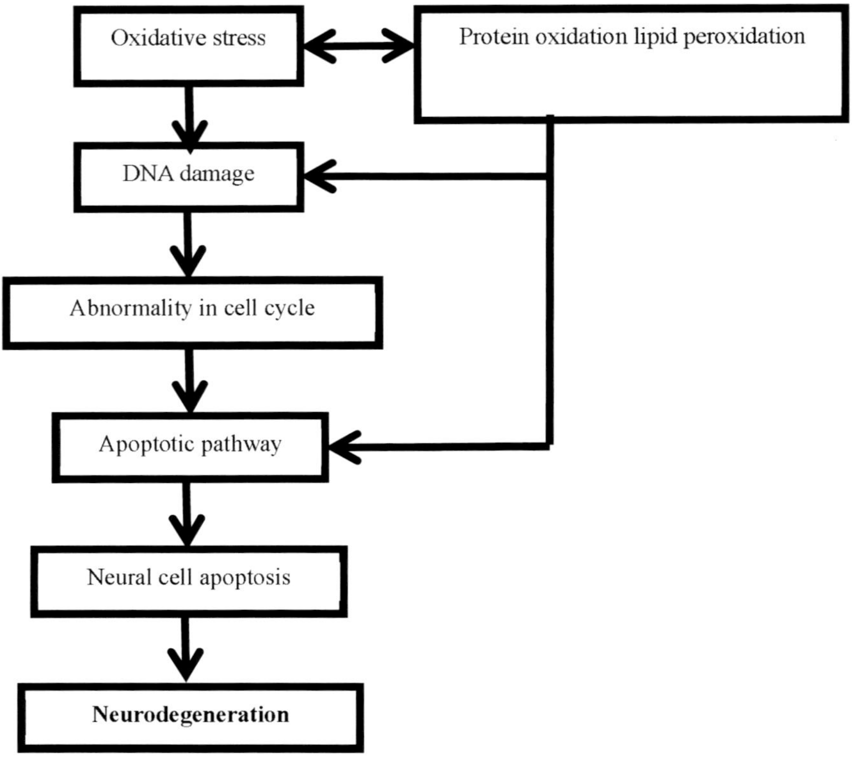

Figure 1. Cellular oxidative stress impact on neuro degeneration (Thanan et al., 2015).

Catechins' Role in Different Neurodegenerative Diseases

The potential neuroprotective effects of catechins in treating neurological disorders, including ALS, Parkinson's disease, Alzheimer's disease, Huntington's disease, frontotemporal dementia, and FASD, are actively being investigated. Catechins are known for their anti-inflammatory properties, which may help reduce neuroinflammation, and their antioxidant effects, which can prevent oxidative stress—a major contributor to these diseases. Research has suggested that catechins might be beneficial in decreasing neurogenesis and preventing beta-amyloid protein aggregation, which is particularly relevant for Alzheimer's disease. Consuming green tea, which is rich in catechins, alongside a healthy diet, may offer neuroprotection against various neurological disorders. However, further studies are needed to fully understand and validate these potential benefits.

Parkinson's Disease

The aggregation of α-synuclein protein is a hallmark of Parkinson's disease, and researchers are exploring various therapeutic approaches by identifying abnormal mitochondrial, lysosomal, and endosomal activities in both sporadic and genetic forms of the disease (Morris et al., 2014). Catechins, particularly due to their ability to reduce oxidative stress, enhance dopamine metabolism, and modulate inflammation and apoptosis pathways, show promise for treating Parkinson's disease (Josiah et al., 2022). Catechins can neutralize free radicals and decrease levels of pro-inflammatory cytokines in the brain (Sharma et al., 2023). The neuroprotective effects of EGCG (epigallocatechin gallate), a major catechin, have been investigated in PC12 cells treated with 6-hydroxydopamine (6-OHDA), a model for studying Parkinson's disease. These studies have highlighted EGCG's potential in mitigating neurotoxic damage and providing neuroprotection.

Protection Against Apoptosis

Apoptosis, whether triggered by intrinsic or extrinsic pathways, plays a significant role in the pathogenesis of Parkinson's disease (Sharma et al., 2023). Evidence of apoptosis has been observed in postmortem nigrostriatal tissues from Parkinson's disease patients, as well as in various cell culture and animal models of the disease. In both *in vitro* and *in vivo* models of Parkinson's disease, EGCG (epigallocatechin gallate) has demonstrated the ability to prevent apoptosis. Specifically, in PC12 cells treated with 6-hydroxydopamine (6-OHDA), EGCG effectively suppressed apoptosis. It achieved this by reducing the expression of several apoptosis-related mRNAs, such as Bad, Bax, and Mdm2, and by decreasing levels of Bcl-w and Bcl (Liu et al., 2022).

Protection Against Oxidative Stress

A growing body of research has identified several sources and mechanisms of oxidative damage in PD, including iron (Fe^{2+}) accumulation, mitochondrial dysfunction, NOX activation, and auto-oxidation of dopamine (Wang et al., 2021). Studies have highlighted the ability of EGCG (epigallocatechin gallate) to reduce the formation of ROS generated by neurotoxins associated with PD in *in vitro* models. EGCG significantly improves cell viability and decreases ROS production induced by MPP+ (1-methyl-4-phenylpyridinium). Additionally, EGCG enhances the up-regulation of protective factors such as Sirtuin 1 (SIRT1), glutathione peroxidase (GPX1), superoxide dismutase 1 (SOD1), peroxisome proliferator-activated receptor gamma (PPARγ), and peroxisome proliferator-activated receptor gamma coactivator 1-alpha (PGC-1α) in response to MPP+. Current studies also show that EGCG reduces lipid peroxidation (LPO) and nitric oxide (NO) levels in rats, thereby reversing neurochemical and motor dysfunctions induced by rotenone (Wang et al., 2022; Tseng et al., 2020).

Catechins and Alpha-Synuclein

Alpha-synuclein, a 140-amino-acid protein, is found in the presynaptic nerve terminals of the brain. Recent research indicates that the aggregation of alpha-synuclein disrupts synaptic regulation, impairs neuronal signaling, and ultimately leads to neuron death. In cell-free *in vitro* systems, EGCG (epigallocatechin gallate) has been shown to significantly inhibit the accumulation of alpha-synuclein protein and prevent the increase of toxic levels in PC12 cell lines. EGCG appears to interact favorably with the naturally unfolded alpha-synuclein polypeptide chain by promoting the formation of unstructured oligomers, which helps to inhibit the generation of harmful beta-sheet structures. By reducing the exposure of hydrophobic groups, EGCG facilitates the formation of small, less toxic fibrils, demonstrating that catechins can mitigate the cytotoxic effects of alpha-synuclein aggregates (Jha et al., 2017; Srinivasan et al., 2021).

Catechins and Dopamine

The nigrostriatal circuits in the midbrain are significantly affected by the loss of more than 80% of dopamine neurons in the substantia nigra pars compacta. This substantial reduction leads to the characteristic motor symptoms of PD, including freezing, postural instability, resting tremors, stiffness, and a lack of voluntary movement (Lee et al., 2021). Dopamine degradation involves two key enzymes: COMT and MAO. Initially, dopamine is metabolized into dopamine-aldehyde (dopal) by MAO. Subsequently, COMT converts dopamine into 3-methoxytyramine, which is further metabolized into homovanillic acid (HVA). These metabolites are then excreted through urine (Wang et al., 2022; Lee et al., 2021).

Huntington's Disease (HD)

HD is a progressive neurological disorder characterized by involuntary movements, progressive dementia, and cognitive impairments. The disease is primarily driven by the aggregation of the huntingtin protein, which is associated with expanded CAG triplet repeats in its polyglutamine region. Targeting these misfolded proteins with small-molecule drugs could offer therapeutic benefits (Sebastiani et al., 2021). Research has identified elevated levels of iron and copper ions in certain brain regions of individuals with HD. EGCG, known for its metal-chelating properties, may help mitigate early symptoms of HD by modulating metal ion levels (Beasley et al., 2019). Studies have explored the potential of EGCG to influence huntingtin protein aggregation and its interaction with lipid membranes. For example, EGCG has been shown to prevent amyloid formation by reducing interactions with phospholipid membranes (Varga et al., 2020). Additionally, a study using a Drosophila model demonstrated that EGCG could reverse neurodegeneration caused by mutant huntingtin protein (Varga et al., 2020). While these initial findings are promising, further human clinical trials are necessary to evaluate the efficacy and safety of EGCG in treating Huntington's disease and related conditions involving protein aggregation.

Multiple Sclerosis

Multiple sclerosis (MS) is a severe autoimmune disease characterized by demyelination, neuronal loss, and scarring (Haki et al., 2024). Research has explored various disease-modifying therapies that aim to slow the progression of MS and prevent relapses. One such approach involves the use of green tea extract, particularly polyphenon E, which contains a high concentration of catechins like epigallocatechin gallate (EGCG). Studies have shown that EGCG can enhance the remyelination process in the cerebral cortex by increasing the levels of proteolipid protein and oligodendrocyte transcription factor 1 (OTF 1), which are crucial for myelin repair (Semnani et al., 2017). In a clinical trial assessing the effects of polyphenon E, which is 50% EGCG, on MS patients, it was found that 800 mg of EGCG increased brain aspartate levels, indicating a potential neuroprotective effect. However, the trial also reported that five out of seven patients had to discontinue the treatment due to abnormal liver function, suggesting that polyphenon E may pose a risk of hepatotoxicity (Lovera et al., 2015). These findings highlight the potential benefits of EGCG in MS treatment but also underscore the need for careful monitoring of liver function and further investigation to fully understand its safety and efficacy.

Amyotrophic Lateral Sclerosis (ALS) and Frontotemporal Dementia (FTD)

FTD and ALS are distinct neurodegenerative disorders but are associated with overlapping pathological mechanisms. Both conditions involve complex molecular and cellular processes, including oxidative stress and mitochondrial dysfunction. Despite current treatments providing only modest symptomatic relief and extending the post-diagnostic lifespan, there remains a significant need for novel therapeutic strategies (Novak et al., 2021). Research on EGCG, a key component of green tea, has shown promising results in relation to these diseases. In ALS, EGCG has been observed to protect motor neurons from oxidative damage and mitochondrial stress. Clinical studies indicate that oral EGCG supplements can improve motor function, extend the lifespan of patients, and delay the onset of symptoms (Xu et al., 2006). Additionally, EGCG appears to enhance the activity of the PI3K/Akt signaling pathway, which is involved in regulating GSK-3, a protein linked to neurofibrillary tangles and neuronal death (Che et al., 2017). By activating this prosurvival pathway, EGCG potentially mitigates neuronal damage and apoptosis associated with elevated GSK-3 levels. Furthermore, EGCG's role in reducing mitochondrial damage is supported by evidence showing that it enhances Akt-mediated phosphorylation of GSK-3, thereby protecting against mitochondrial dysfunction (Koh et al., 2004; Novak et al., 2021). These findings highlight EGCG's potential as a therapeutic agent for both FTD and ALS, though further research is needed to fully elucidate its efficacy and mechanisms of action.

Fetal Alcohol Spectrum Disorders (FASD)

Prenatal alcohol exposure (PAE) is a significant factor in FASD, leading to various neurological and developmental issues. Evidence indicates that PAE disrupts cell growth and can cause heterotopias, malformations, and other neurotoxic effects, many of which are attributed to neuroinflammation (Madeleine et al., 2023). EGCG, a major polyphenol in green tea, has demonstrated potential neuroprotective effects in this context. EGCG enhances antioxidant defenses and reduces oxidative and nitrosative damage, which is critical for mitigating the adverse effects of prenatal alcohol exposure. Research using mouse models has shown that EGCG can counteract developmental abnormalities and placental vascularization issues caused by chronic ethanol exposure. Specifically, EGCG improves fetal development by influencing vascular endothelial growth factor (VEGF-A) and its receptor (VEGF-R1), which are crucial for placental health and fetal growth (Tiwari et al., 2010). Moreover, EGCG administration has been linked to the prevention of maturation delays and loss of mature neurons due to changes in markers such as doublecortin (DCX) and neuronal nuclei (NeuN). It also addresses astrocyte proliferation and disruptions within neural cells related to glial fibrillary acidic protein (GFAP) and brain-derived neurotrophic factor (BDNF). These effects contribute to improvements in behavioral and cognitive deficits, such as memory and learning impairments caused by prenatal alcohol exposure (de la Torre et al., 2016). EGCG's impact on gene expression related to neural differentiation and brain development, including Sox2 and Otx1, further supports its potential therapeutic role. In particular, EGCG's inhibition of over-expressed Dyrk1A protein has been identified as beneficial for neuronal cell plasticity, suggesting that Dyrk1A could be a promising therapeutic target for cognitive disorders and other conditions associated with fetal alcohol spectrum disorders (Almeida et al., 2021).

Alzheimer's Disease

Dementia, characterized by a significant decline in brain function affecting daily life, includes Alzheimer's disease (AD) as the most prevalent form, particularly in individuals aged 65 and older. AD is a progressive neurodegenerative disorder that leads to impaired cognitive abilities such as memory, attention, reasoning, and judgment. While AD itself is not a direct cause of death, it significantly increases vulnerability to other health complications that can ultimately be fatal (Kumar et al., 2023). Currently, there is no cure for Alzheimer's disease. However, treatment options are available that aim to manage symptoms and potentially slow the progression of the disease. Recent advances in research have focused on identifying novel biomarkers for early detection and developing drugs that target these biomarkers to extend the duration and improve the quality of life for individuals with AD (Zetterberg et al., 2021).

Antioxidative Action of Epigallocatechin Gallate

Oxidative stress and AD are interconnected through a feedback loop that exacerbates both conditions. Oxidative stress contributes to the pathogenesis of AD, and the disease, in turn, may further amplify oxidative damage. This complex relationship highlights the potential of targeting oxidative stress as a strategy for preventing or mitigating AD. Antioxidants like green tea catechins, particularly EGCG, have shown promise as therapeutic agents due to their ability to counteract oxidative stress. Catechins act as powerful antioxidant systems, scavenging reactive oxygen and nitrogen species (RONS and RNS) such as NO, peroxyl radicals, peroxynitrite, and lipid radicals. By reducing these harmful molecules, catechins can help protect against oxidative damage (Weinreb et al., 2009). EGCG enhances the activity of antioxidant enzymes such as catalase and SOD, which play crucial roles in reducing oxidative stress (Valverde et al., 2023). Additionally, EGCG has chelating properties due to its hydroxyl groups, which contribute to its antioxidant effects and neuroprotective properties. By decreasing the production of reactive species and 3-hydroxykynurenine, EGCG helps mitigate oxidative damage, offering potential benefits for managing AD (Valverde et al., 2023; Mandel et al., 2004).

Iron Chelation Properties of Epigallocatechin Gallate

The interplay between oxidative damage, AD, and the neuroprotective properties of catechins, particularly EGCG, is further emphasized by EGCG's ability to chelate metal ions like iron and copper. This chelation is significant because altered iron metabolism has been implicated as a contributing factor in several neurological disorders, including AD (Valverde et al., 2023; Wang et al., 2020). Iron chelation, in particular, has been linked to neuroprotective effects through the activation of the hypoxia-inducible factor 1-alpha (HIF-1α) pathway. HIF-1α plays a crucial role in stabilizing HIF-1 and promoting the transcription of genes associated with oxidative stress response and cell survival. In conditions of iron overload, the expression of these protective genes is often downregulated, leading to increased oxidative damage. EGCG, however, acts as a potent activator of HIF-1α, thereby enhancing neuroprotection and supporting cell survival mechanisms (Valverde et al., 2023; Amit et al., 2008; Mandel et al., 2004). Moreover, EGCG's iron-chelating and antioxidant properties have been shown to inhibit ferroptosis, a form of iron-dependent cell death that is notably elevated in the brains of AD patients. Ferroptosis has been linked to neurodegeneration, and its inhibition is considered a potential therapeutic strategy for preventing brain damage, including hemorrhages. Research indicates that EGCG can prevent ferroptosis by modulating pathways such as protein kinase D1 phosphorylation, especially following spinal cord injury (Wang et al., 2020). This inhibition of ferroptosis by EGCG suggests that it may have a protective effect against AD, making it a promising candidate for therapeutic intervention in neurodegenerative diseases associated with iron dysregulation and oxidative stress (Li et al., 2017).

Modulating Impact of EGCG on Pathways Related to Cell Signalling, Survival, and Death

AD and oxidative damage are closely linked to intracellular signaling pathways associated with neuroprotection and cell survival, such as the phosphoinositide 3-kinase (PI3K) pathway (Kumari et al., 2023). These pathways play critical roles in various neural processes, including memory formation, synaptic plasticity, and neurodegeneration. They also influence synaptic architecture and protein synthesis, which are vital for maintaining cognitive functions and preventing neurodegenerative changes (Teleanu et al.,

2022). EGCG has been extensively studied for its ability to modulate neuroprotective effects. It enhances cell survival by activating key signaling pathways like extracellular signal-regulated kinase (ERK), protein kinase B (Akt/PKB), PI3K, and protein kinase C (PKC). These pathways are crucial for promoting cell survival and preventing cell death. Additionally, EGCG inhibits stress-related pathways such as p38 mitogen-activated protein kinases (p38 MAPK) and c-Jun N-terminal kinase (JNK), which are often associated with apoptosis and neurodegeneration. By balancing these pathways, EGCG helps prevent apoptosis and supports neuroprotection, making it a promising compound for therapeutic strategies against AD and related neurodegenerative conditions (Weinreb et al., 2009).

Conclusion

Catechins show great potential as therapeutic agents for a range of neurodegenerative diseases, thanks to their antioxidant, anti-inflammatory, and metal-chelating properties. However, further research is crucial to fully understand their potential and to develop effective treatments.

References

Afzal, O., Dalhat, M. H., Altamimi, A. S. A., Rasool, R., Alzarea, S. I., Almalki, W. H., Murtaza, B. N., Iftikhar, S., Nadeem, S., Nadeem, M. S., & Kazmi, I. (2022). Green Tea Catechins Attenuate Neurodegenerative Diseases and Cognitive Deficits. *Molecules*, 27(21), 7604.

Almeida-Toledano, L., Andreu-Fernández, V., Aras-López, R., García-Algar, Ó., Martínez, L., & Gómez-Roig, M. D. (2021). Epigallocatechin gallate ameliorates the effects of prenatal alcohol exposure in a fetal alcohol spectrum disorder-like mouse model. *International Journal of Molecular Sciences*, 22 (III), 715.

Amit, T., Avramovich-Tirosh, Y., Youdim, M. B., & Mandel, S. (2008). Targeting multiple Alzheimer's disease etiologies with multimodal neuroprotective and neurorestorative iron chelators. *The FASEB Journal*, 22(V), 1296-1305.

Beasley, M., Stonebraker, A. R., Hasan, I., Kapp, K. L., Liang, B. J., Agarwal, G., & Legleiter, J. (2019). Lipid membranes influence the ability of small molecules to inhibit huntingtin fibrillization. *Biochemistry*, 58(43), 4361-4373.

Che, F., Wang, G., Yu, J., Wang, X., Lu, Y., Fu, Q., & Du, Y. (2017). Effects of epigallocatechin 3 gallate on iron metabolism in spinal cord motor neurons. *Molecular medicine reports*, 16(III), 3010-3014.

de la Torre, R., de Sola, S., Hernandez, G., Farré, M., Pujol, J., Rodriguez, J., & Dierssen, M. (2016). Safety and efficacy of cognitive training plus epigallocatechin-3-gallate in young adults with Down's syndrome (TESDAD): a double-blind, randomised, placebo-controlled, phase 2 trial. *The Lancet Neurology*, 15(VIII), 801-810.

Haki, M., Al-Biati, H. A., Al-Tameemi, Z. S., Ali, I. S., & Al-Hussaniy, H. A. (2024). Review of multiple sclerosis: Epidemiology, etiology, pathophysiology, and treatment. *Medicine*, 103(VIII), e37297.

Jha, N. N., Kumar, R., Panigrahi, R., Navalkar, A., Ghosh, D., Sahay, S., & Maji, S. K. (2017). Comparison of α-synuclein fibril inhibition by four different amyloid inhibitors. *ACS chemical neuroscience*, 8(XII): 2722-2733.

Josiah, S. S., Famusiwa, C. D., Crown, O. O., Lawal, A. O., Olaleye, M. T., Akindahunsi, A. A., & Akinmoladun, A. C. (2022). Neuroprotective effects of catechin and quercetin in experimental Parkinsonism through modulation of dopamine metabolism and expression of IL-1β, TNF-α, NF-κB, IκKB, and p53 genes in male Wistar rats. *Neurotoxicology*, 90, 158-171.

Koh, S. H., Kwon, H., Kim, K. S., Kim, J., Kim, M. H., Yu, H. J., & Kim, S. H. (2004). Epigallocatechin gallate prevents oxidative-stress-induced death of mutant Cu/Zn-superoxide dismutase (G93A) motoneuron cells by alteration of cell survival and death signals. *Toxicology*, 202(III), 213-225.

Kumar, A., Sidhu, J., Goyal, A., & Tsao, J. W. (2023). *Alzheimer Disease*. [Updated 2022 Jun 5]. StatPearls [Internet]. Treasure Island (FL): StatPearls Publishing.

Kumari, S., Dhapola, R., & Reddy, D. H. (2023). Apoptosis in Alzheimer's disease: insight into the signaling pathways and therapeutic avenues. *Apoptosis*, 28(VII), 943-957.

Lee, J. H., Kim, H. J., Kim, J. U., Yook, T. H., Kim, K. H., Lee, J. Y., & Yang, G. (2021). A novel treatment strategy by natural products in NLRP3 inflammasome-mediated neuroinflammation in Alzheimer's and Parkinson's disease. *International journal of molecular sciences*, 22(III), 1324.

Li, Q., Han, X., Lan, X., Gao, Y., Wan, J., Durham, F., & Wang, J. (2017). Inhibition of neuronal ferroptosis protects hemorrhagic brain. *JCI insight*, 2(VII), e90777.

Liu, T. W., Chen, C. M., & Chang, K. H. (2022). Biomarker of neuroinflammation in Parkinson's disease. *International journal of molecular sciences*, 23(VIII), 4148.

Liu, Y., Qian, J., Li, J., Xing, M., Grierson, D., Sun, C., & Chen, K. (2022). Hydroxylation decoration patterns of flavonoids in horticultural crops: Chemistry, bioactivity, and biosynthesis. *Horticulture Research*, 9, uhab068.

Lovera, J., Ramos, A., Devier, D., Garrison, V., Kovner, B., Reza, T., & Bourdette, D. (2015). Polyphenon E, non-futile at neuroprotection in multiple sclerosis but unpredictably hepatotoxic: phase I single group and phase II randomized placebo-controlled studies. *Journal of the neurological sciences*, 358(I-II), 46-52.

Madeleine, P. V. M., Isabel, D. I. M., Daniel, O. S., & Esperanza, R. M. A. (2023). Neuroinflammation in fetal alcohol spectrum disorders and related novel therapeutic approaches. *Biochimica et Biophysica Acta (BBA)-Molecular Basis of Disease*, 1870(I), 166854.

Mandel, S., Weinreb, O., Amit, T., & Youdim, M. B. (2004). Cell signaling pathways in the neuroprotective actions of the green tea polyphenol (-)-epigallocatechin-3-gallate: implications for neurodegenerative diseases. *Journal of neurochemistry*, 88(VI), 1555-1569.

Morris, H. R., Spillantini, M. G., Sue, C. M., & Williams-Gray, C. H. (2024). The pathogenesis of Parkinson's disease. *The Lancet*, 403(10423), 293-304.

Novak, V., Rogelj, B., & Župunski, V. (2021). Therapeutic potential of polyphenols in amyotrophic lateral sclerosis and frontotemporal dementia. *Antioxidants*, 10(VIII): 1328.

Ou, J. (2021). Incorporation of polyphenols in baked products. In *Advances in food and nutrition research*, 98, 207-252.

Pervin, M., Unno, K., Ohishi, T., Tanabe, H., Miyoshi, N., & Nakamura, Y. (2018). Beneficial effects of green tea catechins on neurodegenerative diseases. *Molecules*, 23(VI), 1297.

Sebastiani, G., Almeida-Toledano, L., Serra-Delgado, M., Navarro-Tapia, E., Sailer, S., Valverde, O., & Andreu-Fernández, V. (2021). Therapeutic effects of catechins in less common neurological and neurodegenerative disorders. *Nutrients*, 13(VII), 2232.

Semnani, M., Mashayekhi, F., Azarnia, M., & Salehi, Z. (2017). Effects of green tea epigallocatechin-3-gallate on the proteolipid protein and oligodendrocyte transcription factor 1 messenger RNA gene expression in a mouse model of multiple sclerosis. *Folia Neuropathologica*, 55(III), 199-205.

Sharma, P., Kishore, A., De, I., Negi, S., Kumar, G., Bhardwaj, S., & Singh, M. (2023). Mitigating neuroinflammation in Parkinson's disease: Exploring the role of proinflammatory cytokines and the potential of phytochemicals as natural therapeutics. *Neurochemistry International*, 170, 105604.

Srinivasan, E., Chandrasekhar, G., Chandrasekar, P., Anbarasu, K., Vickram, A. S., Karunakaran, R., & Srikumar, P. S. (2021). Alpha-synuclein aggregation in Parkinson's disease. *Frontiers in medicine*, 8, 736978.

Subramaniam, S. R., & Chesselet, M. F. (2013). Mitochondrial dysfunction and oxidative stress in Parkinson's disease. *Progress in neurobiology*, 106, 17-32.

Teleanu, D. M., Niculescu, A. G., Lungu, I. I., Radu, C. I., Vladâcenco, O., Roza, E., & Teleanu, R. I. (2022). An overview of oxidative stress, neuroinflammation, and neurodegenerative diseases. *International journal of molecular sciences*, 23(XI), 5938.

Thanan, R., Oikawa, S., Hiraku, Y., Ohnishi, S., Ma, N., Pinlaor, S., & Murata, M. (2014). Oxidative stress and its significant roles in neurodegenerative diseases and cancer. *International journal of molecular sciences*, 16(I), 193-217.

Tiwari, V., Kuhad, A., & Chopra, K. (2010). Epigallocatechin-3-gallate ameliorates alcohol-induced cognitive dysfunctions and apoptotic neurodegeneration in the developing rat brain. *International Journal of Neuropsychopharmacology*, 13(VIII), 1053-1066.

Tseng, H. C., Wang, M. H., Chang, K. C., Soung, H. S., Fang, C. H., Lin, Y. W., & Tsai, C. C. (2020). Protective effect of (−) epigallocatechin-3-gallate on rotenone-induced parkinsonism-like symptoms in rats. *Neurotoxicity Research*, 37, 669-682.

Valverde-Salazar, V., Ruiz-Gabarre, D., & García-Escudero, V. (2023). Alzheimer's disease and green tea: epigallocatechin-3-gallate as a modulator of inflammation and oxidative stress. *Antioxidants*, 12(VII): 1460.

Varga, J., Dér, N. P., Zsindely, N., & Bodai, L. (2020). Green tea infusion alleviates neurodegeneration induced by mutant Huntingtin in Drosophila. *Nutritional neuroscience*, 23(III): 183-189.

Wang, J., Chen, Y., Chen, L., Duan, Y., Kuang, X., Peng, Z., & Tang, Y. (2020). EGCG modulates PKD1 and ferroptosis to promote recovery in ST rats. *Translational Neuroscience*, 11(I): 173-181.

Wang, L., Yin, Y. L., Liu, X. Z., Shen, P., Zheng, Y. G., Lan, X. R., & Wang, J. Z. (2020). Current understanding of metal ions in the pathogenesis of Alzheimer's disease. *Translational neurodegeneration*, 9: 1-13.

Wang, Y., Gao, L., Chen, J., Li, Q., Huo, L., Wang, Y., & Du, J. (2021). Pharmacological modulation of Nrf2/HO-1 signaling pathway as a therapeutic target of Parkinson's disease. *Frontiers in pharmacology*, 12: 757161.

Wang, Y., Wu, S., Li, Q., Lang, W., Li, W., Jiang, X., & Wang, H. (2022). Epigallocatechin-3-gallate: A phytochemical as a promising drug candidate for the treatment of Parkinson's disease. *Frontiers in pharmacology*, 13, 977521.

Weinreb, O., Amit, T., Mandel, S., & Youdim, M. B. (2009). Neuroprotective molecular mechanisms of (−)-epigallocatechin-3-gallate: a reflective outcome of its antioxidant, iron chelating and neuritogenic properties. *Genes & nutrition*, 4, 283-296.

Xu, Z., Chen, S., Li, X., Luo, G., Li, L., & Le, W. (2006). Neuroprotective effects of (-)-epigallocatechin-3-gallate in a transgenic mouse model of amyotrophic lateral sclerosis. *Neurochemical research*, 31, 1263-1269.

Zetterberg, H., & Bendlin, B. B. (2021). Biomarkers for Alzheimer's disease—preparing for a new era of disease-modifying therapies. *Molecular psychiatry*, 26(I), 296-308.

Chapter 12

Huperzine A: A Natural Cholinesterase Inhibitor

Aditya Kumar[1]
Akash Jain[1]
Arjun Singh[1]
Sonia Kamboj[2]
and Jasmine Chaudhary[1,*]
[1]M. M. College of Pharmacy, M. M. (Deemed to be University), Mullana, Ambala, Haryana, India
[2]Ch. Devi Lal College of Pharmacy, Jagadhri, Yamuna Nagar, Haryana, India

Abstract

Huperzine A (HupA), a sesquiterpenoid alkaloid derived from Huperzia serrata (toothed clubmoss), a traditional Chinese herb in the Lycopodiaceae family, is a potent, specific, and reversible acetylcholinesterase inhibitor (AChE). Its superior oral bioavailability, prolonged duration of action, and enhanced ability to cross the blood-brain barrier make it comparable to other synthetic acetylcholinesterase inhibitors, such as tacrine, rivastigmine, and donepezil. HupA's neuroprotective effects are linked to its ability to mitigate mitochondrial damage by regulating oxidative stress, modulating the expression of anti-apoptotic proteins, and influencing nerve growth factors and their receptors. Additionally, HupA interferes with amyloid precursor protein metabolism and NMDA receptor activity, thereby reducing glutamate toxicity. By activating the MAPK/ERK signaling pathway and regulating

* Corresponding Author's Email: jasmine.jain@mmmullana.org.

In: Natural Solutions for Neurodegenerative Disorders
Editors: Rahul Kumar Sharma, Shailesh Sharma, Ajmer Singh Grewal et al.
ISBN: 979-8-89530-231-6

cell proliferation and differentiation, HupA offers promising potential for managing Alzheimer's-related dementia and promoting neurogenesis. Therefore, this chapter aims to emphasize the role of huperzine A in various neurodegenerative disorders, particularly its function as an acetylcholinesterase inhibitor.

Keywords: huperzine, Alzheimer's, anti-cholinesterase, neuroprotective, Chinese herb, HupA

Abbreviations

AChE	acetylcholinesterase
ADL	Activities of daily living scale
Aβ	Amyloid-beta
CAT	Catalase
GSH	Glutathione
HupA	Huperzine A
HupB	Huperzine B
NMDA	N-methyl D-aspartate
PKC	Protein kinase C
SOD	Superoxide dismutase
TCA	Tricarboxylic acid

Introduction

Huperzia serrata, also known as Lycopodium serratum (Qian Ceng Ta), belongs to the family Huperziaceae and has been traditionally used in Chinese medicine for the treatment of hematological, cardiovascular, and neurological disorders since ancient times (Ishiuchi et al., 2013; Thiet al., 2019). The plant's diverse biological activities are likely attributed to its chemical constituents, including alkaloids, flavanols, triterpenes, and phenolic acids. Among these, the four major alkaloid types—lycodine, fawcettimine, lycopodine, and miscellaneous alkaloids—exhibit acetylcholinesterase (AChE) inhibitory activity. However, lycodine-type alkaloids such as huperzine A (HupA), huperzine B (HupB), huperzinine, and 6-hydroxy huperzine are of particular interest due to their significant potential in managing dementia (memory dysfunction associated with Alzheimer's disease), schizophrenia, and other conditions as AChE inhibitors (Ferreira et al., 2014; Howes et al., 2017). Huperzine A (Figure 1), chemically known as 1-amino-13-ethylidene-11-methyl-6-azatricyclotridecatrienone (Fog. 1), is an unsaturated terpenoidal compound first isolated from Huperzia serrata in China in 1948 (Siengalewicze et al., 2013). The strong AChE inhibitory activity of HupA has led to overharvesting of its natural source, putting the species at risk of becoming endangered (Tun et al., 2012). Efforts to increase the yield of HupA through in-vitro production using tissue culture have been made (Ma and Gang, 2008). Despite the challenges of low yield and the unique pharmacological properties of HupA, researchers have sought alternative sources. The first successful synthesis of HupA was achieved by Kozikowski in 1989, with subsequent improvements by other researchers (Rui et al., 2012). This led to the development of a novel class of hybrid compounds known as "huprines," which combine synthetic AChE drugs with HupA, offering better receptor binding affinity and fewer adverse effects (Ros et al., 2001). In addition to its neuroprotective role, HupA has been found to be effective in treating various conditions, including fever, rheumatism, inflammation, strains, bruising, and myasthenia gravis (Skolnick, 1997). HupA's anxiolytic activity has also been reported in rats (Jaswinder et al., 2017), and it has shown protective effects against isoproterenol-induced myocardial injury in rats through the regulation of the PI3K/Akt signaling pathway (Lili and Wang, 2021). Furthermore, HupA has demonstrated beneficial effects in cases of organophosphorus poisoning (Balali and Sabre, 2012).

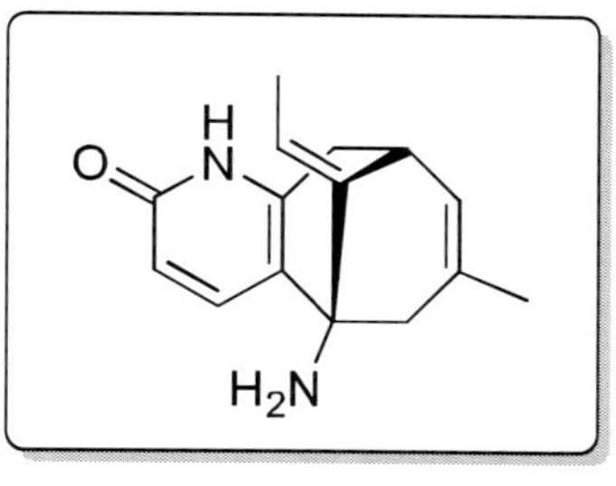

Figure 1. Structure of Huperzine A.

The traditional Chinese medicine HupA gained recognition in the West around 2003 for its ability to enhance cognitive function by maintaining adequate levels of acetylcholine. Low acetylcholine levels are associated with memory impairment and dementia, and HupA works by inhibiting acetylcholinesterase (AChE), the enzyme responsible for breaking down acetylcholine (Howes & Perry, 2011; Kumar et al., 2024). This inhibition helps sustain acetylcholine levels, thereby improving memory and cognitive function (Andrea et al., 2003). HupA is sometimes taken as a dietary supplement to boost cognitive abilities (Xing et al., 2014; Yang et al., 2013). However, when combined with other drugs that increase acetylcholine levels, it may produce additive cholinergic effects, and significant bradycardia has been reported when used with beta-blockers in cardiovascular patients. The primary cholinergic side effects are mild and include nausea, vomiting, diarrhea, hyperactivity, disorientation, and anorexia when taken for 1-3 months at the recommended dosage (Ferreira et al., 2014). Notably, unlike tacrine, HupA has not been associated with hepatotoxicity (Xu et al., 1995).

Acetylcholine and Alzheimer's Disease

Acetylcholine, a neurotransmitter in the parasympathetic nervous system, plays a crucial role in maintaining cognitive functions (Xiao et al., 2002). Alzheimer's disease (AD), a progressive neurodegenerative disorder, primarily leads to dementia, characterized by memory loss, cognitive decline, and behavioral abnormalities. While the exact cause of AD remains unclear, several factors involved in cognitive functions, such as the loss of cholinergic neurons, intracellular neurofibrillary tangles (NFTs), senile plaques with extracellular amyloid-beta (Aβ) deposits, and significant synaptic changes in specific brain regions, are recognized as clinical markers of the disease (Chaudhary et al., 2023). Cholinergic dysfunction, specifically the deficiency of acetylcholine, is identified as a primary factor contributing to the symptoms associated with Alzheimer's. Studies have shown that a decrease in cortical cholinergic activity correlates with lower mental exam scores in Alzheimer's patients (Yang et al., 2013). Consequently, acetylcholinesterase inhibitors (AChEIs) are among the preferred therapeutic options for enhancing cholinergic transmission and have shown significant potential in treating Alzheimer's disease (Chen et al., 2022). Acetylcholinesterase (AChE) is responsible for breaking down acetylcholine into choline in the brain; thus, inhibiting this enzyme leads to increased acetylcholine levels, thereby supporting the normal functioning of the cholinergic system.

Huperzine A: A Naturally Derived Inhibitor of Acetylcholinesterase (AChE)

The cholinergic, or parasympathetic, nervous system relies heavily on the enzyme AChE for its proper functioning. AChE is responsible for catalyzing the hydrolysis of acetylcholine (ACh) into choline and acetate ions, a crucial step in terminating neurotransmission at cholinergic synapses (Figure 2). Structurally, AChE is characterized by a large hydrophobic cavity at its center, which includes specific binding sites such as the esteric (ES) site and an anionic substrate binding site. The positively charged quaternary amine group of acetylcholine binds to the anionic site of AChE. At the bottom of the enzyme's cavity, the esteric site is composed of key amino acids such as Serine 200, Glutamate 327, and Histidine 440, which play a critical role in the catalytic breakdown of ACh. Additionally, AChE possesses an "acyl pocket," which is essential for controlling substrate selectivity, and an "oxyanion hole" that stabilizes the transition state during catalysis by binding to the negatively charged oxygen ions. These specialized regions work together to enhance the overall catalytic efficiency of AChE, making it highly effective at rapidly degrading acetylcholine (Huang et al., 2014). The cholinergic, or parasympathetic, nervous system is primarily dependent on AChE. Acetylcholinesterase is an enzyme catalyzing the conversion of ACh into choline and acetate ions (Figure 2). AChE consists of a large hydrophobic cavity (centre) along with an esteric (ES) and an anionic substrate binding site. The positively charged quaternary amines (cationic substrates) in ACh bind to the anionic site, whereas Ser 200, Glu 327, and His 440 binds to the esteric site at the bottom. Along with these specialized areas, it also has an "acyl pocket" that controls substrate selectivity and an "oxyanion part" that helps AChE bind to negative oxygen ions during catalysis, increasing AChE's overall efficiency (Huang et al., 2014).

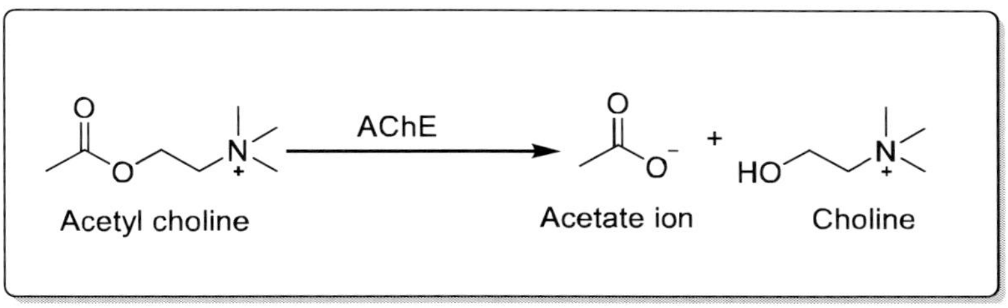

Figure 2. Metabolism of Acetylcholine by AChE.

Numerous studies have validated the neuroprotective effects of HupA in treating AD, primarily through its inhibition of AChE. HupA exhibits both cholinergic and non-cholinergic actions, with its potency and duration of AChE inhibition comparable to other well-known acetylcholinesterase inhibitors like tacrine, galantamine, donepezil, rivastigmine, and physostigmine (Tang and Han, 1999). The mode of action of HupA as an anticholinesterase has been well-documented in various studies (Raves et al., 1997).

Other Pathways Responsible for the Neuroprotective Action of Huperzine A (Qian and Ke, 2014)

Increasing acetylcholine levels at synapses can enhance acetylcholine transport, helping to alleviate cognitive issues associated with Alzheimer's disease. Beyond its role as an AChE inhibitor, HupA offers several additional medicinal benefits. It reduces oxidative stress, promotes the synthesis and release of neural growth factors, and influences the β-amyloid transition, thereby mitigating neuronal death linked to cognitive and memory decline. HupA also inhibits the production of amyloid precursor proteins, preventing amyloid accumulation in cells and enhancing cell viability by boosting antioxidant enzyme activity. Research indicates that overexpression of TP53 and BAX genes contributes to apoptosis, while overexpression of BCL-2 has an anti-apoptotic effect (Orhan et al., 2011). Both HupA and HupB are effective AChE inhibitors. HupB, while being a potent and reversible AChE inhibitor with fewer cholinergic side effects compared to HupA, has slightly less potency. Nonetheless, both HupA and HupB are effective in slowing the onset of dementia and possess notable neuroprotective qualities (Zhang et al., 2000).

Anti-Oxidant and Anti-Apoptotic Effects in Aβ-Stimulated Oxidative Stress and Injury

Oxidative stress, primarily driven by the overexpression of Aβ-protein, is a key factor in neurodegenerative diseases such as Alzheimer's, leading to neurotoxicity and cell death (Xiao et al., 2002). Effective management of oxidative stress—either by inhibiting Aβ-protein production and aggregation or by enhancing its clearance—can be a promising strategy for controlling these conditions. Elevated levels of malondialdehyde (MDA) are commonly used as markers for oxidative stress (Gawel et al., 2004). HupA has been shown to reduce MDA levels in rat pheochromocytoma (PC-12) cells, highlighting its potential in combating oxidative stress (Xiao et al., 1999). HupA demonstrates neuroprotective effects in the context of Aβ-induced oxidative stress through its antioxidant and anti-apoptotic properties, which enhance neuronal cell viability (Michelle et al., 2022). It inhibits Aβ-induced apoptosis by decreasing caspase-3 activity, a critical protein in the apoptotic cascade, thus exerting anti-apoptotic effects (Xiao et al., 2002). Additionally, HupA mitigates Aβ-induced and hydrogen peroxide-induced apoptosis by reversing the upregulation of p53 and Bax, while also increasing Bcl-2 expression (Wang et al., 2001).

NMDA Receptor Antagonistic Effects

Binding HupA to NMDA receptors is another effective strategy for reducing NMDA-induced neuronal damage. HupA inhibits NMDA ion channel activity and the associated calcium ion movement at the PCP and MK-801 ligand sites, thereby mitigating NMDA-induced harm (Zhang and Hu, 2001). It has been shown to suppress NMDA-induced damage in primary neuronal cells (Marx, 2000; Zhang and Tang, 2006). Overexpression of the glutamate receptor, particularly NMDA receptors, is a significant factor contributing to neuronal cell death in neurodegenerative diseases such as Alzheimer's. Excessive glutamate stimulation of NMDA receptors leads to a harmful influx of calcium ions into nerve cells, ultimately causing cell death. HupA's ability to block these glutamate receptors offers neuroprotective effects by preventing this excitotoxicity (Wang et al., 1999).

Improvement in Brain Mitochondrial Dysfunction

Alzheimer's patients frequently experience mitochondrial dysfunction characterized by impaired TCA enzyme complexes, reduced cytochrome c oxidase activity, and diminished ATP production (Cardoso et al., 2001). This dysfunction disrupts mitochondrial membrane integrity and homeostasis, and chronic mitochondrial malfunction contributes to the deposition of amyloid-beta (Aβ), a hallmark of Alzheimer's disease (Yao et al., 2011). Aβ interacts with Aβ-binding alcohol dehydrogenase, a mitochondrial enzyme, leading to oxidative stress and reduced cytochrome c oxidase activity, which results in neurotoxicity (Reddy and Beal, 2008). HupA has been shown to effectively prevent Aβ-induced mitochondrial dysfunction in PC12 cells. It enhances the activity of TCA cycle enzymes, restricts cytochrome c release, and decreases intracellular reactive oxygen species (ROS) generation (Yang et al., 2012). Additionally, HupA alleviates Aβ-induced cellular stress markers, providing protective benefits against mitochondrial dysfunction in isolated rat brains (Gao et al., 2006).

The Enhancement of Non-Amyloidogenic APP Processing

a) Via the WNT-signalling pathway

The Wnt signaling pathway plays a crucial role in the growth and development of the nervous system, and disruptions in this pathway can lead to neurological disorders (Ferrari et al., 2003). In Alzheimer's disease, Aβ-induced neurodegeneration results in the inactivation of Wnt signaling through alterations in key components, including GSK-3β and β-catenin, in mouse models (Farias et al., 2005; Wang et al., 2011). HupA has been shown to stimulate the Wnt signaling pathway in APP/PS1 mouse models of Alzheimer's disease. HupA exerts neuroprotective effects against Aβ fibril-induced damage by suppressing GSK-3β activity and enhancing β-catenin activity, thus promoting the recovery of this critical signaling pathway and protecting against neurodegeneration (Farias et al., 2005; Wang et al., 2011).

b) Via protein kinase C activation

HupA inhibits the non-amyloidogenic processing of amyloid precursor protein (APP) by blocking protein kinase C (PKC). This action alters β-catenin levels and inactivates glycogen synthase kinase-3β (GSK-3β). By interfering with these pathways, HupA can help modulate the processing of APP and potentially reduce the accumulation of amyloid-β (Aβ), contributing to its neuroprotective effects in Alzheimer's disease (Wang et al., 2011).

Regulation of Iron Levels in the Brain

The imbalance of iron levels in the brain is a significant factor in the development of neurodegenerative disorders (Lei et al., 2012). HupA has been shown to effectively reduce the accumulation of amyloid-β (Aβ) peptides and hyperphosphorylated tau protein in the brains of APP/PS1 transgenic mice, which are models for Alzheimer's disease (Huang et al., 2014). HupA also regulates elevated brain iron levels in the cortex and hippocampal regions of these animals, contributing to its neuroprotective effects. Additionally, recent research has demonstrated the neuroprotective effects of HupA-loaded nanoliposomes against chronic intermittent hypoxia-induced neuronal damage (Yang et al., 2023).

Regulation of Nerve Growth Factor (NGF)

NGFs are crucial for neuronal growth and function by activating tropomyosin receptor kinase A (TrkA). This activation triggers intracellular signaling pathways that promote neuronal survival and development (Huang and Reichard, 2003). Research has shown that HupA significantly enhances the mRNA and protein levels of NGF in brain cells, which may contribute to its neurotrophic effects, either directly or indirectly (Tang et al., 2005).

In Vitro Effects and Preclinical Studies on HupA

HupA inhibits acetylcholinesterase (AChE) in a reversible, competitive, strong, and selective manner. *In vitro* studies reveal that HupA shows greater specificity and potency for AChE compared to physostigmine, rivastigmine, tacrine, and galantamine, though it is less potent than donepezil (Cheng et al., 1996; Zhang et al., 2012). After intramuscular injection, acetylcholine levels increase progressively, reaching up to 40% within an hour (Tang et al., 1989). The effect of HupA on acetylcholine levels varies across different brain regions, with the frontal and parietal cortices showing the most significant increase after an hour, while the hippocampus and striatum show moderate increases at thirty minutes (Xing et al., 2014). HupA also increases acetylcholine levels in the brain by inhibiting AChE activity, with effects lasting up to 360 minutes (Tang et al., 1989). It has been shown to reduce memory impairment in various rat models, including elderly, cognitively challenged, and healthy adult rats, and improves spatial memory performance (Grunwald et al., 1994). HupA's cholinergic effects have been compared with synthetic HupA in rat brains, demonstrating its effectiveness (Tang et al., 1994). Additionally, oral HupA administration restores choline acetyltransferase activity in the hippocampus of chronically hypoperfused rats (Wang et al., 2000). HupA has also shown substantial neuroprotection against amyloid ß-peptide exposure in rat cortical neurons (Birks et al., 2006) and protective effects against oxygen-glucose deprivation-induced injury in rat pheochromocytoma cell lines by targeting oxidative energy metabolism (Christodoulou et al., 2006). Furthermore, HupA demonstrates beneficial effects in streptozotocin-induced diabetes with cognitive decline in rats, regulating oxidative stress, inflammation, and apoptosis in a dose-dependent manner (Mao et al., 2014).

Clinical Studies on HupA

The impact of HupA has been investigated in various studies, demonstrating its potential as a cognitive enhancer and therapeutic agent for Alzheimer's disease. The first study assessing HupA involved 34 junior high school students experiencing feelings of inadequacy and forgetfulness. This double-blind, matched-pair trial revealed that administering 0.1 mg of HupA twice daily for one month led to improvements in scores for buildup, recognition, and association (Sun et al., 1999). In the same year, another study found that patients receiving either 50 μg or 100 μg of HupA twice daily for 12 weeks showed improvements in their Mini-Mental State Examination (MMSE) scores. The higher dose group had better scores, with no significant adverse effects reported (Mazurek, 1999). HupA is widely used in China for enhancing cognitive function in Alzheimer's disease management (Chen, 2000). A study with 454 Alzheimer's patients indicated that HupA positively affects cognitive, behavioral, and functional issues with minimal side effects (Li, 2008). Additionally, a study involving 210 Alzheimer's patients with mild to moderate severity found that a dose of 0.4 mg of HupA for 16 weeks improved cognitive function (Rafii, 2011). Xing et al., (2014) conducted a meta-analysis of placebo-controlled RCTs with around 733 Alzheimer patients and observed improvements in MMSE and Activities of Daily Living (ADL) scores. Pharmacokinetic studies show that HupA is rapidly absorbed and distributed in the body, with moderate elimination after oral administration (Wang et al.,

2006). Toxicity studies in various animal species and healthy volunteers have not revealed any unanticipated toxicity (Yan et al., 1987).

Conclusion

HupA, a natural anticholinesterase molecule, is known for its neuroprotective effects due to its ability to enhance the activity of various antioxidant enzymes such as GSH-Px, SOD, and CAT. This enhancement helps protect neurons from Aβ-induced oxidative injury and cell death. HupA also prevents Aβ-induced cell death by reversing the downregulation of BCL-2 and the upregulation of Bax and p53. By blocking NMDA receptors and the subsequent mobilization of Ca2+, HupA mitigates NMDA-induced toxicity. It reduces Aβ-induced mitochondrial dysfunction by improving mitochondrial integrity and energy metabolism while inhibiting ROS production, thus preventing Aβ from penetrating mitochondria. Additionally, HupA promotes the Wnt/β-catenin signaling pathway and increases nerve growth factor levels. These combined actions contribute to HupA's beneficial effects in neurodegenerative disorders.

References

Aloe, L., Rocco, M. L., Branching, P., and Mani, L. (2012). Nerve growth factor: from the early discoveries to the potential clinical use. *Journal of Translational Medicine*, 10: 239.

Andrea, Z. (2003). The psychopharmacology of huperzine A: an alkaloid with cognitive enhancing and neuroprotective properties of interest in the treatment of Alzheimer's disease. *Pharmacology Biochemistry and Behavior*, 75(3): 675-686.

Balali, M. M., and Saber, H. (2012). Recent advances in the treatment of organophosphorous poisonings. *Iranian Journal of Medical Sciences*, 37(2):74-91.

Birks, J. (2006). Cholinesterase inhibitors for Alzheimer's disease. Cochrane Database *Systematic Reviews*, 1: 1-13.

Cardoso, S. M., Santos, S., Swerdlow, R. H., and Oliveira, C. R. (2001). Functional mitochondria are required for amyloid beta-mediated neurotoxicity. *FASEB Journal*, 15: 1439–1441.

Chaudhary, J., Jain, A., Dhingra, A., Chopra, B., Sharma, V., Gupta, J., and Kaushik, A. (2023). 1,3-thiazole Derivatives: A scaffold with considerable potential in the treatment of neurodegenerative diseases. *Current Topics in Medicinal Chemistry*, 23(23): 2185–2196.

Chen, M. J., Gao, Z. X., Deng, H. Y., Liu, F. G., Ma, Y. X. (2000). Huperzine A capsules (upsilon) tablets in the treatment of Alzheimer disease: multicenter studies. *Chinese Journal of New Drugs and Clinical Remedies*, 19: 10-12.

Chen, Z. R., Huang, J. B., Yang, S. L., and Hong, F. F. (2022). Role of cholinergic signaling in Alzheimer's disease. *Molecules*, 27(6): 1816.

Cheng, D. H., Ren, H., Tang, X. C. (1996). Huperzine A, a novel promising acetylcholinesterase inhibitor. *Neuroreports*, 8: 97-101.

Christodoulou, C., Melville, P., Scherl, W. F., Macallister, W. S., Elkins, L. E., and Krupp, L. B. (2006). Effects of donepezil on memory and cognition in multiple sclerosis. *Journal of Neurological Sciences*, 245: 127-136.

De Ferrari, G. V., Chacon, M. A., Barria, M. I., Garrido, J. L., Godoy, J. A., Olivares, G., Reyes, A. E., Alvarez, A., Bronfman, M., Inestrosa, N. C. (2003). Activation of Wnt signaling rescues neurodegeneration and behavioral impairments induced by beta-amyloid fibrils. *Molecular Psychiatry*, 8: 195–208.

Farias, G. G., Godoy, J. A., Vazquez, M. C., Adani, R., Meshulam, H., Avila, J., Amitai, G., and Inestrosa, N. C. (2005). The anti-inflammatory and cholinesterase inhibitor bifunctional compound IBU-PO protects from beta-amyloid neurotoxicity by acting on Wnt signaling components. Neurobiology of Disease, 18: 176–183.

Ferreira, A., Rodrigues, M., Fortuna, A., Falcao, A., and Alves, G. (2014). Huperzine A from *Huperzia serrata*: A review of its sources, chemistry, pharmacology and toxicology. *Phytochemistry Reviews*, 15: 51–85.

Gao, X., and Tang, X. C. (2006). Huperzine A attenuates mitochondrial dysfunction in beta-amyloid-treated PC12 cells by reducing oxygen free radicals accumulation and improving mitochondrial energy metabolism. *Journal of Neuroscience Research*, 83: 1048–1057.

Gaweł, S., Wardas, M., Niedworok, E., and Wardas, P. (2004). Malondialdehyde (MDA) as a lipid peroxidation marker. *Wiadomoscilekarskie*, 57(9-10): 453–455.

Grunwald, J., Raveh, L., Doctor, B. P., and Ashani, Y. (1994). Huperzine A as a pretreatment candidate drug against nerve agent toxicity. *Life Sciences*, 54: 991-97.

Hai, Y. Z., and Xi, C. T. (2006). Neuroprotective effects of huperzine A: new therapeutic targets for neurodegenerative disease. *Trends in Pharmacological Sciences*, 27(12): 619–625.

Howes, M. J., and Perry, E. (2011). The role of phytochemicals in the treatment and prevention of dementia. *Drugs Aging*, 28: 439–468.

Howes, M. R., Fang, R., Houghton, P. J. (2017). Effect of Chinese Herbal Medicine on Alzheimer's Disease. *International Review of Neurobiology*, 135: 29–56.

Huang, E. J., and Reichard, L. F. (2003). TRK receptors: roles in neuronal signal transduction. Annual Reviews in Biochemistry, 72: 609–642.

Huang, X. T., Qian, Z. M., He, X., Gong, Q., Wu, K. C., Jiang, L. R., Lu, L. N., Zhu, Z. J., Zhang, H. Y., Yung, W. H, Ke, Y. (2014). Reducing iron in the brain: a novel pharmacologic mechanism of huperzine A in the treatment of Alzheimer's disease. *Neurobiology of Aging*, 35: 1045–1054.

Ishiuchi, K., Park, J. J., Long, R. M., and Gang, D.R. (2013). Production of huperzine A and other Lycopodium alkaloids in Huperzia species grown under controlled conditions and *in vitro*. *Phytochemistry*, 91: 208–219.

Jaswinder, K., Singh, R., Singh, P., Kaur, J., and Kaur, H. (2017). Anxiolytic and motor coordination activity of Huperzine-A in rats. *International Journal of Pharmaceutical Sciences and Research*, 2017:2560-2566.

Kumar, G., Pratap, G. K., Poornima D. V., Shantaram, M., Ranjita, G. (2024). Natural acetylcholinesterase inhibitors: A multi-targeted therapeutic potential in Alzheimer's disease. *European Journal of Medicinal Chemistry Reports*, 11: 1-16.

Lei, P., Ayton, S., Finkelstein, D. I., Spoerri, L., Ciccotosto, G. D., Wright, D. K., Wong, B. X., Adlard, P. A., Cherny, R. A., Lam, L. Q., Roberts, B. R., Volitakis, I., Egan, G. F., McLean, C. A., Cappai, R., Duce, J. A., and Bush, A. I. (2012). Tau deficiency induces parkinsonism with dementia by impairing APP-mediated iron export. Nature Medicine, 18: 291–295.

Li, J., Wu, H. M., Zhou, R. L., Liu, G. J., and Dong, B. R. (2008). Huperzine A for Alzheimer's disease. *Cochrane Database of Systematic Reviews*, 2: 1-10.

Lili, L., and Fengnian, W. (2021). Protective effect of huperzine A against isoproterenol induced myocardial damage in rats via regulation of PI3K/Akt signaling pathway. *Tropical Journal of Pharmaceutical Research*, 20(5): 953-959.

Ma, X., and Gang, D. R. (2008). *In vitro* production of huperzine A, a promising drug candidate for Alzheimer's disease. *Phytochemistry*, 69: 2022–2028.

Mao, X. Y, Cao, D. F., Li, X., Yin, J. Y., Wang, Z. B., Zhang, Y., Mao, C. X., Zhou, H. H., and Liu, Z. Q. (2014). Huperzine A ameliorates cognitive deficits in streptozotocin-induced diabetic rats. *International Journal of Molecular Sciences*, 15(5): 7667-7683.

Marx, J. (2000). Alzheimer's Congress. Drug shows promise for advanced disease. *Science*, 289: 375–377.

Mazurek A. (1999). An open label trial of huperzine A in the treatment of Alzheimer's disease. *Alternative Therapies in Health and Medicine*, 5: 97-8

Michelle, M. R., Luciclaudio, C. A., Joao, V. O. A., Irivania, F. S. A., Fernanda, G.S. O., Marccia, V. S., Maria, T. C. S. (2022). The promising role of natural products in Alzheimer's disease. *Brain Disorders*, 7: 1-12.

Orhan, I. E., Orhan, G., and Gurkas, E. (2011). An overview on natural cholinesterase inhibitors—A multi-targeted drug class-and their mass production. *Mini Reviews in Medicinal Chemistry*, 11: 836–842

Qian, Z. M. and Ke, Y. (2014). Huperzine A: Is it an effective disease-modifying drug for Alzheimer's disease? *Frontiers in Aging Neuroscience*, 6:216.

Rafii, M. S., Walsh, S., Little, J. T., Behan, K., Reynolds, B., Ward, C., Jin, S., Thomas, R., Aisen, P. S. (2011). A phase II trial of huperzine A in mild to moderate Alzheimer disease. *Neurology*, 76(16): 1389-94.

Raves, M. L., Harel, M., Pang, Y. P., Silman, I., Kozikowski, A. P., and Sussman, J. L. (1997). Structure of acetylcholinesterase complexed with the nootropic alkaloid, (–)-Huperzine A. *Nature Structural & Molecular Biology*, 4: 57–63.

Reddy, P. H., and Beal, M. F. (2008). Amyloid beta, mitochondrial dysfunction and synaptic damage: implications for cognitive decline in aging and Alzheimer's disease. *Trends in Molecular Medicine*, 14: 45–53.

Ros, E., Aleu, J., Gomez de Aranda, I., Munoz-Torrero, D., Camps, P., Badia, A., Marsal, J., and Solsona, C. (2001). The pharmacology of novel acetylcholinesterase inhibitors, (+/-)-huprines Y and X, on the Torpedo electric organ. *European Journal of Pharmacology*, 421(2): 77–84.

Rui, D., Bing, F. S., and Guo, Q. L. (2012). An efficient total synthesis of (−)- Huperzine A. *Organic Letters*, 14(17): 4446–4449.

Siengalewicz, P., Johann, M., and Uwe R. (2013). Chapter One - Lycopodium Alkaloids – Synthetic highlights and recent developments in the alkaloids. *Chemistry and Biology*, 72: 1-151.

Skolnick, A. A. (1997). Old Chinese herbal medicine used for fever yields possible new Alzheimer disease therapy. *JAMA*, 277(10): 776.

Sun, Q. Q., Xu, S. S., Pan, L., Guo, H. M., and Cao, W. Q. (1999). Huperzine-A capsules enhance memory and learning performance in 34 pairs of matched adolescent students. *Acta Pharmacologica Sinica*, 20: 601-03.

Tang, L., Wang, R. and Tang, X. (2005). Effects of huperzine A on secretion of nerve growth factor in cultured rat cortical astrocytes and neurite outgrowth in rat PC12 cells. *Acta Pharmacologica Sinica*, 26: 673–678.

Tang, X. C., and Han, Y. F. (1999). Pharmacological profile of huperzine A, a novel acety1cholinesterase inhibitor from Chinese herb. *CNS Drug Reviews*, 5: 281-300.

Tang, X. C., De Sarno, P., Sugaya, K., and Giacobini E. (1989). Effect of huperzine A, a new cholinesterase inhibitor, on the central cholinergic system of the rat. *Neuroscience Research*, 24: 276-85.

Tang, X. C., Kindel, G. H., Kozikowski, A. P., and Hanin, I. (1994). Comparison of the effects of natural and synthetic huperzine-A on rat brain cholinergic function *in vitro* and *in vivo*. *Journal of Ethnopharmacology*, 44(3): 147-55.

Thi, M. L. T., Thi, H. H. A., Thi, B. L. T., Thi, B. V. T., Van, Q. D., and Hoang C. H. (2019). Isolation of endophytic fungi and screening of Huperzine A-producing fungus from *Huperzia serrata* in Vietnam. *Scientific reports*, 9(1): 1-13.

Tun, M. K., and Herzon, S. B. (2012). The pharmacology and therapeutic potential of (-)-huperzine A. *Journal of Experimental Pharmacology*, 4: 113-23.

Wang, C. Y., Zheng, W., Wang, T., Xie, J. W., Wang, S. L., Zhao, B. L., Amitai, G., and Inestrosa, N. C. (2011). Huperzine A activates Wnt/β-catenin signaling and enhances the nonamyloidogenic pathway in an Alzheimer transgenic mouse model. *Neuropsychopharmacology*, 36: 1073–1089.

Wang, L. M., Yi, F. H., and Xi, C. T. (2000). Huperzine A improves cognitive deficits caused by chronic cerebral hypoperfusion in rats. *European Journal of Pharmacology*, 398(1): 65-72.

Wang, R., Han, Y., Tang, X. (2006). Progress in studies of huperzine A, a natural cholinesterase inhibitor from Chinese herbal medicine. *Acta Pharmacologica Sinica*, 27 (1): 1-26.

Wang, R., Xiao, X. Q., and Tang, X. C. (2001). Huperzine A attenuates hydrogen peroxide-induced apoptosis by regulating expression of apoptosis-related genes in rat PC12 cells. *Neuroreport*, 12(12): 2629–2634.

Wang, X. D., Zhang, M., Yang, H. H., and Hu, G. (1999). Modulation of NMDA receptor by huperzine A in rat cerebral cortex. *Acta Pharmacologica Sinica*, 20: 31-35.

Xiao, X. Q., Yang, J. W., and Tang, X. C. (1999). Huperzine A protects rat pheochromocytoma cells against hydrogen peroxide-induced injury. *Neuroscience letters*, 275(2): 73–76.

Xiao, X. Q., Zhang, H. Y., and Tang, X. C. (2002). Huperzine A attenuates amyloid beta-peptide fragment 25–35-induced apoptosis in rat cortical neurons via inhibiting reactive oxygen species formation and caspase-3 activation. *Journal of Neuroscience Research*, 67: 30–36.

Xing, S. H., Zhu, C. X., Zhang, R., and An, L. (2014). Huperzine a in the treatment of Alzheimer's disease and vascular dementia: a meta-analysis. *Evidence Based Complementary and Alternative Medicine*, 2014: 1-15.

Xu, S. S., Gao, Z. X., Weng, Z., Du, Z. M., Xu, W. A., Yang, J. S., Zhang, M. L., Tong, Z. H., Fang, Y. S., and Chai, X. S. (1995). Efficacy of tablet huperzine-A on memory, cognition, and behavior in Alzheimer's disease. *Acta Pharmacologica Sinica*, 16: 391-95.

Yan, X. F., Lu, W. H., Lou, W., and Tang, X. C. (1987). Effects of huperzine A and B on skeletal muscle and the electroencephalogram (Chinese). *Acta Pharmacologica Sinica*, 8: 117-23.

Yang, G., Wang, Y., Tian, J., and Liu, J. P. (2013). Huperzine A for Alzheimer's disease: a systematic review and meta-analysis of randomized clinical trials. PLoS ONE, 8(9): 1-13.

Yang, L., Ye, C. Y., Huang, X. T., Tang, X. C., and Zhang, H. Y. (2012). Decreased accumulation of subcellular amyloid-beta with improved mitochondrial function mediates the neuroprotective effect of huperzine A. *Journal of Alzheimer Disease*, 31: 131–142.

Yang, X. Y., Geng, L., Li, R., Song, J. X., Jia, C. L., An, J. R., Sun, M. F., Xu, S., Guo, Y. J., Zhao, Y., and Ji, E. S. (2023). Huperzine A-liposomes efficiently improve neural injury in the hippocampus of mice with chronic intermittent hypoxia. *International Journal of Nanomedicine*, 18: 843-859.

Yao, J., Rettberg, J. R., Klosinski, L. P., Cadenas, E., and Brinton, R. D. (2011). Shift in brain metabolism in late onset Alzheimer's disease: Implications for biomarkers and therapeutic interventions. *Molecular Aspects of Medicine*, 32: 247–257.

Zhang, H. V., and Xi, C. T. (2000). Huperzine B, a novel acetylcholinesterase inhibitor, attenuates hydrogen peroxide induced injury in PC12 cells. *Neuroscience Letters*, 292(1): 41-44

Zhang, H. Y. (2012). New insights into huperzine A for the treatment of Alzheimer's disease. *Acta Pharmacologica Sinica*, 33: 1170–1175.

Zhang, J. M., and Hu, G. Y. (2001). Huperzine A, a nootropic alkaloid, inhibits N-methyl-D-aspartate-induced current in rat dissociated hippocampal neurons. *Neuroscience*, 105(3): 663–669.

Chapter 13

Botanical Interventions for Parkinson's Disease

Navjot Kaur[1,*]
Navdeep Kaur[2]
Baljeet Singh[1]
Arvinder Pal Singh[3]
and Simrandeep Singh[4]
[1]Amar Shaheed Baba Ajit Singh Jujhar Singh Memorial College of Pharmacy, Bela, Punjab, India
[2]Rayat Institute of Pharmacy, Railmajra, SBS Nagar, Punjab, India
[3]Maharaja Agrasen School of Pharmacy, Maharaja Agrasen University, Baddi, Solan, Himachal Pradesh, India
[4]UCRD, Chandigarh University, Gharuan, Mohali, Punjab, India

Abstract

Parkinson's disease (PD) is a neurodegenerative disorder that affects approximately 6 million people worldwide. It is characterized by both motor and non-motor symptoms and is associated with Lewy body pathology and the loss of dopaminergic neurons in the substantia nigra, leading to motor dysfunction. Key factors contributing to PD include oxidative stress, neuroinflammation, mitochondrial dysfunction, and α-synuclein aggregation, with the gut-brain axis also playing a role in non-motor symptoms. This chapter explores the potential of natural products in managing the progression of Parkinson's disease. Botanical interventions may influence several pathways, including the Bax/Bcl-2 ratio and caspase activity, the regulation of the TP53-HIPK2-AXIN1 complex, and the modulation of neuroinflammation and oxidative stress.

* Corresponding Author's Email: saini.navjotkaur@gmail.com.

In: Natural Solutions for Neurodegenerative Disorders
Editors: Rahul Kumar Sharma, Shailesh Sharma, Ajmer Singh Grewal et al.
ISBN: 979-8-89530-231-6

They also impact the regulation of dopamine transporters (DAT) and α-synuclein levels. Phytoconstituents with notable effects on Parkinson's disease include coenzyme Q10, flavonoids such as quercetin and epigallocatechin-3-gallate, curcumin, dihydromyricetin, icariin, phenolyl-propanoids, saponins, and non-flavonoid polyphenols. Other beneficial supplements for PD treatment include lipoic acid, vitamins B, C, D3, and E, omega-3 fatty acids, whey protein, melatonin, lycopene, beta-carotene, and cannabinoids. The chapter also provides a list of plants that act through various mechanisms to manage the disease. Recent research has emphasized these plants' potential to modulate cell signaling pathways, scavenge free radicals, and reduce inflammation in animal and cellular models of Parkinson's disease. Botanical compounds are being investigated for their potential as disease-modifying agents or adjuncts to conventional PD therapies. Advances in understanding their mechanisms of action and clinical efficacy suggest that these interventions may play a role in alleviating symptoms and potentially slowing the progression of Parkinson's disease.

Keywords: Parkinson's disease, phytochemicals, antioxidant, neuroprotective, alpha-synuclein, dopamine

Abbreviations

AMPK	AMP-Activated Protein Kinase
AXIN1	Axis Inhibition Protein 1
Bax	BCL2 Associated X
Bcl-2	B-Cell Lymphoma 2
GSK-3β	Glycogen Synthase Kinase 3 Beta
MAPK	Mitogen-Activated Protein Kinase
MPP (+)	1-Methyl-4-Phenylpyridinium Ion
Nrf2	Nuclear Factor Erythroid 2-Related Factor 2
P38 MAPK	P38 Mitogen-Activated Protein Kinase
PD	Parkinson's disease
PI3K/Akt	Phosphoinositide 3-Kinase/Protein Kinase B

Introduction

Parkinson's disease (PD) is a prevalent neurodegenerative disorder, impacting approximately 1.04 million people in the U.S. and 6.1 million globally. It is characterized by motor symptoms such as bradykinesia and tremor, alongside non-motor symptoms like cognitive impairment and depression. Prior to the onset of PD, there is often a prodromal stage, with idiopathic rapid eye movement sleep behavior disorder serving as a red flag symptom in high-risk populations (Armstrong et al., 2020). Monogenic forms of PD, accounting for 5–10% of cases, are classified as idiopathic. Idiopathic PD results from a combination of genetic and environmental factors, leading to α-synuclein deposition in the substantia nigra and the formation of Lewy bodies. Despite current therapies addressing symptoms, they do not offer a cure for the disease. Parkinson's disease was first described by James Parkinson in 1817, and its prevalence is expected to rise, with projections suggesting China alone could have approximately 4.94 million cases by 2030 (Ball et al., 2019). The pathogenesis of PD involves a complex interaction of genetic, environmental, and epigenetic factors. Genes such as SNCA and LRRK2 have been associated with PD, which is characterized by Lewy body pathology and the loss of dopaminergic neurons in the substantia nigra. Contributing factors include oxidative stress, mitochondrial dysfunction, and α-synuclein aggregation (Long et al., 2021). Key molecular signaling pathways involved in PD include PI3K/Akt, Nrf2, P38 MAPK, GSK-3β, JNK, and NF-κB. Additionally, processes like Wnt autophagy play a role in the disease's pathogenesis, highlighting its multifactorial nature and variability among patients (Long et al., 2021). PD presents with both motor symptoms such as tremors and bradykinesia, and non-motor symptoms including mood disorders and cognitive dysfunction. It affects 1–2% of the population, with prevalence increasing with age. The presence of Lewy bodies, comprised of α-synuclein and other proteins, is a hallmark of the disease, which involves a complex interplay of molecular mechanisms leading to neurodegeneration (Ball et al., 2019).

Pathophysiology

Braak Hypothesis and Staged Progression

The Braak hypothesis, proposed by Braak and colleagues, outlines a staged model for the progression of PD. According to this model, the disease initially begins in the olfactory bulb and the enteric nervous system, leading to symptoms such as hyposmia (reduced sense of smell) and gastrointestinal dysfunction. As the pathology progresses, it extends to the medulla and subsequently to the substantia nigra during the pre-symptomatic phase. Motor symptoms, including tremor and bradykinesia, become apparent in the later stages as the disease involves cortical regions. Advanced Parkinson's disease is characterized by widespread involvement of the cerebral cortex, which results in impaired cognition and hallucinations (Iwasaki, 2020).

Dopaminergic Dysfunction and Basal Ganglia Imbalance

PD is characterized by the degeneration of dopaminergic neurons in the substantia nigra, which disrupts the balance between the direct and indirect pathways in the basal ganglia. This imbalance leads to pathological synchronous oscillatory activity, particularly in the β-band of brainwaves. Enhanced β-band oscillations are associated with the dopaminergic "off" state and are linked to motor symptoms such as rigidity and bradykinesia. Moreover, dopaminergic abnormalities may give rise to a lateral premotor loop, further contributing to the motor dysfunction observed in PD (Meoni et al., 2020).

Neuroinflammation

A significant aspect of PD etiology is chronic neuroinflammation. Post-mortem studies have revealed increased levels of pro-inflammatory substances, activated microglia, and T cell infiltration in the brains of PD patients. Microglia, the brain's resident immune cells, play a dual role: they contribute to the progression of the disease but also have the potential to mitigate it. Current immunotherapies targeting α-synuclein rely on microglia to clear and degrade deposits of misfolded proteins, thus highlighting their complex role in both exacerbating and potentially slowing the progression of PD (Liu et al., 2022).

The Role of α-Synuclein in Neuroinflammation

α-Synuclein, a neuronal protein, is closely linked to Parkinson's disease (PD). It is typically found in presynaptic terminals, neuronal nuclei, and mitochondria. Pathologically, α-synuclein accumulates in Lewy bodies (LB) and neurites, contributing to the neuropathology of PD. The prion-like process suggests that misfolded α-synuclein aggregates can propagate between neurons, facilitating the spread of the disease (Lv et al., 2023).

Gut-Brain Axis and Non-Motor Symptoms

The gut-brain axis represents a bidirectional communication pathway between the gut and the brain. During the prodromal phase of PD, non-motor symptoms related to the gastrointestinal tract can emerge. Recent research suggests that these symptoms may indicate the onset of an α-synuclein pathology in the gut, which then travels via the vagus nerve to the brain. Constipation, a common digestive symptom, is considered an early indicator of PD (Schaeffer et al., 2020).

Mitochondrial Dysfunction

PD is closely associated with mitochondrial dysfunction. Research has identified abnormalities in the mitochondria of various tissues in PD patients, including lymphoblasts, platelets, and skeletal muscle. Certain gene mutations linked to mitochondrial function have been connected to dopaminergic cell death. Additionally, mitochondrial failure in PD is compounded by oxidative stress and increased brain iron levels (Li et al., 2022).

Lewy Bodies (LBs) and Microgliosis

LBs, primarily composed of α-synuclein, are both markers of Parkinson's disease pathogenesis and sites of neuronal degeneration. Dysfunction in the ubiquitin-proteasomal system, involving proteins such as parkin and UCH-L1, contributes to altered protein processing in dopaminergic cells. Postmortem studies have shown a decrease in proteasomal enzyme activity, particularly in the substantia nigra (Lazdon et al., 2020).

Neuroinflammation

Neuroinflammation in PD involves a complex interplay between microglia and immune responses. Toll-like receptors (TLRs), nuclear factor kappa B (NF-κB), and NLRP3 inflammasomes are key players in the signaling cascade initiated by α-synuclein. The antioxidant response system, including Nrf2, is implicated in PD, while major histocompatibility complex class II is involved in antigen presentation by microglia, contributing to T cell activation (Gao et al., 2023).

T Cells

In PD, T cells are present in the substantia nigra of affected patients. Various mediators, including gut microbiota, α-synuclein, dopamine, and short-chain fatty acids, can trigger T cell-driven inflammation. Research indicates that T lymphocytes can recognize specific antigenic sites on α-synuclein. The involvement of human leukocyte antigen (HLA) alleles in presenting α-synuclein peptides highlights the link between immune responses and PD (Arlehamn et al., 2020).

Oxidative Stress

The intricate interplay of neuroinflammation, oxidative stress, and dopaminergic degeneration underscores the complexity of PD. Oxidative stress promotes mitochondrial dysfunction, protein misfolding, and lipid peroxidation. Reactive oxygen species further stimulate microglia, exacerbating the inflammatory response (He et al., 2020).

Nonpharmacologic Interventions

Nonmedical interventions, such as nutrition and immunotherapies, play a role in managing PD by addressing oxidative stress and inflammation. Dietary factors, including antioxidants and anti-inflammatory compounds, can help reduce oxidative stress and inflammation. Immunotherapies targeting α-synuclein aim to modulate immune responses and promote the clearance of pathological protein aggregates (Pardo-Moreno et al., 2023).

The Impact of Natural Products on PD Pathophysiology

Natural products are crucial in managing PD due to their effects on various aspects of cellular function. They influence cellular development and apoptosis, modulate anti-inflammatory pathways, and enhance dopamine transmission.

Cellular Developments and Apoptosis

Bax/Bcl-2 Ratio and Caspase Activity

The relationship between the Bax/Bcl-2 ratio and caspase activity is criticalcritical in Parkinson's disease, as it governs cellular development and apoptosis. Bax and Bcl-2, key members of the BCL2 family, regulate apoptotic processes. Pedicularioside A, a natural compound, influences these mechanisms by modulating apoptosis-related genes. It inhibits caspase-3 gene expression and prevents the cleavage of poly (ADP-ribose) polymerase (PARP) in the presence of MPP(+), thereby reducing apoptotic pathways and enhancing the survival of mesencephalic neurons (Li et al., 2008).

Regulation of the TP53-HIPK2-AXIN1 Complex

The TP53-HIPK2-AXIN1 complex is crucial for regulating cellular development and apoptosis. HIPK2, a protein kinase interacting with homeodomains, forms a complex with TP53 and AXIN1. This interaction influences the activity of creatine kinase and initiates TP53 transcription, thereby regulating cell growth and promoting apoptosis (Li et al., 2019).

Anti-Inflammatory Pathway

Neuroinflammation and Oxidative Stress

The transcription factor MAFG promotes neuronal nitric oxide synthase by enhancing NRF1 expression. Botanical interventions can elevate Nrf2 protein levels and its transcriptional activity, which in turn regulates Nrf2-dependent genes. This regulation helps mitigate neuroinflammation and oxidative stress (Li et al., 2019).

Dopamine Transmission

Regulation of Dopamine Transporter and Transporter and α-Synuclein

Natural substances can influence the dopamine transporter, which is responsible for reabsorbing dopamine. α-Synuclein affects both the dopamine transporter and vesicular monoamine transporter 2. For instance, mulberry extract has been shown to reduce the overexpression of α-synuclein and ubiquitin, which are key components of LBs (Gu et al., 2017).

Natural Products Involved in the Treatment of PD

The modulation of key molecular players, such as Bax, Bcl-2, caspases, the TP53-HIPK2-AXIN1 complex, and Nrf2, demonstrates the potential of natural products as medicinal agents (Bhusal et al., 2023). The following are various phytoconstituents that can help improve Parkinson's disease (PD) patients through different mechanisms:

Coenzyme Q10

Coenzyme Q10, a benzoquinone found throughout animal tissues, functions as an electron carrier in the mitochondrial electron transport chain and as an antioxidant. It has shown neuroprotective effects in PD models by reducing dopamine loss and protecting dopaminergic axons. However, its role in the management of PD remains controversial, with mixed results in clinical studies and ongoing debates about its effectiveness in human patients (Jiménez-Jiménez et al., 2022).

Flavonoids

Flavonoids, classified into six subclasses, exhibit a range of beneficial properties, including antioxidative, anti-inflammatory, and neuroprotective effects. Quercetin, a notable flavonoid, has demonstrated anti-inflammatory, antitumor, and neuroprotective properties. Studies suggest that quercetin may improve cognitive functions and reduce oxidative stress in PD patients, indicating its potential therapeutic benefits for managing the disease (Boyinaina et al., 2020).

Epigallocatechin-3-Gallate

Epigallocatechin-3-gallate (EGCG), a compound found in green tea, possesses strong antioxidant properties. It has shown potential in reducing oxidative stress, mitigating lipid peroxidation, and lowering the risk of developing PD (Sergi, 2022).

Curcumin

Curcumin, a rare diketone compound, exhibits neuroprotective effects by counteracting neuronal degeneration linked to mitochondrial dysfunction. It influences signaling pathways such as PI3K/AKT/GSK-3 and PI3K/AKT/CREB/BDNF, which regulate apoptosis and inflammation. Clinical trials have produced mixed outcomes: while some studies indicate cognitive improvement in Alzheimer's disease (AD), others have found no significant cognitive-enhancing effects (Cortés et al., 2021).

Dihydromyricetin (DHM)

DHM provides neuroprotection by preventing neuronal apoptosis through the activation of hemeoxygenase-1 (HO-1). It modulates various signaling pathways, including ERK and AKT, to inhibit oxidative stress and apoptosis. Additionally, DHM's protective effects extend to glucose metabolism and involve the GSK-3β/Nrf2/antioxidant response element (ARE) pathways (Pei et al., 2023).

Icariin (ICA)

ICA, a flavanol, alleviates AD symptoms by boosting insulin-like growth factor (IGF) and brain-derived neurotrophic factor (BDNF), and activating the PI3K/AKT pathway. It promotes hippocampal neural stem cell proliferation through the BDNF-TrkB-ERK/AKT signaling pathway and offers protection against amyloid-beta (Aβ)-induced insulin resistance (Khezri & Ghasemnejad-Berenji, 2022).

Phenylpropanoids

Salidroside provides neuroprotection by exerting antioxidant, anti-inflammatory, and anti-apoptotic effects. It activates the PI3K/AKT pathway, thereby reducing amyloidosis and inflammation in PD models (Li et al., 2022). Arctigenin influences tau protein expression through the PI3K/AKT/GSK-3β pathway, and its bioavailability is enhanced via intranasal administration (Li et al., 2023). Schizandrol A (SchA), a lignan, mitigates apoptosis and oxidative stress by modulating PI3K/AKT signaling, showing potential in PD treatment. It also inhibits ischemia-induced neuronal autophagy through the AMPK/mTOR pathway (Yan et al., 2021).

Saponins

Ginsenosides, compounds from ginseng, enhance synaptic plasticity and reduce apoptosis, making them promising candidates for PD treatment. Specifically, ginsenoside Rg2 inhibits apoptosis induced by Aβ through the PI3K/AKT pathway, while noto ginsenoside R1 provides neuroprotection against Aβ-induced damage by activating the AKT, ERK1/2, and Nrf2 pathways (Gandhi et al., 2023).

Non-Flavonoid Polyphenols

Piceatannol exhibits antioxidant and anti-apoptotic properties by upregulating the PI3K/AKT/BAD signaling pathway. Additionally, polyphenols from Litchi chinensis seeds inhibit hyperphosphorylated Tau protein through the

IRS-1/PI3K/AKT pathway (Gandhi et al., 2023). Zanthoxylum bungeanum Maxim. offers neuroprotection by inhibiting apoptosis and oxidative stress through the PI3K/AKT/Nrf2 pathway. Broussonetia papyrifera enhances neuroprotection by activating the AKT and β-catenin signaling pathways (Huang et al., 2023).

Others in Parkinson's Disease (PD)

Lipoic Acid

Lipoic acid (LA), a naturally occurring antioxidant, alleviates L-DOPA-induced dyskinesia in PD mouse models. It also exhibits anti-inflammatory properties and enhances antioxidant activity, suggesting its potential as a complementary therapy to improve disease outcomes when combined with L-DOPA (Khan et al., 2022).

N-Acetyl-Cysteine

N-Acetyl-cysteine (NAC), known for its antioxidant properties, mitigates oxidative damage, prevents ROS accumulation, and shields against dopamine-induced cell death in animal models. In PD management, NAC enhances mitochondrial complex activities and serves as a precursor to glutathione, contributing to its protective effects (Mursaleen et al., 2020).

Vitamin E

Vitamin E has shown mixed results in clinical trials for PD management. While some studies suggest that it may slow disease progression and that a combination of ascorbate and vitamin E can delay the need for L-DOPA treatment, its neuroprotective role in PD remains contentious and under ongoing scrutiny (İçer et al., 2021).

Carvacrol

Carvacrol, a phenolic monoterpene, exhibits multiple pharmacological properties, including anti-inflammatory, antioxidant, and neuromodulatory effects. In a PD mouse model, carvacrol has been shown to improve cognitive impairments without influencing pain or motor symptoms, highlighting its potential as a therapeutic option for managing PD (Zamanian et al., 2021).

Omega-3 Fatty Acids

Omega-3 fatty acids play a role in lipid metabolism and may contribute to neuroprotection in PD by potentially lowering cholesterol levels. However, further research is necessary to fully establish their efficacy and therapeutic potential (Li & Song, 2022).

Whey Protein

Whey protein, which is rich in cysteine, enhances glutathione synthesis and reduces oxidative stress. Clinical studies have shown a significant increase in plasma reduced glutathione levels in PD patients who received whey protein supplementation. However, it appears that disease modification rates remain unaffected (Pinelli et al., 2023).

Vitamin D3

Vitamin D3, whether produced endogenously or obtained through supplements, has demonstrated neuroprotective properties within the central nervous system. Research indicates that vitamin D3 may play a positive role in managing PD, with benefits extending to muscular and endocrine functions (Pignolo et al., 2022).

Creatine

Creatine, known for its role in providing energy to muscle and nerve cells, exhibits antioxidant properties and offers neuroprotection in PD mouse models. Oral supplementation with creatine has been shown to protect against dopamine depletion caused by neurotoxic agents (Cui et al., 2020).

Melatonin

Produced in the pineal gland, melatonin helps synchronize circadian rhythms and exhibits antioxidant properties. In PD mouse models, melatonin has been shown to prevent neuronal cell death induced by oxidative and nitrative stress, highlighting its potential as a neuroprotective agent (Cui et al., 2020).

Niacin (Vitamin B3)

Niacin, a vital component of human metabolism, plays a crucial role in managing PD due to its neuroprotective and antioxidant properties, even at low doses. Its potential therapeutic effects are linked to its role in addressing mitochondrial dysfunction and cellular energy failure (Chong et al., 2021).

Table 1. Role of natural products in regulation of PD

Biological Source	Family	Phytoconstituents	Mechanism of action	Reference
Acorus calamus	Acoraceae	Beta asarone	Protective function against Parkinson's disease and Alzheimer's disease via controlling autophagy, ER stress, and synaptogenesis via the IRE1/XBP1 ER stress pathways	(Sharma et al., 2022)
Angelica Dahuricae Radix	Umbelliferae	Imperatorin	Anti-apoptotic activity, neuroprotective effects, and increased autophagy	(Wang et al., 2023)
Bacopa monnieri	Plantaginaceae	Bacosides	Antioxidant capacities and mitochondrial ETC complex activation restoration	(Santos et al., 2023)
Carthamustinctorius	Asteraceae	Flavonoids	Enhances the expression of DJ-1 and DA transporter proteins while suppressing the overexpression of α-synuclein.	(Jaiswal et al., 2023)
Centella asiatica	Centalliaceae	Monoterpenes	Inhibits acetylcholinesterase activity and exhibits sedative and antidepressant properties.	(Gofir et al., 2021)
Chrysanthemum indicum Linn	Asteraceae	Flavonoids acacetin, luteolin, apigenin	Minimizes the generation of reactive oxygen species, regulates the Bax/Bcl-2 ratio, stops PARP proteolysis, and blocks the neuroinflammatory NF-κB/IκB-α signaling pathway.	(Nagrik et al., 2020)
Coptis chinensis	Ranunculaceae	Lycopodium alkaloid	AChE inhibition, inhibition of ROS, protection of mitochondrial integrity	(Chen et al., 2022)
Curcuma longa	Zingiberaceae	Curcumin	Prevents the loss of TH-positive neurons brought on by MPTP and lowers inflammatory markers and cytokines.	(Patel et al., 2022)
Erythrina velutina	Fabaceae	Flavonoids	Reduces neurotoxicity caused by 6-OHDA. Potential treatment for Parkinson's disease.	(Canli & Benli, 2023)
Gastrodiaelata blume	Orchidaceae	Gastrodin	Has sedative, anxiolytic, anticonvulsant, analgesic, antioxidant, and anti-inflammatory properties. uses the p38 MAPK/Nrf2 pathway to prevent oxidative stress, protecting dopamine neurons in the process.	(Heese, 2020)
Ginkgo biloba	Ginkgoaceae	Flavonoids, ginkgolic acid, terpenoids	Prevents loss of dopaminergic nerve terminals and protects against MPTP-induced neurotoxicity.	(Yu et al., 2021)
Glycyrrhiza glabra L	Fabaceae	Liquiritigenin	Neuroprotective: it prevents dopamine neuronal cell death by binding to the estrogen receptor beta.	(Karthikkeyan et al., 2020)

Table 1. (Continued)

Biological Source	Family	Phytoconstituents	Mechanism of action	Reference
Hyoscyamus niger	Solanaceae	Hyoscine, hyoscyamine	Anticholinergic properties; used to treat Parkinson's tremor	(Al-Snafi, 2021)
Hypericum perforatum	Hypericaceae.	Naphthodianthrones, phloroglucinols, flavonoids, essential oils.	Lowers Bax levels, decreases neuronal damage, and prevents apoptosis.	(Hajihoseini et al., 2022)
Juglandis semen	Juglandaceae	Polyphenols	Reduces ROS and nitric oxide, blocks monoamine oxidase B (MAO-B) enzyme.	(Mohammad et al., 2023)
Knemala urina	Myristicaceae	Eugonol-type benzofurans	Anti-aging, antioxidant, and anti-inflammatory properties	(Salihu et al., 2023)
Ligusticum chuanxiong Hort	Apiaceae	Volatile oil, phenols, alkaloids and polysaccharides	Neuroprotective effects, including the reduction of cerebral infarct, inflammatory reaction, oxidative stress, and neuronal apoptosis. Boosts neurogenesis, neural stem cell proliferation, and preserves mature neurons	(Qin et al., 2022)
Mucuna pruriens	Fabaceae	L-DOPA and other components	Better long-term treatment than standard L-DOPA therapy, significant neuroprotective properties	(Rai et al., 2020)
Nardostachys jatamansi	Valerianaceae	Sesquiterpenes and coumarins	Reduces neuronal damage, antioxidant effects, modulation of neurotransmitters	(Giri et al., 2020)
Paeonia suffruticosa	Paeoniaceae	Paeonol, paeoniflorin	Neuro-associated activities in PD-like animals, including enhanced cell viability, reduction of ROS formation, and inhibition of neuroinflammation.	(Liu et al., 2023)
Panax ginseng	Araliaceae	Ginsenosides	Protects cells against apoptosis, lowers intracellular reactive oxygen species (ROS).	(Gong et al., 2022)
Passiflora incanata	Passifloraceae	Flavonoids, glycosides, alkaloids, phenolic chemicals.	Reduces jaw movements and improves cognitive abilities in a PD animal model.	(Sharma et al., 2022)
Peganum harmala	Nitrariaceae	β-Carboline and quinazoline alkaloids	Reduces muscle stiffness, protects dopaminergic neurons by reducing angiotensin II activity.	(Rizki et al., 2021)

Biological Source	Family	Phytoconstituents	Mechanism of action	Reference
Pueraria lobata	Fabaceae	Puerarin	Inhibits proteasomal malfunction, protects TH-positive neurons, and recovers DA levels.	(Yu et al., 2022)
Scutellaria baicalensis	Labiatae	Flavonoid	Prevents ROS buildup, apoptosis, and mitochondrial damage. Protects dopaminergic neurons.	(Chand et al., 2022)
Tinospora cordifolia	Menispermaceae	Alkaloids, diterpenoid lactones, glycosides	Investigated for potential anti-Parkinson's efficacy, shows antioxidant action.	(Singh et al., 2023)
Valeriana officinalis	Valerianaceae	Phenolics and flavonoids	Inhibits rotenone-induced cell death, exhibits antioxidant properties	(Mytych & Aebisher, 2022)
Vitis vinifera	Vitaceae	Poly phenolic compounds	Helps with motor impairments, oxidative stress, and loss of TH neurons. minimizes inflammatory indicators and prevents mitochondrial hypertrophy.	(Pazos-Tomas et al., 2020)
Withania somnifera	Solanaceae	Withanolides	Shows antioxidant and neuroprotective effects	(Dar & Ahmad, 2020)

Vitamin C

Vitamin C, known for its crucial physiological roles, acts as a powerful antioxidant that reduces reactive oxygen species (ROS) and oxidative stress. In PD, ascorbic acid supplementation has been shown to decrease ROS derivatives associated with neurotoxicity, suggesting its potential as a protective agent (Chang et al., 2021).

β-Carotene

As a precursor to vitamin A, β-carotene effectively scavenges singlet oxygen. Clinical trials evaluating its antioxidant properties suggest potential benefits in countering free radicals associated with PD (Jamali et al., 2022).

Lycopene

A potent antioxidant among carotenoids, lycopene's capacity to scavenge free radicals suggests its potential as a preventive agent in PD. Found in tomatoes and other fruits, lycopene is responsible for the red color of these foods (Przybylska, 2020).

CBD (Cannabidiol)

They activate the ERK and AKT/mTOR pathways, indicating potential for Parkinson's disease treatment. Ongoing clinical studies on CBD emphasize the need for further research to understand its mechanisms and safety (Rieder, 2020).

These compounds exhibit various mechanisms that contribute to PD treatment, as outlined in Table 1. This underscores the necessity for further research to validate their efficacy and explore their clinical applications.

Conclusion

PD is a common neurodegenerative disorder affecting around 1.04 million people in the U.S. and 6.1 million globally. It presents with both motor symptoms (such as tremors and bradykinesia) and non-motor symptoms (including cognitive impairment and depression). Non-pharmacological interventions, like dietary changes and immunotherapies, are being explored to reduce oxidative stress and inflammation associated with PD. Immunotherapies targeting α-synuclein and inflammatory pathways are under investigation. Additionally, gene therapy, cell transplantation, and deep brain stimulation are emerging as promising surgical options for PD treatment. Natural compounds show potential in modifying PD pathogenesis. These include flavonoids, phenylpropanoids, saponins, and non-flavonoid polyphenols, which impact dopamine transmission, apoptosis, anti-inflammatory pathways, and cellular growth and differentiation. Examples include curcumin, coenzyme Q10, epigallocatechin-3-gallate, quercetin, and omega-3 fatty acids. These substances may offer therapeutic benefits due to their neuroprotective and antioxidative properties. However, further research is needed to elucidate their mechanisms of action, determine optimal dosages, and explore potential interactions with current therapies.

References

Al-Snafi, A. E. (2021). Medicinal plants possessed anti-Parkinsonian effects with emphasis on their mechanisms of action. *GSC Biological and Pharmaceutical Sciences*, 2021(01), 232–237.

Canli, S., & Mehlika, B. (2023). The Potential Role of Plants in the Treatment of Parkinson's Disease: Traditional Review. *Journal of Traditional Medical Complementary Therapies*, 6(2), 184.

Chand, J., Subramanian, G., Jupudi, S., Duyu, T., & Baba, M. Z. (2022). Neuroprotective Effect of Scutellaria baicalensis in Parkinson's disease and Multi-Target Mechanisms Based on Network Pharmacology. Research Square. *Research Square*, PPR566574.

Chen, P., Zhang, J., Wang, C., Chai, Y., Wu, A., Huang, N., & Wang, L. (2022). The pathogenesis and treatment mechanism of Parkinson's disease from the perspective of traditional Chinese medicine. *Phytomedicine*, 100, 154044.

Dar, N. J., & Ahmad, M. (2020). Neurodegenerative diseases and *Withania somnifera* (L.): An update. *Journal of Ethnopharmacology*, 256(112769).

Giri, M. A., Bhalke, R. D., Prakash, K. V., & Kasture, S. B. (2020). Comparative evaluation of and as Nardostachys jatamansi Mucuna pruriens neuroprotective in Parkinson's disease. *Asian Journal of Pharmacy and Pharmacology*, 6(3), 224–230.

Gofir, A., Wibowo, S., & Hakimi, M. (2021). Potential neurological applications of Centella asiatica: a brief review. *Indonesian Journal of Pharmacology and Therapy*, 02(3), 136–143.

Gong, L., Yin, J., Zhang, Y., Huang, R., Lou, Y., Jiang, H., Sun, L., Jia, J., & Zeng, X. (2022). Neuroprotective Mechanisms of Ginsenoside Rb1 in Central Nervous System Diseases. *Frontiers in Pharmacology*, 13.

Hajihoseini, M., Rouzbahani, A. K., Ebrahimi, E., Sadr, S., & Tahermohammadi, H. (2022). Parkinson and Hypericum perforatum: a medical hypothesis. *TMR Integrative Medicine*, 6, e22012.

Heese, K. (2020). Gastrodia elata Blume (Tianma): Hope for Brain Aging and Dementia. *Evidence-Based Complementary and Alternative Medicine*, 2020, 8870148.

Khazdair, M. R., Kianmehr, M., & Anaeigoudari, A. (2021). Effects of Medicinal Plants and Flavonoids on Parkinson's Disease: A Review on Basic and Clinical Evidences. *Advanced pharmaceutical bulletin*, 11(2), 224–232.

Karthikkeyan, G., Altaf, N. M., Pervaje, R., Krishna, P. S., Kumar, M. P., & Subrahmanya, K. P. T. (2020). Identification of Molecular Network Associated with Neuroprotective Effects of Yashtimadhu (Glycyrrhiza glabra L.) by Quantitative Proteomics of Rotenone-Induced Parkinson's. *ACS Publications*, 5(41), 26611–26625.

Liu, J., Li, X., Bai, H., Yang, X., Mu, J., Yan, R., & Wang, S. (2023). Traditional uses, phytochemistry, pharmacology, and pharmacokinetics of the root bark of Paeonia x suffruticosa andrews: A comprehensive review. *Journal of Ethnopharmacology*, 308, 116279.

Mohammad, H. S., Gilavand, H. K., Taherkhani, A., Rafiei, S. K. S., Shahrokhi, M., Faaliat, S., Biabani, M., Abil, E., Ansari, A., Sheikh, Z., Poudineh, M., Khalaji, A. M., Baghini, M. S., Koorangi, M. H., & Deravi, N. (2023). Pharmacotherapeutic potential of walnut (Juglans spp.) in age-related neurological disorders. *IBRO Neuroscience Reports*, 14, 1–20.

Mytych, W., & Aebisher, D. (2022). Valeriana officinalis–a review. *The Central European Journal of Social Sciences and Humanities*, 20(3), 260–265.

Nagrik, S. U., Patil, P. A., Nagrik, D. M., Zagare, V. S., Avchar, P. E., Bahurupi, S. D., & Ambhore, S. G. (2020). Herbal drugs Used on Parkinson Disease. *Journal of Drug Delivery and Therapeutics*, 10(s), 235–239.

Patel, A., Olang, C. A., Lewis, G., Mandalaneni, K., Anand, N., & Rakesh, G. V. (2022). An Overview of Parkinson's Disease: Curcumin as a Possible Alternative Treatment. *Cureus*, 14(5), e25032.

Pazos-Tomas, C. C., Cruz-Venegas, A., Pérez-Santiago, A. D., Sánchez-Medina, A., Matías-Pérez, D., & García-Montalvo, I. (2020). Vitis vinifera: An alternative for the prevention of neurodegenerative diseases. *Journal of Oleo Sciences*, 69(10), 1147–1161.

Qin, Y., Chen, F., Tang, Z., Ren, H., Wang, Q., Shen, N., Lin, W., Xiao, Y., Yuan, M., Chen, H., Bu, T., Li, Q., & Huang, L. (2022). Ligusticum chuanxiong Hort as a medicinal and edible plant foods: Antioxidant, anti-aging and neuroprotective properties in Caenorhabditis elegans. *Frontiers in Pharmacology*, 13, 1049890.

Rai, S. N., Chaturvedi, V. K., Singh, P., Singh, B. K., & Singh, M. P. (2020). Mucuna pruriens in Parkinson's and in some other diseases: recent advancement and future prospective. *3 Biotech*, 10(12), 522.

Rizki, M., Pratama, F., Nasibova, T., Kumar, P., Garaev, E. A., Tohfa, A., Pratiwi, D., & Garaev, A. (2021). Peganum harmala and its alkaloids as dopamine receptor antagonists: in silico study. *Biointerface Research in Applied Chemistry*, 11(3), 10301–10316.

Salihu, A. S., Mohd, W., Hakimi, N., & Salleh, W. (2023). Flavonoids and other constituents of plants from the genus Knema (Myristicaceae) and their pharmacological studies: An updated review. *Vietnam Journal of Chemistry*, 2023(4), 397–411.

Santos, A. F. D., Souza, M. M. Q., Amaral, E. C., Albuquerque, E. R., Bortoloti, D. S., Arquimedes, G. J., Lourenco, E. L. B., Lovato, E. C. W., & Livero, F. A. D. R. (2023). *Bacopa monnieri* in Patients with Parkinson's Disease: A Pilot Study. *Journal of Medicinal Food*, 26(2), 114–119.

Sharma, P., Jain, D. K., Jain, N. K., Jain, A., Singh, U. B., Paliwal, P., & Jain, S. K. (2022). Anti-Parkinson's Potential of Acorus Calamus Linn: A Review. *Journal of Pharmaceutical Negative Results*, 13(05), 2540–2547.

Sharma, V., Bedi, O., Gupta, M., & Deshmukh, R. (2022). A review: traditional herbs and remedies impacting pathogenesis of Parkinson's disease. *Naunyn-Schmiedeberg's Archives of Pharmacology*, 395(5), 495–513.

Singh, R., Bhattacharyya, C., Prashar, V., & Arora, T. (2023). Tinospora cordifolia: A potential neuroprotective agent against various neurodegenerative diseases. *Journal of Herbal Medicine*, 42(100775).

Wang, Q., Li, Y., Wang, S., Xiang, Z., Dong, W., Li, X., Wei, Y., Gao, P., & Dai, L. (2023). A review of the historical records, chemistry, pharmacology, pharmacokinetics and edibility of Angelica dahurica. *Arabian Journal of Chemistry*, 16(8), 104877.

Yu, C. C., Du, Y. J., Li, J., Li, Y., Wang, L., & Kong, L. H. (2022). Neuroprotective mechanisms of puerarin in central nervous system diseases: Update. *Aging and Disease*, 13(4), 1092–1105.

Yu, D., Zhang, P., Li, J., Liu, T., Zhang, Y., Wang, Q., Zhang, J., Lu, X., & Fan, X. (2021). Neuroprotective effects of Ginkgo biloba dropping pills in Parkinson's disease. *Journal of Pharmaceutical Analysis*, 11(2), 220–231.

Chapter 14

Botanicals in Alzheimer's Disease Management

Kavita Munjal[1]
Hitesh Chopra[2,*]
Vinod Kumar Gauttam[3]
Shailendra Sharma[4]
and Rukhsar Syed[5]
[1]Department of Pharmacy, Amity Institute of Pharmacy, Amity University, Noida, Uttar Pradesh, India
[2]Department of Biosciences, Saveetha School of Engineering, Saveetha Institute of Medical and Technical Sciences, Chennai, Tamil Nadu, India
[3]Department of Pharmacognosy, Shiva Institute of Pharmacy, Bilaspur, Himachal Pradesh, India
[4]SN Medical College, MRU, DHR-ICMR, Jodhpur, Rajasthan
5IES Institute of Pharmacy, IES University, Bhopal, Madhya Pradesh, India

Abstract

Cognitive decline and memory loss associated with Alzheimer's disease (AD) present significant public health challenges worldwide. Traditional pharmaceutical treatments have struggled to address the complex neurological processes underlying AD effectively. As a result, there is growing interest in the potential role of botanicals—plant-derived substances—in the treatment of this debilitating condition. Compounds such as curcumin from turmeric, Ginkgo biloba extract, resveratrol from red grapes, and other polyphenols show promise due to their multiple mechanisms of action. These include inhibiting the aggregation of pathogenic proteins like beta-amyloid and reducing the production of

* Corresponding Author's Email: chopraontheride@gmail.com.

In: Natural Solutions for Neurodegenerative Disorders
Editors: Rahul Kumar Sharma, Shailesh Sharma, Ajmer Singh Grewal et al.
ISBN: 979-8-89530-231-6

reactive oxygen species. Botanicals have demonstrated potential in enhancing cognitive function and memory, with some showing disease-modifying benefits. For instance, huperzine-A derived from Huperzia serrate acts as an acetylcholinesterase inhibitor, which may improve mental functioning. However, the effectiveness of botanical therapies varies widely among different substances and populations, and concerns about safety and drug interactions remain. To determine their true efficacy and long-term safety, extensive clinical trials and standardized dosage guidelines are essential. In summary, botanicals offer an exciting new avenue for combating Alzheimer's disease. Their diverse mechanisms—including neuroprotection, cognitive enhancement, and anti-inflammatory effects—suggest significant potential. Nonetheless, further research is crucial before these treatments can be integrated into clinical practice.

Keywords: neurodegenerative, neuroprotective, herbals, botanicals, therapies, cognitive, memory, acetylcholinesterase

Abbreviations

AD	Alzheimer's disease
Aβ	amyloid-beta
EGCG	Epigallocatechin gallate
ROS	reactive oxygen species

Introduction

Alzheimer's disease (AD) poses a significant global health challenge, characterized by progressive cognitive decline, memory loss, and reduced daily functioning. This debilitating condition imposes a heavy emotional and financial burden on patients' families and healthcare systems. Despite numerous medical advancements, a definitive cure for AD has remained elusive for decades. However, recent research suggests that phytochemicals—plant-derived substances—could offer promising avenues for managing and potentially treating this complex illness (Emran et al., 2023; Soliman et al., 2021; Naghavi et al., 2024). This chapter explores the diverse array of phytochemicals, including flavonoids, polyphenols, alkaloids, and terpenoids, and their potential to counteract the degenerative processes associated with

AD. These processes involve oxidative stress, neuro-inflammation, neuronal damage, neurofibrillary tangles, and amyloid-beta plaque accumulation (Hassan et al., 2019). Phytochemicals target these pathogenic pathways through various biological actions, offering a multi-faceted approach to AD. Flavonoids, for instance, have shown neuroprotective benefits by reducing inflammation, regulating oxidative stress, and possibly disrupting amyloid-beta peptide aggregation (Malik et al., 2015; Munjal et al., 2023). Polyphenols from fruits, vegetables, and teas have garnered interest for their antioxidant, neuroprotective, and anti-inflammatory properties (Bansal et al., 2021; Chopra et al., 2022; Singla et al., 2021; Walia et al., 2022a). Additionally, alkaloids and terpenoids from medicinal plants may slow AD progression by influencing neurotransmitter systems (Tayal et al., 2023). The chapter reviews recent studies on phytochemicals, detailing their potential therapeutic uses, mechanisms of action, and the latest developments in phytochemical-based therapies. It also addresses the challenges related to bioavailability, pharmacokinetics, and interactions with the human body. As the volume and complexity of biological data grow, artificial intelligence (AI) may play a crucial role in advancing AD clinical trials (Chopra et al., 2023). Ultimately, phytochemicals represent a promising research frontier in the quest for effective AD management and prevention, offering hope for new therapeutic strategies to combat this devastating neurodegenerative disease.

Flavonoids

Fruits, leaves, vegetables, and other botanical parts are rich in flavonoids, a diverse group of natural compounds that have recently garnered attention as potential treatments for AD (Munjal et al., 2020). These bioactive substances exhibit a range of neuroprotective activities by targeting key pathogenic processes associated with AD, such as oxidative stress, neuro-inflammation, and neuronal damage (Bellavite, 2023). Flavonoids play a crucial role in preventing neuronal damage and cognitive decline caused by oxidative stress, a hallmark of AD. They also possess anti-inflammatory properties, which are vital for managing AD's progression. Chronic neuro-inflammation, marked by microglial activation and pro-inflammatory mediator production, exacerbates neuronal damage and contributes to disease development (Al-Khayri et al., 2022). For instance, apigenin and luteolin have shown promise in mitigating neuro-inflammatory responses by modulating microglial activation and inflammatory mediator release (Rezai-Zadeh et al., 2008; Munjal et al., 2020).

Additionally, flavonoids can disrupt the production and detrimental effects of amyloid-beta (Aβ) aggregates, which are central to AD pathology (Li et al., 2022). Compounds such as fisetin, hesperidin, and kaempferol inhibit Aβ peptide aggregation, potentially preventing the formation of harmful Aβ oligomers and fibrils that lead to synaptic dysfunction and neuronal injury. Some flavonoids also facilitate Aβ clearance, reducing the brain's Aβ load and its neurotoxic effects. Quercetin, a well-studied flavonoid, is noteworthy for its antioxidant and anti-inflammatory properties, which may protect neurons from oxidative stress and inflammation, key factors in AD (Goyal et al., 2023; Khan et al., 2020). Quercetin's ability to neutralize reactive oxygen species and modulate inflammatory pathways could help reduce neuronal damage and support cognitive function. Additionally, it may prevent the formation of Aβ oligomers and enhance Aβ clearance pathways (Alghamdi et al., 2022; Yoon & Jo, 2012). Rutin, another flavonoid, offers significant antioxidant and anti-inflammatory benefits, potentially protecting neurons and slowing AD progression by reducing oxidative stress and inflammation (Xu et al., 2014; Ganeshpurkar & Saluja, 2017). It may also inhibit Aβ aggregation and support Aβ clearance (Sun et al., 2021). EGCG, a polyphenol found in green tea, has gained attention for its neuroprotective properties due to its antioxidant and anti-inflammatory actions, which could mitigate AD-related neuronal damage and cognitive decline (Abu-Elfotuh et al., 2023; Payne et al., 2022). EGCG may also inhibit Aβ plaque formation and facilitate Aβ removal, potentially improving cognitive function (Habashi et al., 2022; Zhang et al., 2022). Apigenin, widely found in parsley, celery, chamomile, and citrus fruits, also demonstrates antioxidant and anti-inflammatory properties, reducing oxidative damage and neuro-inflammation, and potentially preventing Aβ aggregation (Salehi et al., 2019; Huo et al., 2023). The effectiveness of flavonoids in AD therapy depends on overcoming challenges related to their metabolism, absorption, and brain penetration. Researchers are developing strategies to enhance their bioavailability and therapeutic efficacy, including innovative delivery methods and structural modifications (Bhattacharya et al., 2022; Chopra et al., 2021). Overall, flavonoids represent a promising class of compounds with potential neuroprotective effects against AD, offering hope for new therapeutic strategies. Continued research into their mechanisms of action, optimization of administration, and rigorous clinical trials are essential for harnessing their full therapeutic potential.

Alkaloids

Alkaloids, a diverse group of naturally occurring compounds found in plants, fungi, and some mammals, have attracted significant interest for their neuroprotective properties, especially in the context of Alzheimer's disease (AD). One notable alkaloid is huperzine A, derived from the traditional Chinese herb Huperzia serrata. Huperzine A functions as an acetylcholinesterase inhibitor, thereby helping to maintain higher levels of acetylcholine, a neurotransmitter crucial for learning and memory. This action may protect nerve cells and improve memory, potentially delaying cognitive decline associated with AD (Dang et al., 2023; Friedli & Inestrosa, 2021; Tamchès & Decosterd Kerhuel, 2009; Wang et al., 2001, 2003; Wong et al., 2016). Another promising alkaloid is galantamine, found in daffodil and snowdrop plants, which enhances cognitive performance by inhibiting acetylcholinesterase and modulating nicotinic receptors. Clinical trials have shown that galantamine can improve cognitive function and daily living activities in AD patients (Metz & Pavlov, 2021; Buchanan et al., 2017). Both galantamine and rivastigmine are FDA-approved acetylcholinesterase inhibitors for AD. Donepezil, another acetylcholinesterase inhibitor, has demonstrated significant effectiveness in improving cognitive function, behavior, and overall patient outcomes in clinical trials (Gill et al., 2004; Hsieh et al., 2022; Hu et al., 2022). Additionally, hirsutine, an alkaloid from Uncaria rhynchophylla, plays a role in regulating tau phosphorylation, a key pathological feature of AD. Hirsutine and other alkaloids like corynoxine and isocorynoxeine have been shown to penetrate the blood-brain barrier and may exert both central and peripheral effects in AD treatment (Xu et al., 2021; Zeng et al., 2021). While the precise mechanisms of hirsutine's effects are not fully understood, its ability to enter the brain and influence tau phosphorylation suggests potential therapeutic benefits in AD.

Terpenoids

AD is characterized by dementia and various cognitive impairments. Research suggests that Panax ginseng extract may offer symptomatic relief for AD patients. Studies have shown that ginseng extract can mitigate the adverse effects of Aβ oligomer injection on memory in mice and protect against Aβ-induced neurotoxicity in laboratory tests (Seo et al., 2010; Shin et al., 2019).

A 6-month open-label randomized trial demonstrated that Korean red ginseng (KRG) improved cognitive function in AD patients, indicating its potential as a complementary therapy to enhance the effectiveness of existing AD treatments (Heo et al., 2011; Gauttam et al., 2024). Ginseng's active components, ginsenosides, have been linked to improvements in cognitive abilities, including processing speed, working memory, attention, and auditory response time in healthy individuals. These benefits are attributed to ginsenosides' ability to reduce neuroinflammation, protect neurons, and alleviate oxidative stress damage (Figure 1) (Lou et al., 2021; Yang et al., 2023; Yao & Guan, 2022; Yu et al., 2023; Zhao et al., 2022). Ginkgo biloba extract has been widely studied for its potential benefits in both cardiovascular and central nervous system health, with increasing interest in its possible role in preventing AD. A review and meta-analysis indicated that while Ginkgo biloba extract showed limited effectiveness in treating AD in individuals aged around 70 years or older, it demonstrated some positive effects in managing the disease in a younger population (Chong et al., 2020). Clinical trials have yielded mixed results, with some showing benefits and others not. Despite its generally safe profile and minimal reported adverse effects, there is insufficient evidence to conclusively support its efficacy in preventing cognitive decline or dementia.

In the realm of cannabinoid research, compounds like tetrahydrocannabinol (THC) and cannabidiol (CBD) have been explored for their medicinal potential in AD. Combination therapies involving THC and CBD have often proven more effective than single compounds alone. While cannabis use or abuse has been associated with memory and learning impairments due to its high expression in the endocannabinoid system within the hippocampus and cortex, recent studies using AD mouse models have shown that cannabinoids may help alleviate dementia-related symptoms (Walther & Halpern, 2010). Preliminary clinical trials suggest that cannabis may reduce aggressive and agitated behaviors in dementia patients, although research in this area remains limited. Initial evidence indicates that CBD, in particular, may hold therapeutic promise for treating AD.

Conclusion

Investigating phytochemicals as potential treatments for AD represents a promising advancement in the search for effective medicinal solutions. Plant-based substances such as polyphenols, flavonoids, and terpenoids have demonstrated significant antioxidant, anti-inflammatory, and neuroprotective effects in preclinical studies. Despite these encouraging findings, extensive and comprehensive research is needed before these phytochemicals can be applied clinically. Key areas that require further exploration include understanding the specific mechanisms by which phytochemicals interact with the complex pathways involved in AD, determining optimal dosages, and improving bioavailability. Additionally, integrating phytochemical-based treatments into standard AD care requires careful consideration, emphasizing individualized and holistic approaches. As research continues to uncover the medicinal properties of phytochemicals, there is hope that they could contribute to developing new and effective treatments for this devastating neurodegenerative disease.

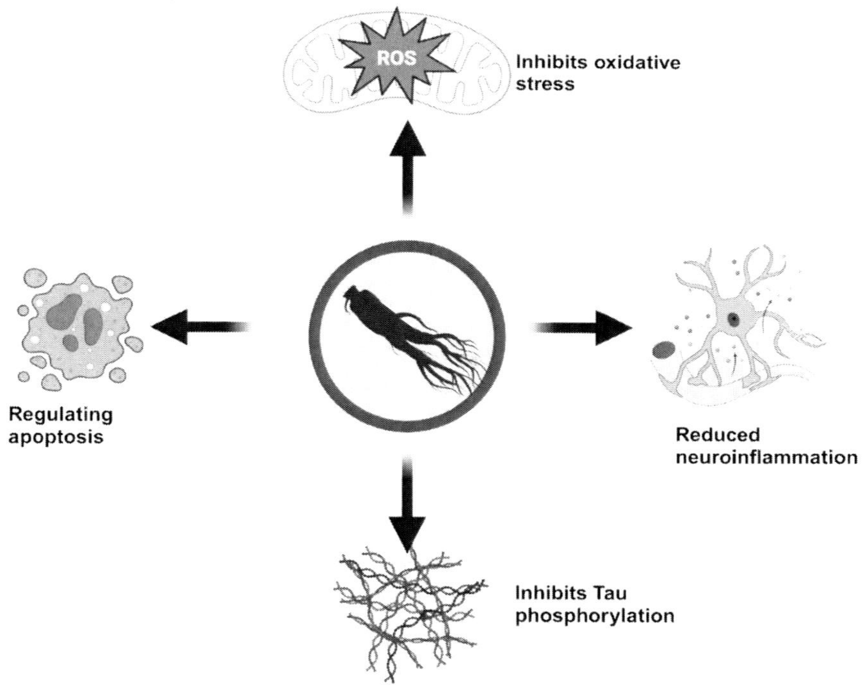

Figure 1. Biological effects of Ginseng on treatment of AD.

References

Abu-Elfotuh, K., Tolba, A. M., Hussein, F. H., Hamdan, A. M., Rabeh, M. A., Alshahri, S. A., Ali, A. A., Mosaad, S. M., Mahmoud, N. A., Elsaeed, M. Y. and Abdelglil, R. M. & Mahran, Y. F. (2023). Anti-alzheimer activity of combinations of cocoa with vinpocetine or other nutraceuticals in rat model: modulation of wnt3/β-catenin/GSK-3β/nrf2/HO-1 and PERK/CHOP/Bcl-2 pathways. *Pharmaceutics*, 15(8), 2063.

Alghamdi, A., Birch, D. J., Vyshemirsky, V., & Rolinski, O. J. (2022). Impact of the Flavonoid Quercetin on β-Amyloid Aggregation Revealed by Intrinsic Fluorescence. *The Journal of Physical Chemistry B*, 126(38), 7229-7237.

Alghamdi, A., Birch, D. J., Vyshemirsky, V., & Rolinski, O. J. (2022). Impact of the Flavonoid Quercetin on β-Amyloid Aggregation Revealed by Intrinsic Fluorescence. *The Journal of Physical Chemistry B*, 126(38), 7229-7237.

Al-Khayri, J. M., Sahana, G. R., Nagella, P., Joseph, B. V., Alessa, F. M., & Al-Mssallem, M. Q. (2022). Flavonoids as potential anti-inflammatory molecules: A review. *Molecules*, 27(9), 2901.

Bansal, H., Singla, R. K., Behzad, S., Chopra, H., Grewal, A. S., & Shen, B. (2021). Unleashing the potential of microbial natural products in drug discovery: focusing on streptomyces as antimicrobials goldmine. *Current Topics in Medicinal Chemistry*, 21(26), 2374-2396.

Bellavite P. (2023). Neuroprotective Potentials of Flavonoids: Experimental Studies and Mechanisms of Action. *Antioxidants*, 12(2), 280.

Bhattacharya, T., Soares, G. A. B. E., Chopra, H., Rahman, M. M., Hasan, Z., Swain, S. S., & Cavalu, S. (2022). Applications of phyto-nanotechnology for the treatment of neurodegenerative disorders. *Materials*, 15(3), 804.

Buchanan, R. W., Kelly, D. L., Weiner, E., Gold, J. M., Strauss, G. P., Koola, M. M., McMahon, R. P. & Carpenter, W. T. (2017). A randomized clinical trial of oxytocin or galantamine for the treatment of negative symptoms and cognitive impairments in people with schizophrenia. *Journal of Clinical Psychopharmacology*, 37(4), 394-400.

Chakrawarti, L., Agrawal, R., Dang, S., Gupta, S., & Gabrani, R. (2016). Therapeutic effects of EGCG: a patent review. *Expert Opinion on Therapeutic Patents*, 26(8), 907-916.

Chong, P. Z., Ng, H. Y., Tai, J. T., & Lee, S. W. H. (2020). Efficacy and safety of Ginkgo biloba in patients with acute ischemic stroke: a systematic review and meta-analysis. *The American Journal of Chinese Medicine*, 48(03), 513-534.

Chopra, H., & Elshikh, M. S. (2023). Introduction to the role of fruits in nutraceutical and functional foods. In *Fruits and Their Roles in Nutraceuticals and Functional Foods* (pp. 1-28). CRC Press.

Chopra, H., Bibi, S., Goyal, R., Gautam, R. K., Trivedi, R., Upadhyay, T. K., Mujahid, M. H., Shah, M. A., Haris, M., Khot, K. B. & Kim, B. (2022). Chemopreventive potential of dietary nanonutraceuticals for prostate cancer: an extensive review. *Frontiers in Oncology*, 12, 925379.

Chopra, H., Dey, P. S., Das, D., Bhattacharya, T., Shah, M., Mubin, S., Maishu, S. P., Akter, R., Rahman, M. H., Karthika, C. & Alamri, B. M. (2021). Curcumin nanoparticles as promising therapeutic agents for drug targets. *Molecules*, 26(16), 4998.

Chopra, H., Mishra, A. K., Baig, A. A., Mohanta, T. K., Mohanta, Y. K., & Baek, K. H. (2021). Narrative review: Bioactive potential of various mushrooms as the treasure of versatile therapeutic natural product. *Journal of Fungi*, 7(9), 728.

Chopra, H., Munjal, K., & Emran, T. B. (2023). Artificial intelligence 2.0: Taking organoid intelligence a step ahead. *International Journal of Surgery Open*, 60, 100693.

Chopra, H., Shin, D. K., Munjal, K., Dhama, K., & Emran, T. B. (2023). Revolutionizing clinical trials: the role of AI in accelerating medical breakthroughs. *International Journal of Surgery*, 109(12), 4211-4220.

Dang, T. K., Hong, S. M., Dao, V. T., Nguyen, D. T., Nguyen, K. V., Nguyen, H. T., Nguyen, K. V., Nguyen, H. T., Ullah, S., Tran, H. T & Kim, S. Y. (2023). Neuroprotective effects of total alkaloids fraction of Huperzia serrata on scopolamine-induced neurodegenerative animals. *Phytotherapy Research*, 37(1), 140-150.

Emran, T. B., Chopra, H., & Dhama, K. (2023). Autophagy and Alzheimer's disease: How far science has to be progressed?- correspondence. *Annals of Medicine and Surgery*, 85(2), 323-325.

Friedli, M. J., & Inestrosa, N. C. (2021). Huperzine A and its neuroprotective molecular signaling in Alzheimer's disease. *Molecules*, 26(21), 6531.

Ganeshpurkar, A., & Saluja, A. K. (2017). The pharmacological potential of rutin. *Saudi Pharmaceutical Journal*, 25(2), 149-164.

Gauttam, V. K., Munjal, K., Chopra, H., Ahmad, A., Rana, M. K., & Kamal, M. A. (2024). A Mechanistic Review on Therapeutic Potential of Medicinal Plants and their Pharmacologically Active Molecules for Targeting Metabolic Syndrome. *Current Pharmaceutical Design*, 30(1), 10-30.

Gauttam, V. K., Munjal, K., Singh, V., Sharma, I., & Sahpuriya, P. (2022). Phytochemicals for metabolic syndrome. In *Natural Products for treatment of metabolic syndrome*. 235-245.

GBD 2021 Causes of Death Collaborators (2024). Global burden of 288 causes of death and life expectancy decomposition in 204 countries and territories and 811 subnational locations, 1990-2021: a systematic analysis for the Global Burden of Disease Study 2021. *Lancet*, 403(10440), 2100–2132.

Gill, S. S., Bronskill, S. E., Mamdani, M., Sykora, K., Li, P., Shulman, K. I., Anderson, G. M., Hillmer, M. P., Wodchis, W. P. & Rochon, P. A. (2004). Representation of patients with dementia in clinical trials of donepezil. *Canadian journal of clinical pharmacology*, 11(2), e274-85.

Goyal, R., Chopra, H., Singh, I., Dua, K., & Gautam, R. K. (2022). Insights on prospects of nano-siRNA based approaches in treatment of Cancer. *Frontiers in Pharmacology*, 13, 985670.

Goyal, R., Mittal, G., Khurana, S., Malik, N., Kumar, V., Soni, A., Chopra, H. & Kamal, M. A. (2024). Insights on Quercetin Therapeutic potential for neurodegenerative diseases and its Nano-technological perspectives. *Current Pharmaceutical Biotechnology*, 25(9), 1132-1141.

Habashi, M., Vutla, S., Tripathi, K., Senapati, S., Chauhan, P. S., Haviv-Chesner, A., Richman, M., Mohand, S. A., Dumulon-Perreault, V., Mulamreddy, R& Rahimipour, S. (2022). Early diagnosis and treatment of Alzheimer's disease by targeting toxic soluble Aβ oligomers. *Proceedings of the National Academy of Sciences*, 119(49), e2210766119.

Han, X., Xu, T., Fang, Q., Zhang, H., Yue, L., Hu, G., & Sun, L. (2021). Quercetin hinders microglial activation to alleviate neurotoxicity via the interplay between NLRP3 inflammasome and mitophagy. *Redox Biology*, 44, 102010.

Han, Y., Zhang, T., Su, J., Zhao, Y., & Li, X. (2017). Apigenin attenuates oxidative stress and neuronal apoptosis in early brain injury following subarachnoid hemorrhage. *Journal of Clinical Neuroscience*, 40, 157-162.

Hassan, M., Raza, H., Abbasi, M. A., Moustafa, A. A., & Seo, S. Y. (2019). The exploration of novel Alzheimer's therapeutic agents from the pool of FDA approved medicines using drug repositioning, enzyme inhibition and kinetic mechanism approaches. *Biomedicine & Pharmacotherapy*, 109, 2513-2526.

He, J., Xu, L., Yang, L., & Wang, X. (2018). Epigallocatechin gallate is the most effective catechin against antioxidant stress via hydrogen peroxide and radical scavenging activity. *Medical Science Monitor*, 24, 8198.

Heo, J. H., Lee, S. T., Oh, M. J., Park, H. J., Shim, J. Y., Chu, K., & Kim, M. (2011). Improvement of cognitive deficit in Alzheimer's disease patients by long term treatment with Korean red ginseng. *Journal of Ginseng Research*, 35(4), 457.

Hsieh, C. F., Tseng, P. T., Chen, T. Y., Lin, P. Y., Chen, Y. W., Ho, B. L., Hsu, C. Y. & Liu, C. K. (2022). The association of changes of sleep architecture related to donepezil: A systematic review and meta-analysis. *Journal of the Formosan Medical Association*, 121(8), 1466-1477.

Hu, Y., Zhang, L., Guan, X., Hou, H., Bi, S., Liu, C., Li. M. & Wang, K. (2022). Gunao-Yizhi decoction combined with donepezil for vascular dementia: A systematic review and meta-analysis. *Medicine*, 101(40), e30971.

Huo, Y., Zhao, C., Wang, Y., Wang, S., Mu, T., & Du, W. (2023). Roles of Apigenin and Nepetin in the assembly behavior and cytotoxicity of prion neuropeptide PrP106-126. *ACS Chemical Neuroscience*, 15(2), 245-257.

Khan, H., Ullah, H., Aschner, M., Cheang, W. S., & Akkol, E. K. (2019). Neuroprotective effects of quercetin in Alzheimer's disease. *Biomolecules*, 10(1), 59.

Kumar, V., & Kundu, S. (2022). Studies on apigenin and its biological and pharmacological activity in brain disorders. *Advanced Pharmaceutical Bulletin*, 12(4), 645.

Lang, G. P., Li, C., & Han, Y. Y. (2021). Rutin pretreatment promotes microglial M1 to M2 phenotype polarization. *Neural Regeneration Research*, 16(12), 2499-2504.

Lee, S. T., Chu, K., Sim, J. Y., Heo, J. H., & Kim, M. (2008). Panax ginseng enhances cognitive performance in Alzheimer disease. *Alzheimer Disease & Associated Disorders*, 22(3), 222-226.

Li, J., Sun, M., Cui, X., & Li, C. (2022). Protective effects of flavonoids against Alzheimer's disease: pathological hypothesis, potential targets, and structure–activity relationship. *International Journal of Molecular Sciences*, 23(17), 10020.

Liao, Z., Cheng, L., Li, X., Zhang, M., Wang, S., & Huo, R. (2020). Meta-analysis of Ginkgo biloba preparation for the treatment of Alzheimer's disease. *Clinical Neuropharmacology*, 43(4), 93-99.

Lou, T., Huang, Q., Su, H., Zhao, D., & Li, X. (2021). Targeting Sirtuin 1 signaling pathway by ginsenosides. *Journal of Ethnopharmacology*, 268, 113657.

Malik, J., Munjal, K., & Deshmukh, R. (2015). Attenuating effect of standardized lyophilized Cinnamomum zeylanicum bark extract against streptozotocin-induced experimental dementia of Alzheimer's type. *Journal of Basic and Clinical Physiology and Pharmacology*, 26(3), 275-285.

Metz, C. N., & Pavlov, V. A. (2021). Treating disorders across the lifespan by modulating cholinergic signaling with galantamine. *Journal of Neurochemistry*, 158(6), 1359-1380.

Munjal, K., Ahmad, S., Gupta, A., Haye, A., Amin, S., & Mir, S. R. (2020). Polyphenol-enriched fraction and the compounds isolated from Garcinia indica fruits ameliorate obesity through suppression of digestive enzymes and oxidative stress. *Pharmacognosy Magazine*, 16(70).

Munjal, K., Gautam, V. K., Goel, Y., Ahamad, J., & Mir, S. R. (2023). Qualitative Diagnostic Features of Alkaloidal Spices. In *Analysis of Food Spices* (pp. 135-150). CRC Press.

Payne, A., Taka, E., Adinew, G. M., & Soliman, K. F. (2023). Molecular mechanisms of the anti-inflammatory effects of epigallocatechin 3-gallate (EGCG) in LPS-Activated BV-2 microglia cells. *Brain Sciences*, 13(4), 632.

Rezai-Zadeh, K., Ehrhart, J., Bai, Y., Sanberg, P. R., Bickford, P., Tan, J., & Shytle, R. D. (2008). Apigenin and luteolin modulate microglial activation via inhibition of STAT1-induced CD40 expression. *Journal of Neuroinflammation*, 5, 1-10.

Sahadevan, R., Singh, S., Binoy, A., & Sadhukhan, S. (2023). Chemico-biological aspects of (−)-epigallocatechin-3-gallate (EGCG) to improve its stability, bioavailability and membrane permeability: Current status and future prospects. *Critical Reviews in Food Science and Nutrition*, 63(30), 10382-10411.

Salehi, B., Venditti, A., Sharifi-Rad, M., Kręgiel, D., Sharifi-Rad, J., Durazzo, A., Lucarini, M., Santini, A., Souto, E. B., Novellino, & Martins, N. (2019). The therapeutic potential of apigenin. *International Journal of Molecular Sciences*, 20(6), 1305.

Sanad, S. M., Farouk, R., Nassar, S. E., Alshahrani, M. Y., Suliman, M., Ahmed, A. E., & Elesawi, I. E. (2023). The neuroprotective effect of quercetin nanoparticles in the therapy of neuronal damage stimulated by acrolein. *Saudi Journal of Biological Sciences*, 30(11), 103792.

Seo, J. S., Yun, J. H., Baek, I. S., Leem, Y. H., Kang, H. W., Cho, H. K., Lyu, Y. S., Son, H. J. & Han, P. L. (2010). Oriental medicine Jangwonhwan reduces Aβ (1–42) level and β-amyloid deposition in the brain of Tg-APPswe/PS1dE9 mouse model of Alzheimer disease. *Journal of ethnopharmacology*, 128(1), 206-212.

Shin, S. J., Jeon, S. G., Kim, J. I., Jeong, Y. O., Kim, S., Park, Y. H., Lee, S. K., Park, H. H., Hong, S. B., Oh, S. & Moon, M. (2019). Red ginseng attenuates Aβ-induced mitochondrial dysfunction and Aβ-mediated pathology in an animal model of Alzheimer's disease. *International Journal of Molecular Sciences*, 20(12), 3030.

Singla, R. K., Behzad, S., Khan, J., Tsagkaris, C., Gautam, R. K., Goyal, R., Chopra, H. & Shen, B. (2022). Natural kinase inhibitors for the treatment and management of endometrial/uterine cancer: preclinical to clinical studies. *Frontiers in pharmacology*, 13, 801733.

Singla, R. K., He, X., Chopra, H., Tsagkaris, C., Shen, L., Kamal, M. A., & Shen, B. (2021). Natural products for the prevention and control of the COVID-19 pandemic: sustainable bioresources. *Frontiers in Pharmacology*, 12, 758159.

Soliman, H. M., Ghonaim, G. A., Gharib, S. M., Chopra, H., Farag, A. K., Hassanin, M. H., Nagah, A., Emad-Eldin, M., Hashem, N. E., Yahya, G., Emam, S. E., Hassan, A. E. A., & Attia, M. S. (2021). Exosomes in Alzheimer's disease: from being pathological players to potential diagnostics and therapeutics. *International Journal of Molecular Sciences*, 22(19), 10794.

Sun, X. Y., Li, L. J., Dong, Q. X., Zhu, J., Huang, Y. R., Hou, S. J., Yu, X. L. & Liu, R. T. (2021). Rutin prevents tau pathology and neuroinflammation in a mouse model of Alzheimer's disease. *Journal of Neuroinflammation*, 18(1), 131.

Tamchès, E., & Kerhuel, G. D. (2009). Mimopezil, A Huperzine A Derivative Undergoing Clinical Development For The Treatment Of Alzheimer's Disease. *Planta Medica*, 75(09), L12.

Tayal, R., Munjal, K., Gauttam, V. K., Popli, P., Khurana, L., & Choudhary, N. (2023). Potential role of hesperidin in lifestyle disorders: A scoping review. *South African Journal of Botany*, 161, 542-554.

Valverde-Salazar, V., Ruiz-Gabarre, D., & García-Escudero, V. (2023). Alzheimer's disease and green tea: epigallocatechin-3-gallate as a modulator of inflammation and oxidative stress. *Antioxidants*, 12(7), 1460.

Walia, V., Kaushik, D., Mittal, V., Kumar, K., Verma, R., Parashar, J., Akter, R., Rahman, M. H., Bhatia, S., Al-Harrasi, A., Karthika, C., Bhattacharya, T., Chopra, H., & Ashraf, G. M. (2022). Delineation of Neuroprotective Effects and Possible Benefits of AntioxidantsTherapy for the Treatment of Alzheimer's Diseases by Targeting Mitochondrial-Derived Reactive Oxygen Species: Bench to Bedside. *Molecular Neurobiology*, 59(1), 657–680.

Walther, S., & Halpern, M. (2010). Cannabinoids and dementia: a review of clinical and preclinical data. *Pharmaceuticals,* 3(8), 2689-2708.

Wang, R., Zhang, H. Y., & Tang, X. C. (2001). Huperzine A attenuates cognitive dysfunction and neuronal degeneration caused by β-amyloid protein-(1–40) in rat. *European Journal of Pharmacology*, 421(3), 149-156.

Wong, J. C., Dutton, S. B., Collins, S. D., Schachter, S., & Escayg, A. (2016). Huperzine a provides robust and sustained protection against induced seizures in Scn1a mutant mice. *Frontiers in Pharmacology*, 7, 357.

Xu, P. X., Wang, S. W., Yu, X. L., Su, Y. J., Wang, T., Zhou, W. W., Zhang, H., Wang, Y. J., & Liu, R. T. (2014). Rutin improves spatial memory in Alzheimer's disease transgenic mice by reducing Aβ oligomer level and attenuating oxidative stress and neuroinflammation. *Behavioural Brain Research*, 264, 173-180.

Xu, Q. Q., Shaw, P. C., Hu, Z., Yang, W., Ip, S. P., Xian, Y. F., & Lin, Z. X. (2021). Comparison of the chemical constituents and anti-Alzheimer's disease effects of Uncaria rhynchophylla and Uncaria tomentosa. *Chinese Medicine*, 16, 1-15.

Yang, Z., Yu, Y., Sun, N., Zhou, L., Zhang, D., Chen, H., Miao, W., Gao, W., Zhang, C., Liu, C& Gao, Y. (2023). Ginsenosides Rc, as a novel SIRT6 activator, protects mice against high fat diet induced NAFLD. *Journal of Ginseng Research*, 47(3), 376-384.

Yao, W., & Guan, Y. (2022). Ginsenosides in cancer: A focus on the regulation of cell metabolism. *Biomedicine & Pharmacotherapy*, 156, 113756.

Yoon, S. S., & Jo, S. A. (2012). Mechanisms of amyloid-β peptide clearance: potential therapeutic targets for Alzheimer's disease. *Biomolecules & Therapeutics*, 20(3), 245.

Yu, T., Tang, Y., Zhang, F., & Zhang, L. (2023). Roles of ginsenosides in sepsis. *Journal of Ginseng Research*, 47(1), 1-8.

Zeng, P., Wang, X. M., Ye, C. Y., Su, H. F., & Tian, Q. (2021). The main alkaloids in Uncaria rhynchophylla and their anti-Alzheimer's disease mechanism determined by a network pharmacology approach. *International Journal of Molecular Sciences*, 22(7), 3612.

Zhang, H., Jiang, X., Ma, L., Wei, W., Li, Z., Chang, S., Wen, J., Sun, J. & Li, H. (2022). Role of Aβ in Alzheimer's-related synaptic dysfunction. *Frontiers in Cell and Developmental Biology*, 10, 964075.

Zhao, A., Liu, N., Yao, M., Zhang, Y., Yao, Z., Feng, Y., Liu, J. & Zhou, G. (2022). A review of neuroprotective effects and mechanisms of ginsenosides from Panax ginseng in treating ischemic stroke. *Frontiers in Pharmacology*, 13, 946752.

Zhao, L., Wang, J. L., Liu, R., Li, X. X., Li, J. F., & Zhang, L. (2013). Neuroprotective, anti-amyloidogenic and neurotrophic effects of apigenin in an Alzheimer's disease mouse model. *Molecules*, 18(8), 9949-9965.

Chapter 15

The Application of Nanophytoherbals in Parkinson's Therapy

Shivanki Joshi[1,*]
Neha Saini[2]
Aakriti Saini[1]
and Swati[1]
[1]Guru Gobind Singh College of Pharmacy, Yamuna Nagar, Haryana, India
[2]Global Research Institute of Pharmacy, Raduar, Yamuna Nagar, Haryana, India

Abstract

Maharishi Charaka described Parkinsonism in Ayurvedic medicine as early as 300 BC in his work, Charaka Samhita. This was followed by James Parkinson's seminal article, An Essay on the Shaking Palsy, which outlined Parkinson's disease (PD) in Western medicine. There is an urgent need for medication therapies that more effectively target the pathobiological pathways of PD while minimizing side effects. Recently, herbal and natural product formulations have emerged as potentially effective therapeutic options, either as stand-alone treatments or as neuroprotective support for existing medications. Nanobiotechnologies offer promising advancements for various applications, including gene therapy, diabetes, cancer treatment, antiviral and antifungal medications, and chronic lung ailments. The use of specialized nanomaterials in drug delivery has resulted in several benefits, such as improved blood circulation half-lives, increased solubility, and reduced impact on healthy cells. Phytochemicals integrated into nanotechnological approaches are proving to be valuable for PD therapy. However, creating

* Corresponding Author's Email: shivankijoshi1@gmail.com.

In: Natural Solutions for Neurodegenerative Disorders
Editors: Rahul Kumar Sharma, Shailesh Sharma, Ajmer Singh Grewal et al.
ISBN: 979-8-89530-231-6

nanophytomedicines for PD treatment presents challenges. Future development should focus on engineering smart nanoparticle drug delivery systems to achieve more efficient and customized drug delivery. This involves optimizing pharmacokinetics, controlling biodistribution, and preventing drug release at non-target sites to enhance therapeutic effectiveness and minimize side effects. Although human trials of nanophytomedicines are limited, *in vivo* studies in animal models have shown promising results in mitigating Parkinson's-related processes, indicating that these approaches may eventually serve as viable therapeutic agents for PD.

Keywords: Parkinson's disease, neuroprotective, nanophytomedicines, clinical trials, stability

Abbreviations

6-OHDA	6-hydroxydopamine
AuNPs	Gold nanoparticles
BEND3 BEN	Domain Containing 3
H_2O_2	Hydrogen Peroxide
HBMEC	Human brain microvessel endothelial cells
MAO-B	Monoamine Oxidase B
mPEG-PLGA	Methyoxy poly(ethylene glycol)-block-poly((D,L)-lactico-glycolic acid)
MPP+	(1-Methyl-4-Phenylpyridinium)
NIR	Near infrared spectroscopy
NPs	Nanoparticles
P188	Poloxamer 188
PCL	Poly(ε-caprolactone)
PD	Parkinson's Disease
PEG	Poly(ethylene glycol)
PLGA	Co-polymer poly(lactic-co-glycolic acid)
PS80	Polysorbate 80
ROS	Reactive Oxygen Species
SO	Sesame Seed Oil

Introduction

Maharishi Charaka described Parkinsonism in Ayurvedic medicine in his Charaka Samhita as early as 300 BC (Borah et al., 2017). This was followed by James Parkinson's seminal work, "An Essay on the Shaking Palsy," which provided a Western medical description of Parkinson's disease (PD) (Parkinson, 2002). PD is characterized by motor symptoms such as bradykinesia, resting tremor, postural instability, and rigidity, alongside various non-motor symptoms including depression, cognitive decline, hyposmia, psychosis, gastrointestinal dysfunction, sleep disturbances, and autonomic dysfunction (Armstrong & Okun, 2020). The long-term progression of these symptoms leads to significant disability and care needs, adversely affecting the patient's quality of life. Neuropathological features of PD include toxic α-synuclein protein accumulations in Lewy bodies and Lewy neurites, and dopaminergic degeneration of the substantia nigra pars compacta, resulting in reduced dopamine levels in the striatum (Kouli et al., 2018). The pathobiological microenvironment of PD involves multiple processes. Post-translational modifications and genetic variants that cause α-synuclein overexpression contribute to protein aggregation (Kim et al., 2017). This aggregation leads to neurotoxicity and neuronal degeneration (Chiba et al., 2006). Additionally, oxidative stress plays a crucial role in neuronal degeneration in PD, as evidenced by the oxidation of DNA, lipids, and proteins in the presence of depleted antioxidants such as glutathione (Dias et al., 2013). Levodopa remains the current gold standard for PD treatment. It crosses the blood-brain barrier (BBB) and is converted to dopamine, helping to restore dopamine levels in the striatum. The development of this medication was based on Arvid Carlsson's experiments from the 1950s. However, while levodopa provides temporary relief of motor symptoms, it does not halt disease progression or prevent dopaminergic neuron death. Moreover, adverse effects such as dyskinesias, impulse control disorders, and drug-induced toxicity are frequently associated with its use (Connolly et al., 2014). Its short half-life also results in variable plasma levels and clinical responses, often requiring combination with other medications (Poewe & Antonini, 2015). Other approved treatments include monoamine oxidase B (MAO-B) inhibitors, dopamine agonists, and anticholinergics, though these also have significant side effects (Sivanandy et al., 2022). Non-pharmaceutical options such as deep brain stimulation have shown promising results but are not suitable for all patients. There is a critical need to develop drug therapies for PD that more precisely target the pathobiological pathways while minimizing side effects. Recent interest in herbal and natural product formulations has highlighted their potential as therapeutic options for PD, either as stand-alone treatments or as neuroprotective adjuncts to conventional medications. Plant-derived medications offer several advantages over synthetic treatments, including lower costs, fewer side effects, ease of use, and greater public acceptability. However, challenges such as structural instability, acidic pH sensitivity, and difficulties in crossing the blood-brain barrier can limit their effectiveness. Nanoplatforms have emerged as effective solutions to these challenges, enhancing the pharmacological activity, stability, solubility, and bioavailability of plant-derived medicines. This advancement facilitates the application of these therapies in areas such as PD (Burns et al., 2023).

Nanotechnology in Medicine

The potential advantages of nano-biotechnologies offer promising prospects for various medical applications, including gene therapy, diabetes management, cancer treatments, antiviral and antifungal medications, and chronic lung diseases (Wanisa, 2019). At the single-cell and molecular levels, nanotechnologies enhance medical diagnosis capabilities (Hulla et al., 2015). Commonly utilized nanoparticles, such as quantum dots, gold, and silver nanoparticles, are making significant impacts. Notably, they hold promise for biomarker discovery, early cancer diagnosis, and infectious germ detection, though their potential diagnostic applications extend beyond these areas (Brown, 2014).

Phytotherapy in PD

Numerous studies have shown tea polyphenols to protect against brain damage in various animal models of PD. Albizia adianthifolia (Leguminosae) leaf aqueous extract has antioxidant capacity and may be able to help treat PD-related neurological abnormalities. Environmental pollution, on the one hand, and the adverse consequences of pharmaceutical medications, on the other, may be the cause of the global propensity in favour of using alternative natural products and herbal medicines. A growing trend towards the usage of these plants and the resurgence of traditional medicine are caused by the rising incidence of nervous system illnesses. Promising findings from recent studies have also been published, highlighting the benefits of herbal treatments for the prevention or treatment of a wide range of illnesses, including depression, Alzheimer's disease, and many other ailments. In many animal models of PD, plants and plant-based active components such as astragaloside IV, berberine, tinospora cordifolia, and sesame seed oil (SO) are employed (Rabiei et al., 2019). It is evident that employing phytomedicine and nanomedicine to treat PD is an appealing new treatment strategy. An exciting area of development is nanosurgery, which is actively being researched. This field benefits from advancements in nanodiagnosis and targeted nanotherapy, founded on nanopharmacology. Nano-surgical instruments are being developed as practical applications of nano-biotechnology in this domain. Additionally, new biomaterials derived from nanotechnology are showing promise in orthopaedic treatments, despite the complexity of bone tissue and its diverse functions in the body. The use of specialized nanomaterials in drug delivery has numerous advantages, such as extended drug half-lives in the bloodstream, enhanced solubility, and reduced impact on healthy cells. Liposomes, which are phospholipid vesicles with a bilayered membrane structure, are a significant class of nanomaterials used in delivering anticancer medications. For example, PEGylated liposomes can be functionalized with fluorophores or gadolinium for imaging and can encapsulate drugs like doxorubicin for treatment (Lawrence & Lawrence, 2004).

Nanoplatforms and Phytomedicines for PD

Twelve out of the 27 publications reviewed focused on *in vitro* research related to Parkinson's disease (PD). All but one study employed the neuroblastoma cell line SH-SY5Y, with the exception of a study using PC-12 cells (Nellore et al., 2012). Nine studies used the neurotoxin MPP+ to model PD, while two studies utilized both MPP+ and H2O2, and the remaining two employed α-synuclein overexpression models using 6-OHDA95 or an SNCA plasmid. The phytochemicals tested included curcumin (from Curcuma longa), ginkgolide B, schisantherin A, naringenin, puerarin, paeoniflorin, and resveratrol, all showing potential as therapeutic agents for PD. The studies varied in their use of nanoparticles (NPs) for delivery. One study used lipid-based NPs, another used metallic-based NPs, and seven used polymeric NPs (Chen et al., 2016, 2017, 2019; Zhang et al., 2018; Liu et al., 2020, 2022; Zhao et al., 2020; Xiong et al., 2020, 2021; Katila et al., 2022; Md et al., 2019). Types of NPs included gold nanoparticles (AuNPs) (Nellore et al., 2012), nanocrystals (Chen et al., 2016), methoxy poly(ethylene glycol)-block-poly((D,L)-lactide-co-glycolic acid) (mPEG-PLGA) (Chen et al., 2017), and N-(N-(3-triethoxysilyl)propylsuccinamoyl) (Zhang et al., 2018). Other materials used were chitosan (Chen et al., 2019), poly(ethylene glycol) (PEG), poly(ε-caprolactone) (PCL) (Xiong et al., 2020), hydroxypropyl methylcellulose (Liu et al., 2022), and graphene oxide (Xiong et al., 2021). All treatments effectively reduced the toxic effects, with curcumin demonstrating reduced apoptosis, decreased reactive oxygen species (ROS) levels, decreased α-synuclein aggregates, and preserved cellular structure (Nellore et al., 2012; Zhang et al., 2018; Liu et al., 2020). Puerarin and ginkgolide B increased respiration rates, mitochondrial membrane potential, and ATP levels (Chen et al., 2019; Liu et al., 2022; Zhao et al., 2020; Xiong et al., 2020). Encapsulation of phytochemicals in nanoparticles notably enhanced their neuroprotective effects compared to their unencapsulated forms. This improvement is attributed to increased blood-brain barrier (BBB) permeability provided by the nanoparticles (Xiong et al., 2021; Xiong et al., 2020; Katila et al., 2022). Studies using HBMEC or BEND3 cell lines, which closely mimic the BBB, demonstrated that graphene oxide, PLGA, and black phosphorus-incorporated NPs increased BBB permeability of encapsulated phytomedicines by 1-, 2-, and 2-fold, respectively. Functionalization of NPs with lactoferrin further enhanced permeability by 7-, 2-, and 17.5-fold compared to NPs without lactoferrin (Xiong et al., 2020; Katila et al., 2022; Md et al., 2019).

Studies of Nano-Phytomedicines Against PD

Neurotoxins, primarily MPP+ (Chen et al., 2016; Liu et al., 2022; Xiong et al., 2021; Katila et al., 2022) or rotenone, were used to induce Parkinsonism or Parkinson's disease (PD)-related symptoms in various *in vivo* models, including rats, mice, zebrafish, and Drosophila melanogaster. Three studies investigated the therapeutic effects and release characteristics of the drugs across multiple animal models. Resveratrol (5 to 40 mg/kg) and curcumin (15 to 50 mg/kg) were the most commonly used phytochemicals in these studies (Zhang et al., 2018; Liu et al., 2020). Comparisons between phytomedicines and phyto-nanomedicines revealed that nanoparticles (NPs) significantly enhanced the pharmacokinetic properties of the phytochemicals. Specifically, these studies demonstrated that NPs increased both the exposure levels of the phytochemicals and their removal from the brain (Chen et al., 2016; Chen et al., 2017; Liu et al., 2022; Zhao et al., 2020; Xiong et al., 2020). Most studies that involved NP functionalization used lactoferrin, along with near-infrared (NIR) light and P188 (Xiong et al., 2021; Xiong et al., 2020; Katila et al., 2022). Lactoferrin functionalization led to a 25-fold increase in comparison to the control group and a three-fold increase compared to non-lactoferrin-functionalized NPs (Xiong et al., 2021). Additionally, applying NIR resulted in a three-fold increase over NPs without NIR and lactoferrin functionalization, and a two-fold increase compared to the control (Xiong et al., 2020). Studies that used surfactants such as PS80 or P188 also demonstrated neuroprotective effects, indicating that these NPs could effectively cross the blood-brain barrier (BBB). However, these studies did not compare the efficiency of these surfactants to that of the controls.

Phytochemical Effects on PD-Related Implicit Disease Processes

In the later stages of PD, the condition spreads to other brain regions due to the progressive loss of dopaminergic neurons in the substantia nigra pars compacta. This degeneration involves multiple biological mechanisms, including inflammation, oxidative stress, α-synuclein aggregation, and mitochondrial failure. However, not all models fully capture the complex pathology of PD. For instance, one study found that the MPP+ toxin can cause mitochondrial dysfunction, lipid peroxidation, decreased antioxidant activity, and reduced cell viability. Phytomedicines discussed in this chapter target these pathways and have shown potential neuroprotective effects. Notably, turmeric/curcumin (Chen et al., 2017), schisantherin A (Chen et al., 2016), naringenin (Md et al., 2019), puerarin (Zhang et al., 2018), paeoniflorin (Xiong et al., 2021), ginkgolide B (Xiong et al., 2020), resveratrol (Katila et al., 2022; Pangeni et al., 2014), epigallocatechin gallate, *Bacopa monnieri* (Joy et al., 2022), and fisetin have demonstrated neuroprotective benefits, such as reduced apoptosis and necrosis, elevated ATP levels, improved cell survival pathways, and enhanced cell viability. These phytomedicines have been shown to reduce oxidative stress (e.g., turmeric/curcumin, resveratrol, hypericum hookerianum, puerarin, paeoniflorin, lutein, piperine, *Bacopa monnieri*), mitigate lipid peroxidation (e.g., puerarin, resveratrol, paeoniflorin, turmeric/curcumin), and ameliorate mitochondrial dysfunction (e.g., curcumin, ginkgolide B, resveratrol, puerarin). Additionally, they reduce α-synuclein aggregation (e.g., curcumin, resveratrol) and inflammation levels (e.g., curcumin, epigallocatechin gallate). These compounds also enhance levels of tyrosine hydroxylase and dopamine (e.g., curcumin, resveratrol, hypericum hookerianum, schisantherin A, epigallocatechin gallate, paeoniflorin, ginkgolide B, lutein, puerarin, piperine, fisetin). Ultimately, phytomedicines such as fisetin, *Bacopa monnieri*, resveratrol, puerarin, curcumin, lutein, ginkgolide B, paeoniflorin, and schisantherin A have been effective in alleviating motor symptoms in animal models. The use of NPs as a drug delivery system further enhances the permeability of the blood-brain barrier and improves the efficacy of these phytomedicines.

Preclinical Studies on Nanophytoherbals for Parkinson's Therapy

In vitro and preclinical (*in vivo*) research has shown that combining plant-based medications with nanomaterials can improve their targeted delivery to specific cells or tissues. However, many herbal treatments fail to replicate their efficacy *in vitro* or *in vivo*, hindering their advancement to clinical trials. To address this, it is essential to develop integrated approaches using consistent *in vitro* and *in vivo* methods. Preclinical studies focusing on the pharmacodynamics and pharmacokinetics of these phytoconstituents are crucial, given their proven safety and effectiveness. Additionally, research into systemic toxicity is necessary to uncover potential adverse effects and facilitate their future use. Future research should concentrate on identifying critical process variables, refining methodologies, and overcoming challenges to advance nano-phytopharmaceuticals effectively (Lim et al., 2022).

Clinical Trials and Case Studies

As of 2023, there are 70 Phase I studies, 70 Phase II trials, and 20 Phase III trials underway for novel PD treatments (McFarthing et al., 2013). Among these, two botanical-based drugs, hypoestoxide and WIN-1001X, are currently being tested in Phase II trials (Prasad et al., 2021). Hypoestoxide, a naturally occurring diterpene phytochemical from Hypoestes rosea, has demonstrated potential in altering PD characteristics and reducing inflammatory pathway activity (Ojo-Amaize et al., 2016). WIN-1001X, which includes extracts from

Dimocarpus longan, Polygala tenuifolia, and Angelica tenuissima Nakai, targets antioxidant and autophagy mechanisms while aiming to reduce neuroinflammation (Kim et al., 2014). In a clinical investigation, WIN-1001X is being tested in doses of 400, 800, and 1200 mg for early-stage PD patients; however, subject recruitment is ongoing, and results have not yet been reported (Prasad et al., 2021). There is a pressing need for new therapeutic approaches for PD that more effectively address the underlying pathobiological pathways and have fewer side effects.

Conclusion

The development of nanophytomedicines for treating disorders like PD faces substantial challenges. While preclinical results are promising, translating these findings into clinical practice has been slow. Nanomedicine holds potential for overcoming the limitations of traditional pharmacokinetics, including those associated with phytomedicines. The use of nano-phytomedicines in PD treatment shows promise, but further studies and clinical trials are necessary. Future research should concentrate on engineering advanced nanoparticles to enable more effective and targeted drug delivery. Key areas for optimization include enhancing pharmacokinetic properties, controlling biodistribution, and ensuring drug release is confined to target sites to maximize efficacy and minimize side effects. Although human trials on nanophytomedicines are currently limited, promising *in vivo* results in animal models suggest that these innovations could eventually become valuable tools in the management of PD.

References

Armstrong, M. J., & Okun, M. S. (2020). Diagnosis and treatment of Parkinson disease: A review. *JAMA*, 323(6), 548–560.

Borah, A., Choudhury, A., Paul, R., Mazumder, M. K., & Chetia, S. (2017). Neuroprotective effect of Ayurvedic preparations and natural products on Parkinson's disease. In *Neuroprotective natural products: Clinical aspects and mode of action* (pp. 91–105).

Brown, E. M. B. (2014). Nanomedicine advancements in cancer diagnosis and treatment. In *Horizons in clinical nanomedicine*, 67.

Burns, J., Buck, A. C., Souza, S. D., Dube, A., & Bardien, S. (2023). Nanophytomedicines as therapeutic agents for Parkinson's disease. *ACS Omega*, 8, 42045–42061.

Chen, T., Li, C., Li, Y., Yi, X., Lee, S. M. Y., & Zheng, Y. (2016). Oral delivery of a nanocrystal formulation of Schisantherin A with improved bioavailability and brain delivery for the treatment of Parkinson's disease. *Molecular Pharmaceutics*, 13(11), 3864–3875.

Chen, T., Li, C., Li, Y., Yi, X., Wang, R., Lee, S. M. Y., & Zheng, Y. (2017). Small-sized MPEG-PLGA nanoparticles of Schisantherin A with sustained release for enhanced brain uptake and anti-Parkinsonian activity. *ACS Applied Materials & Interfaces*, 9(11), 9516–9527.

Chen, T., Liu, W., Xiong, S., Li, D., Fang, S., Wu, Z., Wang, Q., & Chen, X. (2019). Nanoparticles mediating the sustained puerarin release facilitate improved brain delivery to treat Parkinson's disease. *ACS Applied Materials & Interfaces*, 11(48), 45276–45289.

Chiba-Falek, O., Lopez, G. J., & Nussbaum, R. L. (2006). Levels of alpha-synuclein mRNA in sporadic Parkinson disease patients. *Movement Disorders*, 21(10), 1703–1708.

Connolly, B. S., & Lang, A. E. (2013). Pharmacological treatment of Parkinson disease: A review. *JAMA*, 311(16), 1670–1683.

Da Rocha Lindner, G., Bonfanti Santos, D., Colle, D., Gasnhar Moreira, E. L., Daniel Prediger, R., Farina, M., Khalil, N. M., & Mara Mainardes, R. (2015). Improved neuroprotective effects of resveratrol-loaded polysorbate 80-coated poly(Lactide) nanoparticles in MPTP-induced parkinsonism. *Nanomedicine*, 10(7), 1127–1138.

Dias, V., Junn, E., & Mouradian, M. M. (2013). The role of oxidative stress in Parkinson's disease. *Journal of Parkinson's Disease*, 3(4), 461.

Fernandes, E. J., Poetini, M. R., Barrientos, M. S., Bortolotto, V. C., Araujo, S. M., Santos Musachio, E. A., De Carvalho, A. S., Leimann, F. V., & Gonçalves, O. H. (2021). Exposure to lutein-loaded nanoparticles attenuates Parkinson's model-induced damage in Drosophila melanogaster: Restoration of dopaminergic and cholinergic system and oxidative stress indicators. *Chemical Biology & Interactions*, 340, 109431.

Hulla, J. E., Sahu, S. C., & Hayes, A. W. (2015). Nanotechnology: History and future. *Human & Experimental Toxicology*, 34(12), 1318-1321.

Joy, D., Jose, J., Bibi, S., Bandiwadekar, A., Gopan, G., Goncalves Lima, C. M., Emran, T. B., Alhumaydhi, F. A., Ashtekar, H., S, S., & Conte-Junior, C. A. (2022). Development of microneedle patch loaded with *Bacopa monnieri* solid lipid nanoparticles for the effective management of Parkinson's disease. *Bioinorganic Chemistry and Applications*, 2022, 9150205.

Katila, N., Duwa, R., Bhurtel, S., Khanal, S., Maharjan, S., Jeong, J. H., Lee, S., Choi, D. Y., & Yook, S. (2022). Enhancement of blood-brain barrier penetration and the neuroprotective effect of resveratrol. *Journal of Controlled Release*, 346, 1–19.

Kim, J., Li, H., Kim, H., & Yang, H. (2014). Protective effect of WIN1001X, an herbal extract, on Parkinson's disease experimental model via autophagy enhancement. *Planta Medica*, 80(16), P1L98.

Kim, W. S., Kagedal, K., & Halliday, G. M. (2014). Alpha-synuclein biology in Lewy body diseases. *Alzheimer's Research & Therapy*, 6(1), 73.

Kouli, A., Torsney, K. M., & Kuan, W. L. (2018). Parkinson's disease: Etiology, neuropathology, and pathogenesis. In *Parkinson's Disease: Pathogenesis and Clinical Aspects* (pp. 3–26). Exon Publications.

Lawrence, R. M., & Lawrence, R. A. (2004). Breast milk and infection. *Clinics in Perinatology*, 31(3), 501–528.

Lim, C. L., Raju, C. S., Mahboob, T., Kayesth, S., Gupta, K. K., Jain, G. K., Dhobi, M., Nawaz, M., Wilairatana, P., de Lourdes Pereira, M., & Patra, J. (2022). Precision and advanced nano-phytopharmaceuticals for therapeutic applications. *Nanomaterials*, 12(2), 238.

Liu, L., Li, Y., Peng, H., Liu, R., Ji, W., Shi, Z., Shen, J., Ma, G., & Zhang, X. (2020). Targeted exosome coating gene-chem nanocomplex as "nanoscavenger" for clearing α-synuclein and immune activation of Parkinson's disease. *Science Advances*, 6(50), eaba3967.

Liu, Y., Liu, W., Xiong, S., Luo, J., Li, Y., Zhao, Y., Wang, Q., Zhang, Z., Chen, X., & Chen, T. (2020). Highly stabilized nanocrystals delivering ginkgolide B in protecting against Parkinson's disease. *International Journal of Pharmaceutics*, 577, 119031.

McFarthing, K., Buff, S., Rafaloff, G., Fiske, B., Mursaleen, L., Fuest, R., Wyse, R. K., & Stott, S. R. W. (2023). Parkinson's disease drug therapies in the clinical trial pipeline: 2023 update. *Journal of Parkinson's Disease*, 13(4), 427–439.

Md, S., Alhakamy, N. A., Aldawsari, H. M., & Asfour, H. Z. (2019). Neuroprotective and antioxidant effect of naringenin-loaded nanoparticles for nose-to-brain delivery. *Brain Sciences*, 9(10), 275.

Nellore, J., Pauline, C., Amarnath, K., & Shilpa, P. N. (2019). Antioxidant effect of gold nanoparticles synthesized from Curcuma longa restrains 1-methyl-2-phenyl pyridinium ion-induced stress in PC12 cells. *Journal of Nanoneuroscience*, 2(1), 63–74.

Ojo-Amaize, E. A., & Cottam, H. B. (2016). Short review of current research on the development of hypoestoxide as a therapeutic agent for Parkinson's disease. *Journal of Neurology & Neurophysiology*, 7(4), 1000385.

Palle, S., & Neerati, P. (2018). Improved neuroprotective effect of resveratrol nanoparticles as evidenced by abrogation of rotenone-induced behavioral deficits and oxidative and mitochondrial dysfunctions in a rat model of Parkinson's disease. *Naunyn-Schmiedeberg's Archives of Pharmacology*, 391(4), 445–453.

Pangeni, R., Sharma, S., Mustafa, G., Ali, J., & Baboota, S. (2014). Vitamin E loaded resveratrol nanoemulsion for brain targeting for the treatment of Parkinson's disease by reducing oxidative stress. *Nanotechnology*, 25(48), 485102.

Parkinson, J. (2002). An essay on the shaking palsy. *Journal of Neuropsychology & Clinical Neuroscience*, 14(2), 223.

Poewe, W., & Antonini, A. (2015). Novel formulations and modes of delivery of levodopa. *Movement Disorders*, 30(1), 114–120.

Prasad, E. M., & Hung, S.-Y. (2021). Current therapies in clinical trials of Parkinson's disease: An update. *Pharmaceuticals*, 14(8), 717.

Rabiei, Z., Solati, K., & Amini-Khoei, H. (2019). Phytotherapy in treatment of Parkinson's disease: A review. *Pharmaceutical Biology*, 57(1), 355–362.

Ramires Junior, O. V., Alves, B. da S., Barros, P. A. B., Rodrigues, J. L., Ferreira, S. P., Monteiro, L. K. S., Araujo, G. de M. S., Fernandes, S. S., Vaz, G. R., Dora, C. L., & Hort, M. A. (2021). Nanoemulsion improves the neuroprotective effects of curcumin in an experimental model of Parkinson's disease. *Neurotoxicology Research*, 39(3), 787–799.

Sivanandy, P., Leey, T. C., Xiang, T. C., Ling, T. C., Wey Han, S. A., Semilan, S. L. A., & Hong, P. K. (2022). Systematic review on Parkinson's disease medications, emphasizing on three recently approved drugs to control Parkinson's symptoms. *International Journal of Environmental Research and Public Health*, 19(1), 364.

Tian, X. H., Lin, X. N., Wei, F., Feng, W., Huang, Z. C., Wang, P., Ren, L., & Diao, Y. (2011). Enhanced brain targeting of temozolomide in polysorbate-80 coated polybutylcyanoacrylate nanoparticles. *International Journal of Nanomedicine*, 6, 445.

Wanisa, M. A. (2019). Review of therapeutic applications of nanotechnology in the medicine field and its side effects. *Journal of Chemical Reviews*, 3(1), 243-251.

Xiong, S., Li, Z., Liu, Y., Wang, Q., Luo, J., Chen, X., Xie, Z., Zhang, Y., Zhang, H., & Chen, T. (2020). Brain-targeted delivery shuttled by black phosphorus nanostructure to treat Parkinson's disease. *Biomaterials*, 260, 120339.

Xiong, S., Liu, W., Li, D., Chen, X., Liu, F., Yuan, D., Pan, H., Wang, Q., Fang, S., & Chen, T. (2019). Oral delivery of puerarin nanocrystals to improve brain accumulation and anti-Parkinsonian efficacy. *Molecular Pharmaceutics*, 16(4), 1444–1455.

Xiong, S., Luo, J., Wang, Q., Li, Z., Li, J., Liu, Q., Gao, L., Fang, S., Li, Y., & Pan, H. (2021). Targeted graphene oxide for drug delivery as a therapeutic nanoplatform against Parkinson's disease. *Biomaterials Science*, 9(5), 1705–1715.

Yue, D., Zeng, C., Okyere, S. K., Chen, Z., & Hu, Y. (2021). Glycine nano-selenium prevents brain oxidative stress and neurobehavioral abnormalities caused by MPTP in rats. *Journal of Trace Elements in Medicine and Biology*, 64, 126680.

Zhang, N., Yan, F., Liang, X., Wu, M., Shen, Y., Chen, M., Xu, Y., Zou, G., Jiang, P., & Tang, C. (2018). Localized delivery of curcumin into brain with polysorbate 80-modified cerasomes by ultrasound-targeted microbubble destruction for improved Parkinson's disease therapy. *Theranostics*, 8(8), 2264–2277.

Zhao, Y., Xiong, S., Liu, P., Liu, W., Wang, Q., Liu, Y., Tan, H., Chen, X., Shi, X., Wang, Q., & Chen, T. (2020). Polymeric nanoparticles-based brain delivery with improved therapeutic efficacy of ginkgolide B in Parkinson's disease. *International Journal of Nanomedicine*, 15, 10453–10467.

Chapter 16

Adverse Effects of Botanical Interventions

Nitin Pandey
Ahsan Ahmed Khan*
Kuldeep Singh
Arun Kumar
Mohemmed Faraz Khan
Syed Mehndi Hasan Zaidi
and Maaz Khan
Faculty of Pharmacy, Integral University, Dashauli, Kursi Road, Lucknow, Uttar Pradesh, India

Abstract

Modern healthcare increasingly recognizes the value of botanical treatments, which build on a long tradition of using plants and plant-derived chemicals for medicinal purposes. Despite their potential benefits, these therapies can pose risks. Adverse effects may arise from plant-drug interactions, allergic reactions, toxin contamination, and improper dosage or administration. Known allergic reactions to certain plants highlight the need for comprehensive patient evaluation and allergen screening. Herb-drug interactions can be particularly dangerous when herbal remedies influence the metabolism and effectiveness of conventional medications. Contamination with toxic substances, such as heavy metals and pesticide residues, remains a significant issue in the production and sale of botanical products, underscoring the importance of stringent quality control. Incorrect dosing and administration can

* Corresponding Author's Email: ahsankhan@iul.ac.in.

In: Natural Solutions for Neurodegenerative Disorders
Editors: Rahul Kumar Sharma, Shailesh Sharma, Ajmer Singh Grewal et al.
ISBN: 979-8-89530-231-6

cause a range of negative effects, from mild gastrointestinal disturbances to severe poisoning. Pharmacovigilance programs and clinical trials are crucial for monitoring and reporting side effects. Medical practitioners must stay informed about botanical medicine and work closely with patients to make well-informed decisions about botanical therapies. While botanical interventions offer promising healthcare benefits, managing their potential adverse effects is essential. This chapter underscores the need for a holistic approach that integrates traditional knowledge with modern scientific evaluation to maximize benefits and minimize risks.

Keywords: adverse effect, contamination, plant-drug interaction, pharmacovigilance, traditional medications

Abbreviations

IGE	Immunoglobulin E
IgG	Immunoglobulin G
IgM	Immunoglobulin M
P450 enzymes	Cytochrome P450 enzymes.

Introduction

The use of plants and plant-derived materials for medicinal purposes, or botanical treatments, has a long history and is deeply rooted in traditional medical practices. Modern healthcare increasingly acknowledges the broad applications of botanical therapies. However, like any medical strategy, botanical treatments are not without potential side effects. This discussion highlights the importance of recognizing and managing these potential negative effects. The complexity of integrating botanical therapies into contemporary medicine necessitates a nuanced understanding of their risks, including herb-drug interactions, allergic reactions, pesticide residue, heavy metal contamination, and dosage issues. It is crucial to explore these aspects to ensure the safe and effective use of botanical interventions. Understanding the dual nature of these therapies—grounded in historical practices and evolving in modern healthcare—is essential for a balanced approach. This chapter aims to provide researchers, practitioners, and enthusiasts with a comprehensive resource on the potential side effects of botanical treatments.

By merging traditional knowledge with contemporary scientific research, we strive to foster an informed and equitable approach to botanical therapies. Our goal is to navigate this landscape, optimizing the benefits of botanical treatments while minimizing their inherent risks, acknowledging the interplay between historical practices and the evolving field of evidence-based medicine (Mosihuzzaman, 2012).

Botanical Intervention

Plant-derived materials, including herbs, extracts, and plant-based chemicals, are utilized in botanical interventions for therapeutic or preventive purposes. These interventions encompass various methods: herbal medicines often use parts of plants such as leaves, roots, or seeds and are consumed as teas, tinctures, or pills; plant extracts are concentrated preparations derived from plants, standardized for specific active compounds, and used for their medicinal properties; and phytochemical supplements, which contain isolated plant chemicals like flavonoids or polyphenols, are taken for their potential health benefits. Botanical therapies, with their extensive history in traditional medicine across numerous cultures, are increasingly integrated with conventional medical treatments to address specific conditions or enhance overall health (Che et al., 2019). For these therapies to provide reliable therapeutic benefits, it is crucial to standardize and maintain consistent levels of active compounds. Additionally, scientific research focusing on evidence-based applications is essential to validate the effectiveness and safety of botanical interventions for specific medical conditions. As with any medical treatment, botanical therapies should be used cautiously, considering individual health needs, potential interactions, and guidance from medical professionals.

Mechanisms of Adverse Effects

Understanding the mechanisms underlying the adverse effects of botanical therapies is crucial for their safe integration into medical practice. Despite their natural origins, botanicals can indeed cause unintended reactions. This section delves into the intricate processes that contribute to these adverse responses, highlighting the need for thorough evaluation and monitoring to mitigate potential risks (Rieder et al., 1994).

Allergic Reactions

Allergic responses can vary significantly in severity, ranging from mild to severe. Understanding the different types of allergic reactions is crucial for timely identification and appropriate management.

- Type 1 hypersensitivity (immediate hypersensitivity): The signs and symptoms of Type I hypersensitivity, also known as immediate hypersensitivity, include wheezing, hives, itching, nasal congestion, and, in severe cases, anaphylaxis. The mechanism of Type I hypersensitivity involves the reaction of an allergen with IgE antibodies, which triggers mast cells and basophils to release histamine and other mediators. Natural substances like latex from rubber trees can induce this type of hypersensitivity. Although latex is not a medication, it can cause a range of adverse effects, from mild skin irritation to severe allergic reactions. Awareness of natural allergens is crucial, as they can lead to significant allergic responses (Niggemann and Beyer, 2014).
- Type II hypersensitivity (cytotoxic hypersensitivity): Hemolytic anemia and thrombocytopenia are examples of tissue-specific reactions that can manifest as symptoms of Type II hypersensitivity. This type of hypersensitivity is caused by IgG or IgM antibodies binding to antigens on the surface of cells, leading to cell destruction. Occasionally, natural extracts can be implicated in Type II adverse drug reactions, which are immune responses triggered by medications. It is important for patients and healthcare providers to be vigilant about potential adverse reactions related to natural substances and to monitor for any signs that might indicate an immunological response (Leite et al., 2010).
- Type III hypersensitivity (immune complex-mediated hypersensitivity): Signs of Type III hypersensitivity involve the formation and deposition of immune complexes in tissues, leading to inflammation and tissue damage. These immune complex-mediated reactions occur when antibodies bind to medications to form

complexes, which can result in Type III adverse drug events. Natural compounds, such as hydralazine—derived from plants and used to treat hypertension—can also contribute to such reactions (Böhm et al., 2018).

- Type IV hypersensitivity (delayed-type hypersensitivity): Signs of Type IV hypersensitivity, also known as cell-mediated responses, develop slowly and include reactions such as contact dermatitis or skin test responses to tuberculin. This hypersensitivity mechanism involves the recruitment and activation of T cells, which trigger an inflammatory response. Although synthetic medications are commonly associated with these reactions, natural chemicals, such as hydralazine derived from plants used to treat hypertension, can also contribute (Alkhatib et al., 2022).
- Contact dermatitis: Symptoms of Type IV hypersensitivity, such as contact dermatitis, include skin irritation, redness, and itching after exposure to allergens like certain metals, plants, or cosmetics. This reaction involves T-cell activation. A naturally occurring substance like urushiol, which is found in plants such as poison ivy, can induce contact dermatitis, even though it is not a prescription drug (Agosta et al., 2021).
- Drug allergies: Symptoms of drug allergies include rash, itching, swelling, and, in severe cases, anaphylaxis following exposure to specific medications. The mechanism behind drug allergies involves various immunological pathways, such as direct stimulation of T cells or IgE-mediated responses. Chamomile, a common yet infrequent allergen, is a natural plant used in beverages and supplements. It can trigger skin rashes and respiratory issues. Awareness of potential allergies to both synthetic and natural medications is crucial (Bégin et al., 2020).
- Food allergies: Signs of food allergies can be immediate or delayed and may range from anaphylaxis to hives and gastrointestinal issues. Food allergies are primarily IgE-mediated, although non-IgE pathways can also play a role. Peanuts, for example, are known to cause severe allergic reactions due to their proteins. Unlike medication reactions, food allergies involve reactions to proteins found in food. Caution is essential for individuals prone to allergies, particularly concerning both food and medication (Calvani et al., 2020).

- Allergic rhinitis (hay fever): Symptoms such as sneezing in response to mold or pollen, along with a runny nose and itchy eyes, are typical of type I hypersensitivity reactions. These symptoms are often associated with environmental allergies, such as hay fever or allergic rhinitis, rather than with natural extracts used as medications. However, certain natural substances, like quercetin found in fruits and vegetables, can also trigger allergic reactions. Although quercetin is a supplement rather than a medication, it may have anti-allergic effects. Individuals with hay fever should manage their allergen exposure and consult with medical professionals before starting any new natural supplements, especially if they are already on other medications.

Types of Herb-Drug Interactions

Herb-drug interactions are complex interactions between traditional medicines and botanical remedies that can significantly impact the efficacy and safety of medication therapy. Healthcare professionals need to recognize the various types of interactions that can occur. Here are some common categories (Gouws et al., 2020):

- Pharmacokinetic interactions: The absorption of certain herbs can affect the bioavailability and metabolic process of medications by altering how well drugs are absorbed in the digestive system. For instance, some herbs might inhibit or enhance the absorption of drugs, thereby impacting their effectiveness. Additionally, herbs can influence drug metabolism in the liver by modifying the activity of enzymes responsible for drug breakdown. This can lead to either increased or decreased drug levels in the body. Furthermore, herb-drug interactions can also impact drug distribution, affecting how pharmaceuticals are distributed throughout the body and their concentration in specific tissues (Rombolà et al., 2020).
- Pharmacodynamic interactions: Synergistic or additive effects occur when herbs and medications with similar pharmacological actions are used together, potentially enhancing the therapeutic benefits of the treatment. This can result in a more pronounced effect than when each is used separately. Conversely, some herbs may neutralize or reduce

the effects of certain medications, which could diminish the intended therapeutic benefits and potentially lead to suboptimal treatment outcomes (Choi et al., 2017).

- Herb-induced changes in drug transporters: Certain herbs can alter the function of drug transporters, which affects how medications are absorbed, distributed, and eliminated in the body. These interactions can influence the efficiency of drug delivery and the overall pharmacokinetics of medications (Parvez et al., 2019).
- Herb-induced changes in drug metabolizing enzymes: Herbs can either induce or inhibit cytochrome P450 enzymes, which significantly affects the metabolism of drugs and consequently alters their concentration in the bloodstream (Ueng et al., 2002).
- Pharmacokinetic changes in herb absorption and metabolism: When medications and herbs are administered together, it can alter the absorption and metabolism of the herbs, potentially impacting their overall bioavailability (Kidd, 1999).
- Electrolyte imbalance: Certain herbs can cause electrolyte imbalances, which may affect the therapeutic efficacy of drugs that depend on specific electrolyte levels for optimal performance (Head, 2008).
- Herbs with blood-thinning properties: Certain plants possess inherent anticoagulant properties that can amplify the effects of blood thinners, increasing the risk of bleeding (Panaro et al., 2022; Wang et al., 2020).
- Impact on drug excretion: Herbs may influence how medications are excreted by the kidneys, potentially altering the medication's half-life and overall effectiveness (Rahman et al., 2021; Hanfi et al., 2020; Costa, 2010; Gil et al., 2016).

Contamination Concerns

When herbal treatments for neurodegenerative diseases contain contaminants, toxins, or unexpected chemicals, it raises significant concerns regarding their safety and efficacy.

Heavy Metals and Adulterants

Potential side effects of using botanical therapies for neurodegenerative diseases include the risk of adulterants and heavy metal contamination. Botanical products can become contaminated with heavy metals such as lead, mercury, and cadmium during manufacturing or from soil absorption. Prolonged exposure to these metals may exacerbate neurodegenerative conditions. Additionally, adulterants—chemicals added intentionally to mislead consumers or reduce production costs—can include synthetic additives, non-therapeutic chemicals, or unlisted botanical ingredients. To enhance the safety and efficacy of plant-based remedies for neurodegenerative diseases, regular testing for contaminants and clear product labeling are essential. Providing detailed information about the source and processing of these interventions supports informed decision-making for those seeking alternative therapies (Deng et al., 2009).

Dosage and Administration

It is crucial to exercise caution and seek advice from trained healthcare professionals when determining the dosage and administration of botanical therapies for neurodegenerative diseases, as this is a complex task. Adverse outcomes can vary depending on the specific botanical product, the individual's health status, and potential drug interactions.

Dosage

Individualized approaches: When determining the appropriate dosage of botanical therapies for neurodegenerative diseases, it's crucial to consider factors such as the patient's age, weight, overall health, and the severity of their condition (Shaw et al., 2012).

Start low and go slow: Start the therapy at a lower dose and gradually increase it while monitoring for any side effects. This approach minimizes the risk of adverse effects and helps in identifying the lowest effective dosage (Bandaranayake, 2006).

Consultation with healthcare professionals: Always consult medical professionals with expertise in botanical medicine, such as doctors or herbalists. They can provide personalized guidance based on the patient's specific health profile (Adams et al., 2002).

Administration

- Formulation: There are several types of botanical interventions, including extracts, tinctures, teas, and capsules. The method of administration can be influenced by the specific formulation used.
- Consistency in administration: It is important to advise patients to take botanical medicine exactly as directed and consistently. Inconsistent administration can affect the effectiveness of the intervention.
- Timing of administration: While taking some botanicals on an empty stomach may enhance their effectiveness, others might need to be taken with meals. The timing of administration can significantly impact the effects and absorption of the botanical intervention.
- Monitoring and adjustment: It is essential to regularly monitor the patient's response and any potential side effects. If adverse effects occur, the medical practitioner may need to adjust the dosage, change the formulation, or discontinue the botanical intervention.
- Interaction with conventional drugs: It's crucial to consider any traditional medications the patient may be taking for potential interactions. Pharmaceutical medications and botanical therapies can have negative interactions or adverse side effects (Bast et al., 2002).

Improper Dosage

When botanical therapies for neurodegenerative illnesses are administered incorrectly, there can be significant negative consequences and health risks. It is crucial to emphasize the importance of following dosage recommendations and consulting medical authorities before starting any herbal treatment. Potential adverse effects of incorrect dosage include:

Toxicity: In large dosages, certain botanicals may contain toxic substances. Overindulgence in these plants can lead to poisoning and various adverse health effects. It is essential to adhere to recommended dosages and seek professional medical advice to avoid such risks and ensure safe and effective use of botanical therapies.

Allergies and reactions: Some individuals may be allergic to specific botanicals. Excessive use of these supplements can trigger allergic reactions, ranging from mild skin rashes to severe anaphylaxis. It is crucial to be aware of any potential allergies and to monitor for symptoms when using botanical therapies.

Drug interactions: An incorrect dose may increase the risk of drug interactions for individuals taking medication for other health issues or neurological conditions. Such interactions can affect both the effectiveness of prescribed medications and the efficacy of botanical treatments.

Cardiovascular effects: Incorrect doses of certain plants can alter heart rate and blood pressure, potentially leading to cardiovascular issues, particularly in individuals with pre-existing heart conditions.

Liver and kidney damage: When consumed in excess, several botanicals can have hepatotoxic or nephrotoxic effects, potentially causing damage to the liver or kidneys.

Central nervous effects: When some botanical therapies are taken in excess, they may cause neurological symptoms such as headaches, dizziness, or disorientation (Heinrich et al., 2020).

Gastrointestinal distress: Certified botanicals can induce gastrointestinal problems, including nausea, vomiting, diarrhea, or abdominal discomfort, when taken in excess.

Ethical and Safety Considerations

Exploring botanical therapies for neurodegenerative illnesses requires a thorough evaluation of safety and ethical considerations, particularly in light of potential adverse effects. Informed consent is crucial, as it ensures patients are educated about botanical therapies, including their potential health benefits, risks, adverse effects, drug interactions, and allergies. Professional guidance from qualified medical personnel, such as doctors or herbalists, is essential for tailoring treatments to each patient's unique health conditions and medical history, given the complexity and variability of neurodegenerative diseases (Parveen et al., 2015). Quality control through comprehensive testing and precise labeling is necessary to ensure product purity and build consumer trust. Monitoring and reporting adverse events are critical for maintaining safety and effectiveness, allowing for timely adjustments to treatments. Clinicians should prioritize the benefits of botanical interventions, using robust evidence to support their use while avoiding those with harmful effects or potential interactions (Shetti et al., 2011). Cultural sensitivity is also important in patient-centered care, respecting individual beliefs and aligning treatments with cultural practices. Transparency and accountability in discussing risks, uncertainties, and scientific evidence are vital for informed decision-making and patient safety, emphasizing evidence-based practices (Choudhury et al., 2023).

Overcoming Challenges

Healthcare professionals must carefully address the issues associated with botanical interventions for neurodegenerative illnesses. It is crucial to consult with licensed experts, tailor dosages to individual circumstances, start with a low dose, and gradually increase as needed. Ensuring the purity of botanical products, establishing a robust system for reporting adverse events, and educating patients about informed consent are essential. Additionally, assess potential interactions with prescription medications, prioritize evidence-based treatments, and conduct regular follow-ups. Maintain transparency about uncertainties, adhere to quality standards, and continuously evaluate the risk-benefit ratio to optimize patient safety and treatment efficacy (Ghosh et al., 2023).

Future Aspects

Exploring and improving botanical therapies for neurodegenerative illnesses requires a focus on minimizing side effects. Advanced research and clinical trials are essential for evaluating the safety and efficacy of these therapies. Employing rigorous methodologies, such as randomized controlled trials and longitudinal studies, combined with advanced techniques like biomarker analysis and neuroimaging, provides accurate results and aids in developing personalized treatments (Enioutina et al., 2020; Efferth et al., 2017). Identifying biomarkers is crucial for tailoring herbal treatments to predict patient responses and reduce adverse effects. Precision medicine enhances this approach by considering individual genetic and lifestyle factors, optimizing treatment effectiveness while mitigating risks. Innovations in formulation improve bioavailability and efficacy, reducing side effects. Bioinformatics and big data analytics help analyze large datasets to understand patient variability and personalize treatments (Bhatt, 2016; Lin and Wang, 2019). Robust regulatory frameworks ensure the consistency, quality, and safety of botanical products. Patient-centered approaches involve patients in treatment decisions and risk-benefit evaluations, fostering transparency and collaboration. Global cooperation promotes sharing of research findings and standardization of practices, integrating traditional medicine into mainstream healthcare (Rahman et al., 2011; Bradley et al., 2019). Long-term safety monitoring, through adverse event reporting and information-sharing networks, is vital for detecting and managing potential side effects. Public health initiatives should educate the public on proper herbal treatment use and emphasize collaboration between patients and healthcare providers to ensure safe and personalized interventions (Moreira et al., 2014).

Conclusion

In conclusion, exploring herbal treatments for neurodegenerative diseases presents both benefits and challenges, especially regarding potential side effects. While botanical substances offer therapeutic potential, the risk of adverse effects highlights the need for careful management, thorough investigation, and thoughtful integration into medical practices. To apply botanical therapies more effectively, it is crucial to identify side effects, understand their mechanisms, and assess associated risk factors.

References

Abdel-Rahman, A., Anyangwe, N., Carlacci, L., Casper, S., Danam, R. P., Enongene, E., & Walker, N. J. (2011). The safety and regulation of natural products used as foods and food ingredients. *Toxicological Sciences*, 123(2), 333-348.

Adams, K. E., Cohen, M. H., Eisenberg, D., & Jonsen, A. R. (2002). Ethical considerations of complementary and alternative medical therapies in conventional medical settings. *Annals of Internal Medicine*, 137(8), 660-664.

Alkhatib, A. J. (2022). Types of Hypersensitivities (Updates). In *The Role of Microbes in Autoimmune Diseases: New Mechanisms of Microbial Initiation of Autoimmunity* (pp. 21-28). Singapore: Springer Nature Singapore.

Bandaranayake, W. M. (2006). Quality Control, Screening, Toxicity, and Regulation of Herbal Drugs. In *Modern Phytomedicine: Turning Medicinal Plants into Drugs*; 25-57.

Bast, A., Chandler, R. F., Choy, P. C., Delmulle, L. M., Gruenwald, J., Halkes, S. B. A., & Vermeer, I. T. (2002). Botanical health products, positioning and requirements for effective and safe use. *Environmental Toxicology and Pharmacology*, 12(4), 195-211.

Bégin, P., Chan, E. S., Kim, H., Wagner, M., Cellier, M. S., Favron-Godbout, C., & Goetghebeur, M. M. (2020). CSACI guidelines for the ethical, evidence-based and patient-oriented clinical practice of oral immunotherapy in IgE-mediated food allergy. *Allergy, Asthma & Clinical Immunology*, 16, 1-45.

Bhatt, A. (2016). Phytopharmaceuticals: A new drug class regulated in India. *Perspectives in clinical research*, 7(2), 59-61.

Böhm, R., Proksch, E., Schwarz, T., & Cascorbi, I. (2018). Drug hypersensitivity: diagnosis, genetics, and prevention. *Deutsches Ärzteblatt International*, 115(29-30), 501.

Bradley, R., Harnett, J., Cooley, K., McIntyre, E., Goldenberg, J., & Adams, J. (2019). Naturopathy as a model of prevention-oriented, patient-centered primary care: a disruptive innovation in health care. *Medicina*, 55(9), 603.

Calvani, M., Anania, C., Caffarelli, C., Martelli, A., Del Giudice, M. M., Cravidi, C., & Marseglia, G. L. (2020). Food allergy: An updated review on pathogenesis, diagnosis, prevention and management. *Acta Bio Medica: Atenei Parmensis*, 91(Suppl 11), e2020012.

Che, C. T., & Zhang, H. (2019). Plant natural products for human health. *International journal of molecular sciences*, 20(4), 830.

Choi, S., Oh, D. S., & Jerng, U. M. (2017). A systematic review of the pharmacokinetic and pharmacodynamic interactions of herbal medicine with warfarin. *PloS one*, 12(8), e0182794.

Choudhury, A., Singh, P. A., Bajwa, N., Dash, S., & Bisht, P. (2023). Pharmacovigilance of herbal medicines: Concerns and future prospects. *Journal of Ethnopharmacology*, 309, 116383.

Costa, G. (2010). Shift work and health: current problems and preventive actions. *Safety and Health at Work*, 1(2), 112-123.

Deng, G. E., Frenkel, M., Cohen, L., Cassileth, B. R., Abrams, D. I., Capodice, J. L., Courneya, K. S., Dryden, T., Hanser, S., Kumar, N., Labriola, D., Wardell, D. W., Sagar, S., & Society for Integrative Oncology (2009). Evidence-based clinical practice guidelines for integrative oncology: complementary therapies and botanicals. *Journal of the Society for Integrative Oncology*, 7(3), 85-120.

Di Agosta, E., Salvati, L., Corazza, M., Baiardini, I., Ambrogio, F., Angileri, L., & Rossi, O. (2021). Quality of life in patients with allergic and immunologic skin diseases: in the eye of the beholder. *Clinical and Molecular Allergy*, 19, 1-17.

Efferth, T., Saeed, M. E., Mirghani, E., Alim, A., Yassin, Z., Saeed, E., & Daak, S. (2017). Integration of phytochemicals and phytotherapy into cancer precision medicine. *Oncotarget*, 8(30), 50284.

Enioutina, E. Y., Job, K. M., Krepkova, L. V., Reed, M. D., & Sherwin, C. M. (2020). How can we improve the safe use of herbal medicine and other natural products? A clinical pharmacologist mission. *Expert Review of Clinical Pharmacology*, 13(9), 935-944.

Ghosh, S., Bishal, A., Ghosh, S. K., Jana, K., Gayen, B., Sahu, S., & Debnath, B. (2023). Herbal medicines: A potent approach to human diseases, their chief compounds, formulations, present status, and future aspects. *International Journal of Membrane Science and Technology*, 10, 442-464.

Gil, F., Hernández, A. F., & Martín-Domingo, M. C. (2021). Toxic contamination of nutraceuticals and food ingredients. In *Nutraceuticals* (pp. 1145-1158). Academic Press.

Gouws, C., & Hamman, J. H. (2020). What are the dangers of drug interactions with herbal medicines? *Expert opinion on drug metabolism & toxicology*, 16(3), 165-167.

Hanfi, M. Y., Mostafa, M. Y., & Zhukovsky, M. V. (2020). Heavy metal contamination in urban surface sediments: sources, distribution, contamination control, and remediation. *Environmental monitoring and assessment*, 192, 1-21.

Head, K. A. (2008). Natural approaches to prevention and treatment of infections of the lower urinary tract. *Alternative Medicine Review*, 13(3), 227-244.

Heinrich, M., Appendino, G., Efferth, T., Fürst, R., Izzo, A. A., Kayser, O., & Viljoen, A. (2020). Best practice in research–overcoming common challenges in phytopharmacological research. *Journal of Ethnopharmacology*, 246, 112230.

Kidd, P. M. (1999). A review of nutrients and botanicals in the integrative management of cognitive dysfunction. *Alternative Medicine Review*, 4(3), 144-161.

Leite, F. H. A., Taranto, A. G., dos Santos Junior, M. C., Branco, A., De Araujo, M. T., & de M. Carneiro, J. W. (2010). Search for new antimalarial compounds obtained from natural sources by molecular modeling. *International Journal of Quantum Chemistry*, 110(11), 2057-2066.

Liu, L., & Wang, H. (2019). The recent applications and developments of bioinformatics and omics technologies in traditional chinese medicine. *Current Bioinformatics*, 14(3), 200-210.

Moreira, D. D. L., Teixeira, S. S., Monteiro, M. H. D., De-Oliveira, A. C. A., & Paumgartten, F. J. (2014). Traditional use and safety of herbal medicines. *Revista Brasileira de Farmacognosia*, 24(2), 248-257.

Mosihuzzaman, M. (2012). Herbal medicine in healthcare-an overview. *Natural product communications*, 7(6), 1934578X1200700628.

Niggemann, B., & Beyer, K. (2014). Factors augmenting allergic reactions. *Allergy*, 69(12), 1582-1587.

Panaro, M. A., & Porro, C. (2022). Bioactive Natural Compounds for Therapeutic and Nutraceutical Applications in Neurodegeneration. *Nutrients*, 14(11), 2216.

Parveen, A., Parveen, B., Parveen, R., & Ahmad, S. (2015). Challenges and guidelines for clinical trial of herbal drugs. *Journal of Pharmacy and Bioallied Sciences*, 7(4), 329-333.

Parvez, M. K., & Rishi, V. (2019). Herb-drug interactions and hepatotoxicity. *Current drug metabolism*, 20(4), 275-282.

Rahman, M. H., Bajgai, J., Fadriquela, A., Sharma, S., Trinh, T. T., Akter, R., Jeong, Y. J., Goh, S. H., Kim, C. S., & Lee, K. J. (2021). Therapeutic Potential of Natural Products in Treating Neurodegenerative Disorders and Their Future Prospects and Challenges. *Molecules*, 26(17), 5327.

Rieder, M. J. (1994). Mechanisms of unpredictable adverse drug reactions. *Drug Safety*, 11(3), 196-212.

Rombolà, L., Scuteri, D., Marilisa, S., Watanabe, C., Morrone, L. A., Bagetta, G., & Corasaniti, M. T. (2020). Pharmacokinetic interactions between herbal medicines and drugs: their mechanisms and clinical relevance. *Life*, 10(7), 106.

Shaw, D., Graeme, L., Pierre, D., Elizabeth, W., & Kelvin, C. (2012). Pharmacovigilance of herbal medicine. *Journal of ethnopharmacology*, 140(3), 513-518.

Shetti, S., Kumar, C. D., Sriwastava, N. K., & Sharma, I. P. (2011). Pharmacovigilance of herbal medicines: Current state and future directions. *Pharmacognosy Magazine*, 7(25), 69.

Ueng, Y. F., Don, M. J., Peng, H. C., Wang, S. Y., Wang, J. J., & Chen, C. F. (2002). Effects of Wu-chu-yu-tang and its component herbs on drug-metabolizing enzymes. *Japanese journal of pharmacology*, 89(3), 267-273.

Wang, Z., He, C., & Shi, J. S. (2020). Natural products for the treatment of neurodegenerative diseases. *Current medicinal chemistry*, 27(34), 5790-5828.

Chapter 17

Phytochemicals and Nutraceuticals of *Moringa oleifera* Lam.: Treating Neurodegenerative Disorders

Varsha Nigam*

Department of Botany, Guru Nanak Khalsa College, Yamuna Nagar, Haryana, India

Abstract

The nutritional value of *Moringa oleifera* Lam. is exceptionally high, with its various parts containing essential vitamins, minerals, and biomolecules. These include vitamin A, thiamin, riboflavin, niacin, vitamin C, calcium, copper, magnesium, phosphorus, zinc, potassium, protein, and carbohydrates. Additionally, the leaves and pods are rich in amino acids such as arginine, histidine, lysine, and tryptophan. As a result, Moringa is a straightforward and accessible solution for addressing malnutrition. Beyond its nutritional benefits, *Moringa oleifera* leaves and seeds extracts exhibit neuroprotective and memory-enhancing properties, making them valuable in combating several neurodegenerative disorders. Key neuroprotective phytochemicals isolated from Moringa oleifera, including quercetin, chlorogenic acid, myricetin, isoquercetin, and cryptochlorogenic acid, have shown efficacy against Alzheimer's disease (AD), Parkinson's disease (PD), amnesia, ischemia-reperfusion injury (IRI), depression, epilepsy, multiple sclerosis (MS), Huntington's disease, cognitive impairment (CI), oxidative stress, and other related conditions. The aim of this study is to provide a comprehensive overview of the phytochemicals, nutritional quality, and applications of *Moringa oleifera* in the context of

---

* Corresponding Author's Email: varshanigam29@gmail.com.

In: Natural Solutions for Neurodegenerative Disorders
Editors: Rahul Kumar Sharma, Shailesh Sharma, Ajmer Singh Grewal et al.
ISBN: 979-8-89530-231-6

neurodegenerative disorders. This will aid in assessing future research opportunities and exploring potential advancements in this area.

Keywords: *Moringa oleifera,* nutraceutical use, phytochemicals, neurodegenerative disorder, antioxidants

Abbreviations

AD	Alzheimer's disease
CI	Cognitive impairment
IRI	Ischemia-reperfusion injury
MS	Multiple sclerosis
PD	Parkinson's disease

Introduction

Moringa oleifera Lam., commonly known as the "wonder tree," belongs to the Moringaceae family and is also known by various names, including its Hindi name, Sahajan. The Moringa tree is native to the tropical regions of Southeast Asia, with India being the world's largest grower of moringa. The tree is also utilized for agricultural and medicinal purposes in the Philippines, Africa, Central America, Indonesia, Pakistan, Nepal, and Taiwan. This study aims to provide current and organized information on the phytochemicals, nutritional value, and therapeutic uses of *Moringa oleifera* to evaluate possibilities for future research and explore its medicinal potential. According to the World Health Organization, 80% of the global population depends on medicinal plants (El-Saadony et al., 2023). Moringa leaves and seeds have been used for thousands of years to treat serious diseases and improve wound healing. Despite their widespread use in food and medicine, the effectiveness of Moringa leaves and other products in treating malnutrition and their therapeutic effects on humans have not been well-documented (Dhakad et al., 2019). The use of different parts of the Moringa tree, such as seeds, leaves, seed oils, gum, bark, roots, and flowers, is extensive in herbal remedies. Moringa leaves are reported to contain antioxidants, including flavonoids, phenolics, and carotenoids, and are noted for their optimal nutritional balance of vitamins, minerals, amino acids, and fatty acids (Abdull Razis et al., 2014; Vongsak et al., 2014). Moringa has been used medicinally for ages and across numerous cultures worldwide to treat a wide range of ailments, including acne, blood impurities, bronchial inflammation, sinusitis, chest congestion, cholera, fevers, ulcers, convulsions, high cholesterol, kidney problems, and hyperglycemia (Singh et al., 2012; Sharma et al., 2012).

Botanical Description of *Moringa oleifera*

Moringa tree typically grows to a height of 2-8 meters and features grey bark, tripinnately compound leaves, and oval leaflets. At the base of each leaf, where it joins the branch or stem, are swellings called pulvini. The leaves are 20-70 cm long, greenish, and droop when young, with glands present at the base of the petioles. Each leaf bears two pairs of opposing ovate leaflets and one at the apex, all 1-2 cm long. Moringa produces pleasantly fragrant clusters of flowers, each with five white or cream petals, 2.5 cm wide, adorned with yellow dots at the base. The petals encircle five stamens and five staminodes in the androecium, held to one side. The fruits of Moringa plants are capsules, hanging and 22-45 cm long, angled, and dagger-like, which dehisce explosively to release white-brown seeds. Each seed has three papery white wings that facilitate airborne dispersal (Morton, 1991; Raja et al., 2016).

Phytochemicals of *Moringa oleifera*

Numerous bioactive compounds, including flavonoids, tannins, phenolic acids, alkaloids, glucosinolates, and terpenes, are found in *Moringa oleifera*. The diversity of these phytochemicals supports a wide range of pharmacological applications.

Flavonoids

The majority of the flavonoids found in this genus are glycosides and flavanols. Common flavonoids include myricetin, apigenin, rhamnetin, kaempferol, quercetin, and isoquercetin (see Figures 1A and 1B). According to Rani et al., (2018), the high concentration of flavonoids in the Moringa genus is a key factor contributing to its potent antioxidant activity.

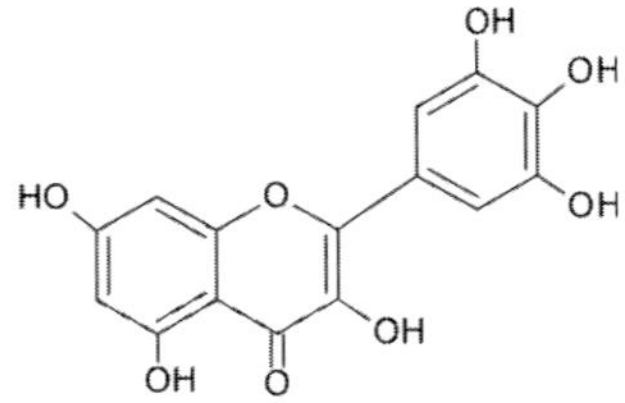

Figure 1A. Structure of myricetin.

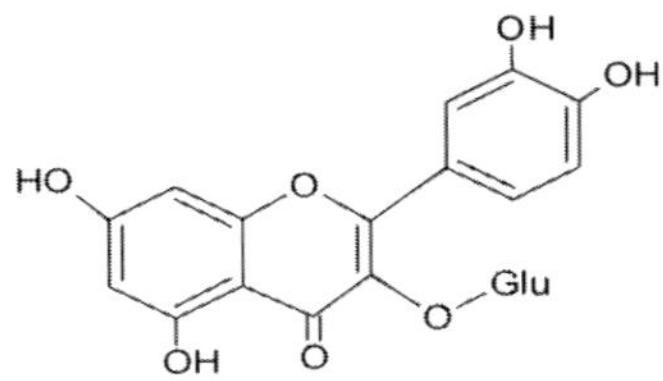

Figure 1B. Structure of isoquercetin.

Phenolic Acids

The main phenolic acids present in *Moringa oleifera* leaves include ferulic acid, ellagic acid, chlorogenic acid, and cryptochlorogenic acid, with gallic acid being the predominant phenolic acid (Vongsak et al., 2014; Leone et al., 2015) (Figure 2A, 2B).

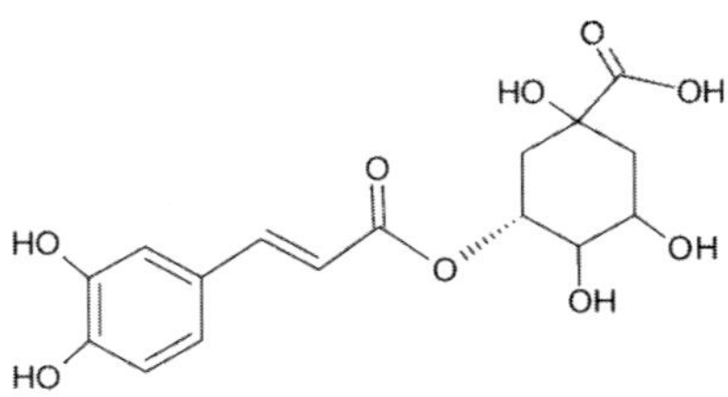

Figure 2A. Structure of chlorogenic acid.

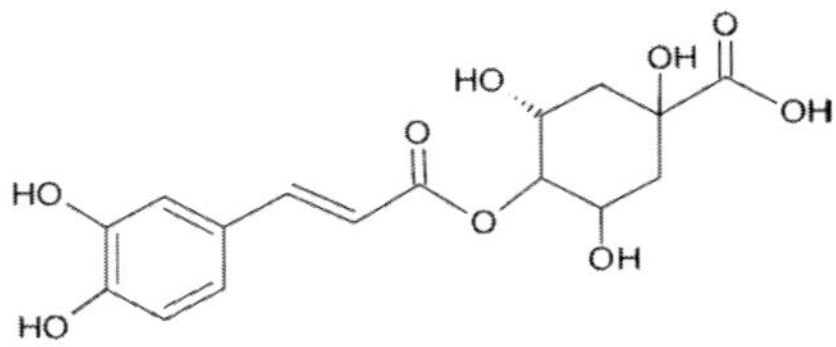

Figure 2B. Structure of crypto-chlorogenic acid.

Alkaloids

Alkaloids are naturally occurring bioactive compounds primarily composed of basic nitrogen, hydrogen, carbon, and oxygen atoms (Figure 3). Several alkaloids, including 1,3-dibenzyl urea and 4-(α-L-rhamnopyranosyloxy), have been isolated from the leaves, seeds, roots, and other parts of the plant. These compounds are known for their ability to scavenge free radicals and provide protection against cardiovascular issues (Abd Rani et al., 2018).

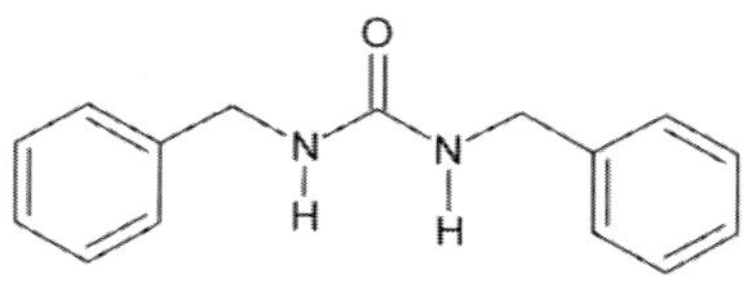

Figure 3. Structure of 1,3-dibenzyl urea.

Vitamins

Moringa oleifera fresh leaves are reported to contain approximately 11,300–23,000 IU of vitamin A. They are also rich in carotenoids with pro-vitamin A and vitamin C, making them an excellent source of these nutrients. Vitamin C plays a crucial role in the synthesis and metabolism of various molecules, including tryptophan, tyrosine, folic acid, and proline, and is involved in the hydroxylation of glycine, proline, lysine, carnitine, and catecholamines. Additionally, it enhances iron absorption in the gut by converting ferric to ferrous state and promotes the conversion of cholesterol into bile acids, thereby reducing blood cholesterol levels (Figure 4A, 4B). As an antioxidant, vitamin C also protects the body from the harmful effects of toxins, pollutants, and free radicals (Leone et al., 2015).

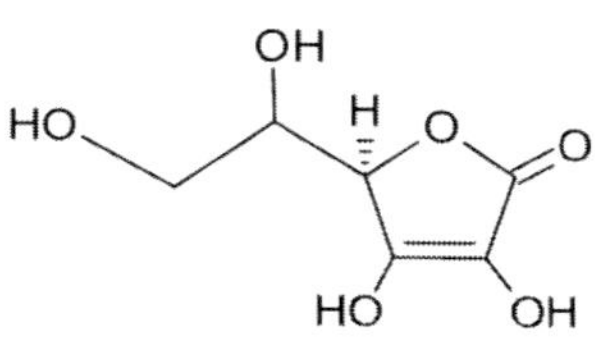

Figure 4A. Structure of L-Ascorbic acid.

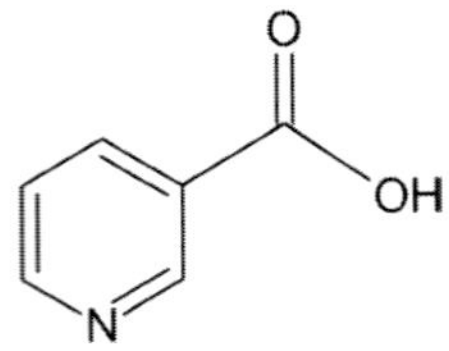

Figure 4B. Structure of Niacin.

Glucosinolates

The concentrations of glucosinolates are influenced by the plant's physiological stage and the maturity of the leaves. In *Moringa oleifera*, the most abundant leaf glucosinolates are identified as 4-O-(α-L-rhamnopyranosyloxy)-benzyl glucosinolate and 4-hydroxybenzyl glucosinolate (Amaglo et al., 2010), as shown in Figure 5.

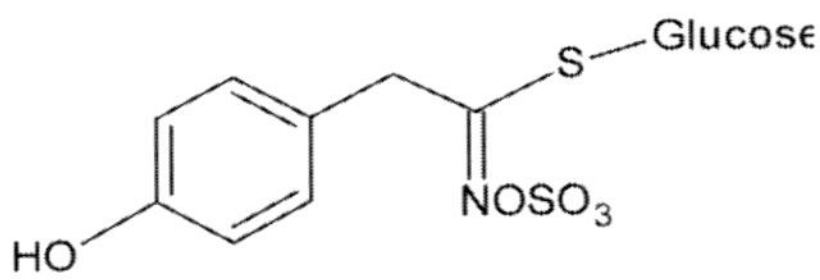

Figure 5. Structure of 4 Hydroxybenzyl glucosinolate (Sinalbin).

Terpenes

Lutein has been identified as the primary terpene in *Moringa oleifera* leaves (Teixeira et al., 2014; Saini et al., 2014), as depicted in Figure 6.

In addition, various other phytochemicals present in this plant are depicted in Figure 8.

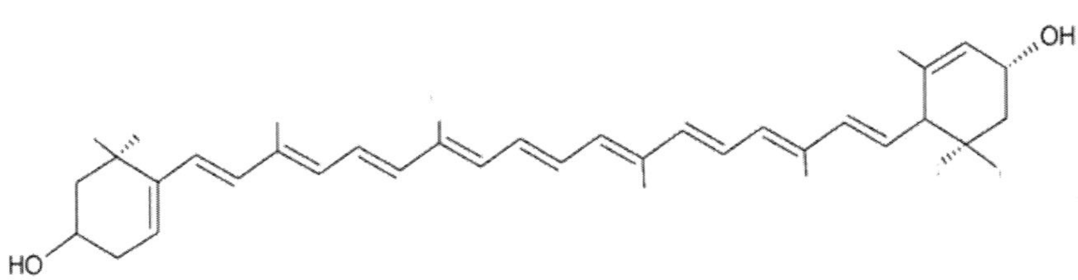

Figure 6. Structure of All-E- Lutein.

Table 1. Different Amino Acids present in *Moringa oleifera* and their use (Abrams et al.,1993; Akram et al., 2011)

Sr. No	Amino acids	Uses in the Human body
1	Ar (Arginine)	Anti-ageing, skin is kept smooth, firm, and plump.
2	His (Histidine)	Use in the biosynthesis of protein
3	Lys (Lysine)	Necessary for human health but the human body cannot make it have to get it in the form of food.
4	Trp (Tryptophan)	Helps in the making of melatonin and serotonin. Serotonin helps to regulate sleep, appetite, mood, and pain.
5	Phe (Phenylalanine)	Helps to regulate the production of many hormones and chemicals. Improve memory, and mood, and decrease anxiety.
6	Met (Methionine)	Antioxidants protect the cell from oxidative stress and help in the growth of new blood vessels.
7	Thr (Theroine)	An essential amino acid, that can be taken by diet only, Boost immune system, important for the formation of collagen, elastin, and tooth enamel
8	Leu (Leucine)	Essential amino acids, regulate protein synthesis, tissue regeneration, metabolism
9	Ile (Isoleucine)	Branched-chain amino acid is necessary as a stress reliever, energy-producing, and important for healthy muscle.
10	Val (Valine)	Promotes muscle growth and tissue repair, enhancing energy.

Moringa leaves contain all essential amino acids, which are fundamental components of proteins (Mahmood et al., 2011). The two most important amino acids present in Moringa leaves are arginine and histidine, which are crucial for young children who cannot synthesize protein adequately for their development and growth. Researchers estimate that 30% of children in sub-Saharan Africa suffer from protein deficiencies, and drumstick leaves can be a significant source of nutrition for these children (Fuglie, 2001; Manzoor, 2007). Other amino acids in Moringa leaves and pods include lysine, tryptophan, phenylalanine, methionine, threonine, leucine, isoleucine, and valine. The amount of amino acids is always higher in dried leaves compared to green leaves and legumes. Moringa leaves (100 grams of dried leaves) contain ten times more carotene than carrots, twelve times more vitamin C than oranges, seventeen times more calcium than milk, double the protein content of cow's milk, and fifteen times more potassium than bananas (Table 1). Additionally, they are an outstanding source of vitamin B and other micronutrients (Razis et al., 2014). Moreover, Moringa contains a variety of unusual sugar-modified glucosinolates, including a group of sugar and rhamnose, which have been discovered in the plant (Amaglo et al., 2010). Reports suggest that these compounds have unique chemopreventive efficacy by triggering apoptosis (Brunelli et al., 2010).

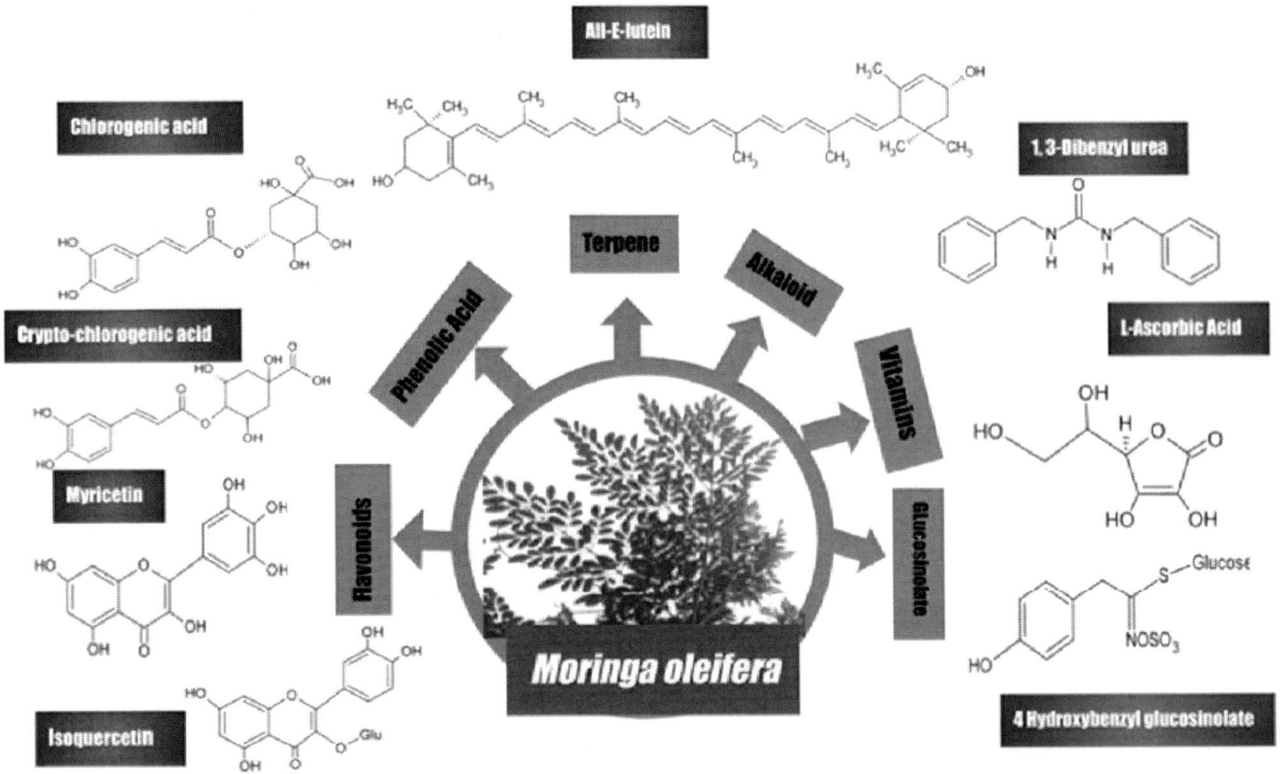

Figure 7. Phytochemical structure of *Moringa oleifera.*

The Application of Moringa Leaves and Seed Extract in Neurodegenerative Disorders

Neurodegeneration is recognized as the key pathophysiological change in most brain-related disorders (Merelli et al., 2013). The onset and progression of neurodegeneration are influenced by specific genes, as well as the timing and extent of the degeneration (Van den Heuvel & Sporns, 2013). While most neurons originate in the brain, they are distributed throughout the body (Pino et al., 2017). Neural stem cells produce the majority of neurons during childhood, but their numbers decrease significantly in adulthood (Ganat et al., 2006). Neurons are perishable, and their gradual loss, along with the deterioration of their structure and function, is known as neurodegeneration (Basics, 2002). Neurodegeneration is linked to synaptic dysfunction, disruption of neural networks, and the accumulation of physically and chemically modified protein variants in the brain (Scott et al., 2010; Kovacs, 2019). Common neurodegenerative diseases include Alzheimer's disease, Parkinson's disease, prion disease, amyotrophic lateral sclerosis, motor neuron disease, Huntington's disease, spinal muscular atrophy, depression, and spinocerebellar ataxia (Klockgether et al., 2019; Lamptey et al., 2022). Recent investigations suggest that *Moringa oleifera* exhibits neuroprotective effects against Alzheimer's disease (AD), dementia, Parkinson's disease (PD), stroke, and neurotoxicity-related issues. Several neuroprotective phytochemicals isolated from *Moringa oleifera,* including quercetin, chlorogenic acid, myricetin, isoquercetin, and cryptochlorogenic acid, have shown efficacy against various brain-related conditions such as AD, PD, ischemia-reperfusion injury (IRI), depression, epilepsy, multiple sclerosis (MS), Huntington's disease, cognitive impairment (CI), and oxidative stress (Ghimire et al., 2021; Hashim et al., 2021) as depicted in Figure 8. According to Bollen and Prickaerts (2012), many neurodegenerative disorders are associated with cyclic nucleotide intracellular signaling, with cyclic nucleotide phosphodiesterases (PDEs) playing a crucial role in this process. Abnormal PDE expression and function, leading to disrupted cyclic nucleotide signaling, may contribute to neurodegenerative disorders. Alterations in the expression of PDE4, PDE7, and PDE8 in the brain may be associated with Alzheimer's disease, while changes in PDE4 and PDE11 expression may contribute to major depressive disorders. Additionally, neurodegenerative disorders such as Huntington's disease and Parkinson's disease are linked to abnormal expression of PDE1B and PDE10. Recent research reveals that oxidative stress is a primary cause of neurodegenerative disorders. The exceptional antioxidant activity of Moringa species can be attributed to their high phenolic content, which stabilizes free radicals generated in cells (Rani et al., 2018). Extracts from both mature and young *Moringa oleifera* leaves have shown potent antioxidant activity, protecting against oxidative damage (Mahmood, 2010). Raza et al., (2024) observed that PD, a leading neurodegenerative disorder affecting 1 to 3% of the older population, is largely driven by oxidative stress, leading to dopaminergic neuron loss, neuroinflammation, and mitochondrial dysfunction. In their study, they experimented with rotenone-mediated motor function impairments in a PD mouse model. Mice were treated with two types of *Moringa oleifera* seed extract: ethanolic and aqueous. The brains of Parkinson's disease mice were examined, and those treated with Moringa seed extract showed a significant reduction in motor dysfunction compared to the rotenone-treated mice. AD is characterized by cognitive and behavioral deterioration due to cholinergic nervous system dysfunction (Scarpini, 2003). Jhou et al., (2018) investigated the neuropharmacological effects of 70% ethanolic *Moringa oleifera* seed extract (MSE) on cognitive impairment induced by scopolamine injection in mice. Mice were administered 250 or 500 mg/kg of Moringa seed extract orally for 7 or 14 days. The results indicated that Moringa seed extract has anti-amnesic effects and induces cognitive improvement through the enhancement of the cholinergic neurotransmission system and neurogenesis. Additionally, Moringa leaves exhibit nootropic activity and protection against oxidative stress in AD (Mohan, 2005). Ekong et al., (2017) reported that *Moringa oleifera* leaf extract protects against aluminum-induced temporal cortical degeneration in male albino Wistar rats, reducing serum aluminum concentration and combating aluminum-induced neurohistopathology. Another study found that incubating embryonic hippocampal neurons with *Moringa oleifera* leaf extract promoted axodendritic maturation and neuroprotection (Hannan et al., 2014). Furthermore, *Moringa oleifera* has been tested against hyperhomocysteinemia-induced AD-like pathology in rats, showing prevention of oxidative stress and cognitive impairments induced by homocysteine, and reducing tau hyperphosphorylation and Aβ production in the AD rat model (Mahaman et al., 2018; Ahmad et al., 2021). Dementia is a serious neurodegenerative disorder in elderly people characterized by loss of global cognitive ability along with memory impairment, attention deficits, language difficulties, and problem-solving issues. Sutalangka et al., (2013) demonstrated that Moringa leaf extract enhances memory, cholinergic function, and reduces oxidative stress, further improving dopaminergic function by increasing regional blood flow and suppressing monoamine oxidase (MAO).

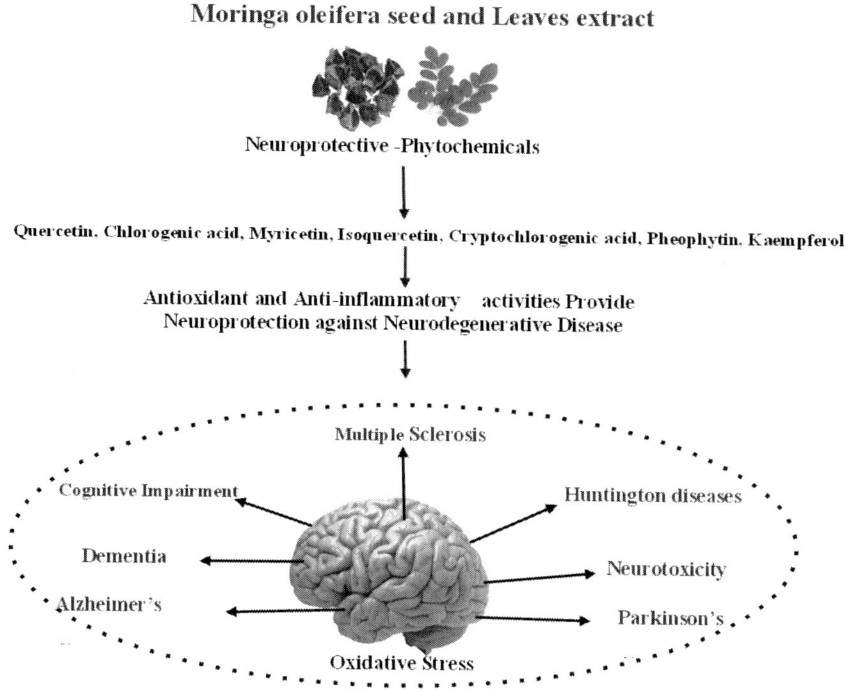

Figure 8. Neuroprotective activity of *M. oleifera* (Ghimire et al., 2021; Hashim et al., 2021).

Conclusion

Moringa oleifera is a highly affordable and reliable source of nutritious food. Its remarkable nutritional value is evident in all parts of the plant, including the leaves, fruit, seeds, and stem, which are beneficial for treating various diseases. Several phytochemicals isolated from *Moringa oleifera* exhibit antioxidant properties, making them promising candidates for applications in neurodegenerative diseases. However, further research is needed to develop preventive strategies against these disorders and to identify specific active ingredients with potential neuroprotective capacities.

Acknowledgments

The author would like to thank Dr. Daljeet Kaur, and Dr. Prabhjot Kaur for their motivation, help and support.

References

Abrams, B., Duncan, D., & Hertz-Picciotto, I. (1993). A prospective study of dietary intake and acquired immune deficiency syndrome in HIV-seropositive homosexual men. *JAIDS Journal of Acquired Immune Deficiency Syndromes*, *6*(8), 949-958.

Ahmad, S. S., Khalid, M., Kamal, M. A., & Younis, K. (2021). Study of Nutraceuticals and Phytochemicals for the Management of Alzheimer's Disease: A Review. *Current Neuropharmacology*, *19*(11), p.1884.

Akram, M., Asif, H. M., Uzair, M., Akhtar, N., Madni, A., Shah, S. A., Hasan, Z. U., & Ullah, A., (2011). Amino acids: A review article. *Journal of medicinal plants research*, *5*(17), pp. 3997-4000.

Amaglo, N. K., Bennet R. N., Curto RBL, et al., (2010). Profiling selected phytochemicals and nutrients in different tissues of the multipurpose tree *Moringa oleifera* L., grown in Ghana. *Journal of Food Chemistry*, 122, 1047-54.

Basics, B. (2002). The life and death of a neuron. *Office of Communications and Public Liaison, National Institute of Neurological Disorders and Stroke: Bethesda, MD, USA*.

Bollen, E., & Prickaerts, J. (2012). Phosphodiesterases in neurodegenerative disorders. *IUBMB life*, *64*(12), 965-970.

Brunelli, D., Tavecchio, M., Falcioni, C., Frapolli, R., Erba, E., Iori, R., Rollin, P., Barillari, J., Manzotti, C., Morazzoni, P., & D'Incalci, M. (2010). The isothiocyanate produced from glucomoringin inhibits NF-kB and reduces myeloma growth in nude mice *in vivo*. *Biochemical Pharmacology*, 79, 1141-1148.

Chambial, S., Dwivedi, S., Shukla, K. K., John, P. J., & Sharma, P. (2013). Vitamin C in disease prevention and cure: An overview. *Indian Journal of Clinical Biochemistry*, 2013, 28, 314–328.

Dhakad, A. K., Ikram, M., Sharma, S., Khan, S., Pandey, V. V., & Singh, A. (2019). Biological, nutritional, and therapeutic significance of *Moringa oleifera* Lam. *Phytotherapy Research*, *33*(11), 2870-2903.

Ekong, M. B., Ekpo, M. M., Akpanyung, E. O., & Nwaokonko, D. U. (2017). Neuroprotective effect of *Moringa oleifera* leaf extract on aluminium-induced temporal cortical degeneration. *Metabolic Brain Disease*, *32*, 1437-1447.

El-Saadony, M. T., Zabermawi, N. M., Burollus, M. A., Shafi, M. E., Alagawany, M., Yehia, N., Askar, A. M., Alsafy, S. A., Noreldin, A. E., & Khafaga, A. F. (2023). Nutritional aspects and health benefits of bioactive plant compounds against infectious diseases: A review. *Food Reviews International*, 39(4), 2138-216.

Foidl N., Makkar H. P. S., & Becker K. (2001). The potential of *Moringa oleifera* for agricultural and industrial uses, 2001. *Dar Es Salaam.*

Fuglie, L. J. (2001) The Miracle Tree: *Moringa oleifera*: Natural Nutrition for the Tropics. *Training Manual. 2001*. Church World Service, Dakar, Senegal.

Ganat, Y. M., Silbereis, J., Cave, C., Ngu, H., Anderson, G. M., Ohkubo, Y., Ment, L. R., & Vaccarino, F. M. (2006). Early postnatal astroglial cells produce multilineage precursors and neural stem cells *in vivo*. *Journal of Neuroscience*, *26*(33), 8609-8621.

Ghimire, S., Subedi, L., Acharya, N., & Gaire, B. P. (2021). Moringa oleifera: A tree of life as a promising medicinal plant for neurodegenerative diseases. *Journal of Agricultural and Food Chemistry*, *69*(48), 14358-14371.

Hannan, M. A., Kang, J. Y., Mohibbullah, M., Hong, Y. K., Lee, H., Choi, J. S., Choi, I. S., & Moon, I. S. (2014). *Moringa oleifera* with promising neuronal survival and neurite outgrowth promoting potentials. *Journal of Ethnopharmacology*, 152(1), 142-150.

Hashim, J. F., Vichitphan, S., Boonsiri, P., & Vichitphan, K. (2021). Neuroprotective assessment of *Moringa oleifera* leaves extract against oxidative-stress-induced cytotoxicity in SHSY5Y neuroblastoma cells. *Plants*, *10*(5), 889.

Klockgether, T., Mariotti, C., & Paulson, H. L. (2019). Spinocerebellar ataxia. *Nature Reviews Disease Primers*, *5*(1), 24.

Kovacs, G. G. (2019). Molecular pathology of neurodegenerative diseases: principles and practice. *Journal of Clinical Pathology*, *72*(11), 725-735.

Lamptey, R. N., Chaulagain, B., Trivedi, R., Gothwal, A., Layek, B., & Singh, J. (2022). A review of the common neurodegenerative disorders: current therapeutic approaches and the potential role of nanotherapeutics. *International Journal of Molecular Sciences*, *23*(3), 1851.

Leone, A., Spada, A., Battezzati, A., Schiraldi, A., Aristil, J., & Bertoli, S. (2015). Cultivation, genetic, ethnopharmacology, phytochemistry and pharmacology of *Moringa oleifera* leaves: An overview. *International Journal of Molecular Sciences*, 16(6), 12791-12835.

Mahaman, Y. A. R., Huang, F., Wu, M., Wang, Y., Wei, Z., Bao, J., Salissou, M. T. M., Ke, D., Wang, Q., Liu, R., Wang, J. Z., Zhang, B., Chen, D., & Wang, X. (2018). *Moringa oleifera* alleviates homocysteine-induced Alzheimer's disease-like pathology and cognitive impairments. *Journal of Alzheimer's Disease*, *63*(3), 1141-1159.

Mahmood, K. T., Mugal, T., & Haq, I. U. (2010). Moringa oleifera: a natural gift-A review. *Journal of Pharmaceutical Sciences and Research*, *2*(11), 775.

Manzoor, M., Anwar, F., Iqbal, T., & Bhanger, M. I. (2007). Physico-chemical characterization of Moringa concanensis seeds and seed oil. *Journal of the American Oil Chemists' Society*, *84*, 413-419.

Merelli, A., Czornyj, L., & Lazarowski, A. (2013). Erythropoietin: a neuroprotective agent in cerebral hypoxia, neurodegeneration, and epilepsy. *Current Pharmaceutical Design*, *19*(38), 6791-6801.

Mohan, M., Kaul, N., Punekar, A., Girnar, R., Junnare, P., & Patil, L. (2005). Nootropic activity of *Moringa oleifera* leaves. *Journal of Natural Remedies*, *5*(1), 59-62.

Morton, J. F. (1991). The Horseradish Tree, Moringa pterygosperma (Moringaceae) - A Boon to Arid Lands? *Economic Botany*, 45, 318-333.

Nigam, V., & Sodhi, J. S. (2014). Some medicinal plants with antioxidant activity: a review. *International Journal of Pharmacy and Biological Sciences*, *4*, 173-8.

Pino, A., Fumagalli, G., Bifari, F., & Decimo, I. (2017). New neurons in adult brain: distribution, molecular mechanisms and therapies. *Biochemical Pharmacology*, *141*, 4-22.

Popoola, J. O., & Obembe, O. O. (2013). Local knowledge, use pattern and geographical distribution of *Moringa oleifera* Lam. (Moringaceae) in Nigeria. *Journal of Ethnopharmacology*, 150, 682–691.

Raja, R. R., Sreenivasulu, M., Vaishnavi, S., Muni Navyasri, D., Samatha, G., & Geethalakshmi, S. (2016). Moringa oleifera: An overview. *RA Journal of Applied Research*, 2(9), 620-624.

Rani, N. Z., Husain, K., & Kumolosasi, E. (2018). Moringa genus: a review of phytochemistry and pharmacology. *Frontiers in pharmacology*, *9*, 108.

Raza, C., Mohsin, S., Faheem, M., Hanif, U., Alkhathlan, H. Z., Shaik, M. R., Riaz, H. A., Anjum, R., Jurrat, H., & Khan, M. (2024). *In Vivo* Study of *Moringa oleifera* Seed Extracts as Potential Sources of Neuroprotection against Rotenone-Induced Neurotoxicity. *Plants*, *13*(11), 1479.

Razis, A. F., Ibrahim, M. D., & Kntayya, S. B. (2014). Health benefits of Moringa oleifera. *Asian pacific journal of cancer prevention*, *15*(20), 8571-8576.

Saini, R. K., Shetty, N. P., & Giridhar, P. (2014). Carotenoid content in vegetative and reproductive parts of commercially grown *Moringa oleifera* Lam. cultivars from India by LC–APCI–MS. *European Food Research and Technology*, 238(7), 971–978.

Scarpini, E., Scheltens, P., & Feldman, H. (2003). Treatment of Alzheimer's disease: current status and new perspectives. Lancet Neurology, 2, 539–547.

Scott, D. A., Tabarean, I., Tang, Y., Cartier, A., Masliah, E., & Roy, S. (2010). A pathologic cascade leading to synaptic dysfunction in α-synuclein-induced neurodegeneration. *Journal of Neuroscience*, *30*(24), 8083-8095.

Sharma, V., Paliwal, R., Janmeda, P., & Sharma, S. (2012). Renoprotective effects of *Moringa oleifera* pods in 7,12-dimethylbenz[a]anthracene-exposed mice. *Journal of Chinese Integrative Medicine*, 10, 1171–1178.

Singh, G. P., & Sharma, S. K. (2012). Antimicrobial evaluation of leaf extract of *Moringa oleifera* Lam. *International Research Journal of Pharmacy*, 3, 1–4.

Sutalangka, C., Wattanathorn, J., Muchimapura, S., & Thukham-mee, W. (2013). *Moringa oleifera* mitigates memory impairment and neurodegeneration in animal model of age-related dementia. *Oxidative Medicine and Cellular Longevity*, *2013*(1), 695936.

Teixeira, E. M., Carvalho, M. R., Neves, V. A., Silva, M. A., & Arantes-Pereira, L. (2014). Chemical characteristics and fractionation of proteins from *Moringa oleifera* Lam. leaves. *Food Chemistry*, 147, 51–54.

Van den Heuvel, M. P., & Sporns, O. (2013). Network hubs in the human brain. *Trends in Cognitive Sciences*, *17*(12), 683-696.

Vongsak, B., Sithisam, P., & Gritsanapan, W. (2014). Simultaneous HPLC quantitative analysis of active compounds in leaves of *Moringa oleifera* Lam. *Journal of Chromatographic Science*, 52(6), 641–645.

Yabesh, J. E., Prabhu, S., & Vijayakumar, S. (2014). An ethnobotanical study of medicinal plants used by traditional healers in silent valley of Kerala, India. *Journal of Ethnopharmacology*, 154, 774–789.

Zaffer, M., Ahmad, S., Sharma, R., Mahajan, S., Gupta, A., & Agnihotri, R. K. (2014). Antibacterial activity of bark extracts of *Moringa oleifera* Lam. Against some selected bacteria. *Pakistan Journal of Pharmaceutical Sciences*, 27, 1857–1862.

Zhou, J., Yang, W. S., Suo, D. Q., Li, Y., Peng, L., Xu, L. X., Zeng, K. Y., Ren, T., Wang, Y., Zhou, Y., & Zhao, Y. (2018). *Moringa oleifera* seed extract alleviates scopolamine-induced learning and memory impairment in mice. *Frontiers in Pharmacology*, 9, 389.

About the Editors

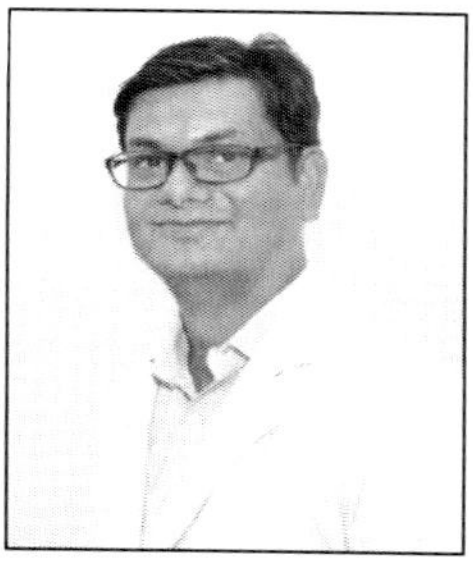

Dr. Rahul Kumar Sharma, Assistant Professor, ASBASJSM College of Pharmacy, Bela, Ropar, Punjab has 12 years of teaching experience. He holds a B. Pharmacy from Dr. Bhimrao Ambedkar University, Agra (2008, First Division), M. Pharmacy (Pharmacology) from Jaipur National University, Jaipur, Rajasthan (2012, First Division), and a PhD in Pharmacy from Sunrise University, Alwar, Rajasthan (2019). With 12 years of teaching experience, 3 years in research, and 8 months in the industry, Dr. Sharma has guided 45 undergraduate and 12 postgraduate student projects. His research areas include antidiabetic, cardiovascular disorders, and neurobehavioral activities. He has published 15 articles in national and international journals of repute, authored 2 books, published 3 patents, and secured 8 copyrights. He is a life member of IGPA and is affiliated with the Indian Hospital Pharmaceutical Association (IHPA), Alcohol Free Society, and Art of Living. His other notable achievements include serving as a mentor in the CSIR online training program in 2020 and acting as a panel expert for designing a laboratory for Shri Guru Gobind Singh Skill Institute, Shri Chamakaur Sahib.

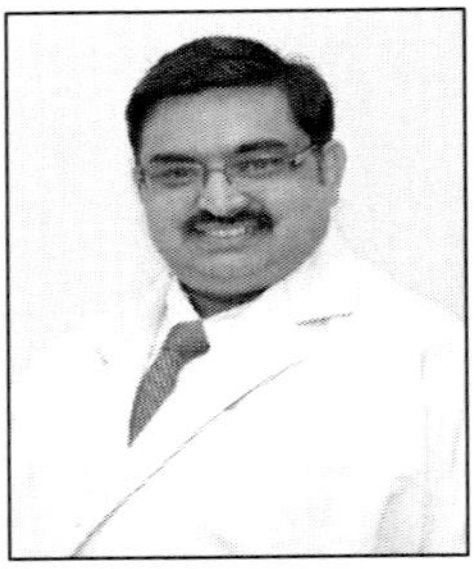

Dr. Shailesh Sharma, Director & Professor, ASBASJSM College of Pharmacy, Bela, Ropar, Punjab is an accomplished pharmaceutical researcher and educator. He holds a PhD in Pharmacy from Punjab Technical University, Jalandhar (Punjab), M. Pharmacy (Pharmaceutics) from B. N. College of Pharmacy, Udaipur (Gold Medalist), and B. Pharmacy from B. R. Nahata College of Pharmacy, Mandsaur. With over 18 years of experience, he has supervised research for PhD and postgraduate students and taught various pharmaceutics subjects at both undergraduate and postgraduate levels. He specializes in the development and evaluation of conventional dosage forms and novel drug delivery systems, with expertise in solubility, tablet technology, taste masking, polymeric films, osmotic controlled delivery, and more. He has contributed to the pharmaceutical field through numerous publications, and as a key player in the accreditation processes (NBA, and NAAC). His technical proficiency extends to handling advanced pharmaceutical instruments and software. Additionally, he has received multiple awards, including Best Oral Paper Award, Young Scientist Award, and Best Teacher Award, and is an active member of various professional societies such as ISTE, APTI, and SPIC MACAY.

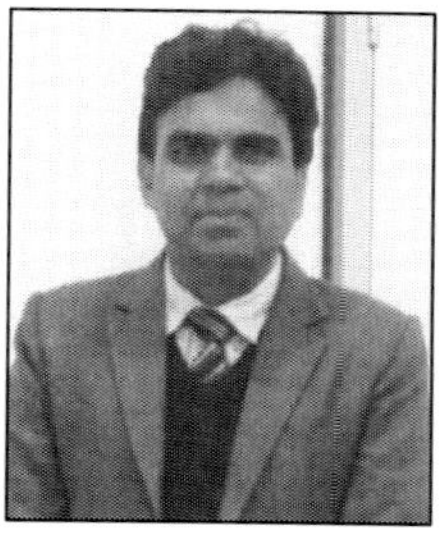

Dr. Ajmer Singh Grewal, Professor (Pharmaceutical Chemistry), Guru Gobind Singh College of Pharmacy, Yamuna Nagar, Haryana (India), has 12+ years of experience in medicinal chemistry. He hascompleted a PhD in Pharmaceutical Sciences in the subject area of Computational and Medicinal Chemistry from I. K. Gujral Punjab Technical University, Jalandhar, Punjab (India) in 2020. His present areas of research include structure-based drug design and medicinal chemistry of MMP2 and MMP9 inhibitors as anticancer agents, antibacterial drug resistance (NDM-1), GK activators as anti-diabetic agents, AR inhibitors for diabetic complications, PPAR agonists for metabolic syndrome, multi-potent anti-Alzheimer's agents, selective PDE4 & 7 inhibitors as anti-inflammatory agents and environmental chemistry. He owns to his credit more than 100 publications in national and international journals of repute, 20 book chapters, 14 books, and 6 patents (3 granted). He serves as a reviewer for reputed international journals published by Elsevier, Springer, Wiley, SAGE, and Frontiers. He is a life member of the Indian Society for Technical Education (ISTE). He has worked on various sophisticated analytical instruments including UV-Vis and FTIR spectrophotometer, Flash chromatography, and HPLC; and also, on various molecular modeling softwares including ChemSketch, ChemDraw and Marvin Sketch; Open Babel and Frog2 for structure optimization; PyMOL for molecular graphics, Glide (Schrodinger), AutoDock Tools, AutoDock Vina, Discovery Studio (Dassault Systemes BIOVIA), Omega and Open Eye for in silico molecular docking studies.

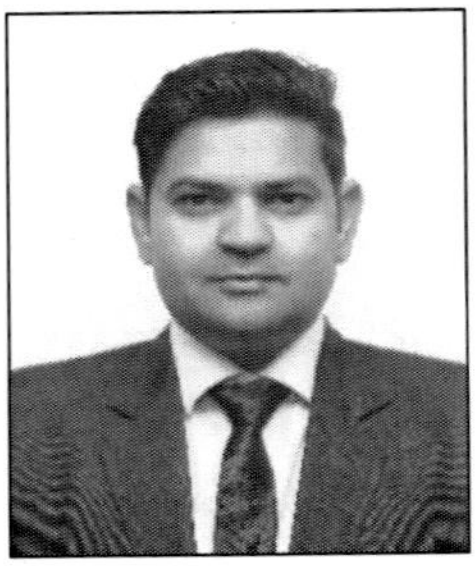

Dr. Ashwani K. Dhingra, is a principal and professor, at the Global Research Institute of Pharmacy, Radaur, Yamuna Nagar, Haryana (India), and has 15+ years of experience in medicinal and pharmaceutical chemistry. He has completed a PhD in Pharmaceutical Sciences in the subject area of Pharmaceutical Chemistry from I.K. Gujral Punjab Technical University, Jalandhar, Punjab (India) in 2017. His present areas of research include the medicinal chemistry of antimicrobial and anti-inflammatory agents and drug discovery from natural products. He owns to his credit a total of 90 publications in national and international journals of repute, 15 book chapters, 10 books, 6 patents, 10 design patents, 8 copyrights and various poster presentations at several conferences. He was awarded "Highly Cited Research" in Fitoterapia by Elsevier. He is a life member of the Association of Pharmaceutical Teachers of India and the Indian Society for Technical Education. He has worked on various sophisticated analytical instruments including UV-Visible spectrophotometer, and HPLC.

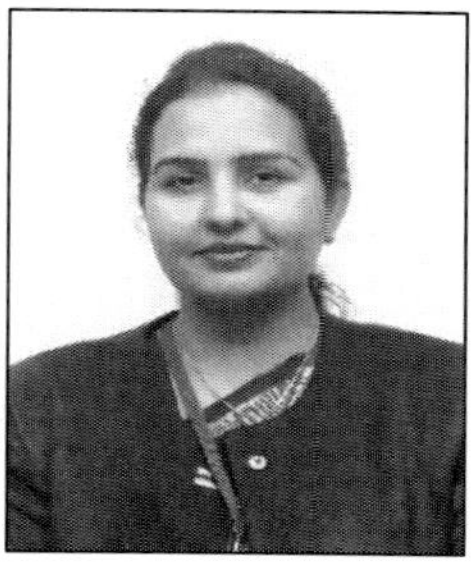

Dr. Geeta Deswal is presently working as Professor (Pharmacognosy) at Guru Gobind Singh College of Pharmacy, Yamuna Nagar, Haryana (India). Additionally, she is coordinating the Internal Quality Assurance Cell (IQAC) and NBA, ensuring the highest standards of academic excellence and quality assurance. She has obtained a PhD from M. M. Deemed to be University, Mullana, Haryana (India) in Quality Audit of Herbal Formulations in 2017. She is an expert in bioactivity-guided extraction and isolation of phytoconstituents, standardization of drugs and herbal formulations, and phytochemical screening of medicinal plants and plant tissue culture. She is also working on the formulation and evaluation of herbal products as antimicrobial agents. She has worked on UV spectrophotometer, HPLC, Soxhlet Apparatus, Clevenger Apparatus, Sonicator, Rota evaporator, and Thin Layer Chromatography and Column Chromatography. She owns to her credit 32 publications in national and international journals of repute, 10 book chapters and 9 books, 6 patents (2 granted), 6 designs and 6 copyrights. She is also a Life member of the Association of Pharmaceutical Teachers of India (APTI), the Indian Society for Technical Education (ISTE), the Indian Pharmacy Graduates Association (IPGA). She received the "Young Achiever Award" on the occasion of "Pharma Vision 2K25" by Shree Balaji Books (New Delhi) and Innovational Ambassador by the Innovational Cell, MHRD, AICTE, New Delhi.

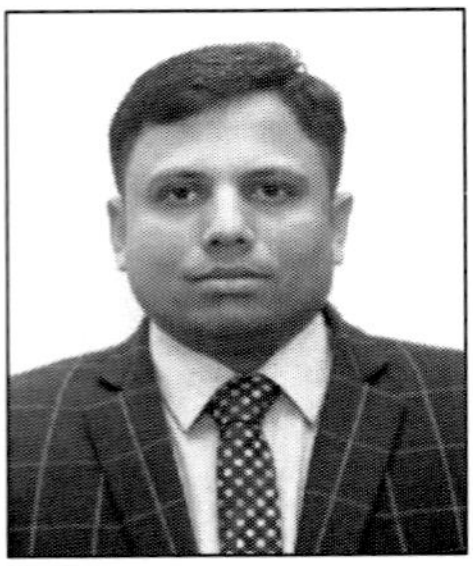

Dr. Kumar Guarve is an accomplished education professional with over 18 years of experience in the field. He has been serving as the Principal at Guru Gobind Singh College of Pharmacy, Yamuna Nagar, Haryana (India) since 2017. He has a specialized expertise in maintaining and achieving prestigious accreditations like NAAC and NBA, demonstrating a commitment to top-tier educational standards. Throughout his career, he has been instrumental in creating robust policies for revenue generation and successfully developing incubation centres within educational institutions. As an innovative leader, he has a proven track record of leveraging strategic planning and decision-making to drive institutional growth and academic excellence. He is renowned for his ability to transform colleges into thriving educational centres by implementing a visionary approach and ensuring its execution. He excels in fostering a culture of innovation, driving profitability, and launching start-up initiatives within colleges to enhance revenue and improve the overall educational experience. He has made significant contributions to academic research, with faculty under his guidance publishing numerous Scopus-indexed papers. He has also played a key role in patenting innovative products and securing copyrights for various educational processes and curricular frameworks. He is an active member of the Association of Pharmaceutical Teachers of India, the Indian Pharmacy Graduates Association, the Indian Society for Technical Education (ISTE), and the Association of Registered Pharmacists (ARP).

Index

A

B

C

D

E

F

G

H

I

M

N

O

P

R

S

T

V

W